Integrative Medicine and Rehabilitation

Editors

DAVID X. CIFU
BLESSEN C. EAPEN

PHYSICAL MEDICINE AND REHABILITATION CLINICS OF NORTH AMERICA

www.pmr.theclinics.com

Consulting Editor
SANTOS F. MARTINEZ

November 2020 • Volume 31 • Number 4

ELSEVIER

1600 John F. Kennedy Boulevard • Suite 1800 • Philadelphia, Pennsylvania, 19103-2899

http://www.theclinics.com

PHYSICAL MEDICINE AND REHABILITATION CLINICS OF NORTH AMERICA Volume 31, Number 4
November 2020 ISSN 1047-9651, 978-0-323-79092-5

Editor: Lauren Boyle
Developmental Editor: Nicole Congleton

Reprints. For copies of 100 or more of articles in this publication, please contact the Commercial Reprints Department, Elsevier Inc., 360 Park Avenue South, New York, NY 10010-1710. Tel.: 212-633-3874; Fax: 212-633-3820; E-mail: reprints@elsevier.com.

Physical Medicine and Rehabilitation Clinics of North America (ISSN 1047-9651) is published quarterly by Elsevier Inc., 360 Park Avenue South, New York, NY 10010-1710. Months of issue are February, May, August, and November. Business and Editorial Offices: 1600 John F. Kennedy Blvd., Suite 1800, Philadelphia, PA 19103-2899. Customer Service Office: 3251 Riverport Lane, Maryland Heights, MO 63043. Periodicals postage paid at New York, NY and additional mailing offices. Subscription price per year is $313.00 (US individuals), $633.00 (US institutions), $100.00 (US students), $366.00 (Canadian individuals), $833.00 (Canadian institutions), $100.00 (Canadian students), $429.00 (foreign individuals), $833.00 (foreign institutions), and $210.00 (foreign students). Foreign air speed delivery is included in all *Clinics* subscription prices. All prices are subject to change without notice. **POSTMASTER:** Send address changes to *Physical Medicine and Rehabilitation Clinics of North America*, Customer Service Office: Elsevier Health Sciences Division, Subscription Customer Service, 3251 Riverport Lane, Maryland Heights, MO 63043. **Customer Service: 1-800-654-2452 (US). From outside of the United States, call 314-447-8871. Fax: 314-447-8029. E-mail: JournalsCustomer Service-usa@elsevier.com (for print support); JournalsOnlineSupport-usa@elsevier.com (for online support).**

Physical Medicine and Rehabilitation Clinics of North America is indexed in *Excerpta Medica, MEDLINE/ PubMed (Index Medicus), Cinahl, and Cumulative Index to Nursing and Allied Health Literature.*

Contributors

CONSULTING EDITOR

SANTOS F. MARTINEZ, MD, MS
Diplomate of the American Academy of Physical Medicine and Rehabilitation, Certificate of Added Qualification Sports Medicine, Assistant Professor, Department of Orthopaedics, Campbell Clinic Orthopaedics, University of Tennessee, Memphis, Tennessee

EDITORS

DAVID X. CIFU, MD
Associate Dean of Innovation and System Integration, Herman J. Flax, MD Professor and Chair, Department of Physical Medicine and Rehabilitation, Virginia Commonwealth University School of Medicine, Senior TBI Specialist, U.S. Department of Veterans Affairs, Principal Investigator, Long-term Impact of Military-Relevant Brain Injury Consortium - Chronic Effects of Neurotrauma Consortium (LIMBIC-CENC), Hunter Holmes McGuire VA Medical Center, Richmond, Virginia

BLESSEN C. EAPEN, MD
Chief, Physical Medicine and Rehabilitation Service, VA Greater Los Angeles Healthcare System, Associate Clinical Professor, Department of Medicine, Division of Physical Medicine and Rehabilitation, David Geffen School of Medicine at UCLA, Health Sciences Associate Clinical Professor, University of California, Los Angeles, Los Angeles, California

AUTHORS

LISA ALTMAN, MD
Associate Chief of Staff, Healthcare Transformation, VA Greater Los Angeles Health Care System, Health Sciences Clinical Professor, University of California, Los Angeles, Los Angeles, California

WILLIAM CARNE, PhD
Department of Physical Medicine and Rehabilitation, Virginia Commonwealth University School of Medicine, Hunter Holmes McGuire VA Medical Center, Richmond, Virginia

DAVID X. CIFU, MD
Associate Dean of Innovation and System Integration, Herman J. Flax, MD Professor and Chair, Department of Physical Medicine and Rehabilitation, Virginia Commonwealth University School of Medicine, Senior TBI Specialist, U.S. Department of Veterans Affairs, Principal Investigator, Long-term Impact of Military-Relevant Brain Injury Consortium - Chronic Effects of Neurotrauma Consortium (LIMBIC-CENC), Hunter Holmes McGuire VA Medical Center, Richmond, Virginia

ISABELLE CIFU, BA
Department of Anthropology, University of Virginia, Richmond, Virginia

CAMILLA CINQUINI, DPT
Senior Physical Therapist, Kaiser Permanente Rehabilitation, The Permanente Medical Group, Santa Rosa, California

NATHAN D. CLEMENTS, MD
Academic Chief Resident, Department of Rehabilitation Medicine, The University of Texas Health Science Center at San Antonio, San Antonio, Texas

BRIAN RYDER CONNOLLY, MD
Academic Chief Resident, Department of Rehabilitation Medicine, The University of Texas Health Science Center at San Antonio, San Antonio, Texas

DAVID COSIO, PhD, ABPP
Clinical Health Psychologist, Jesse Brown VA Medical Center, Chicago, Illinois

JOVAUNA CURREY, MD
Physician, Department of Sports and Physical Medicine, Kaiser Permanente, The Permanente Medical Group, Santa Rosa, California

JORGE CUZA, MD
Resident Physician, Department of Physical Medicine and Rehabilitation, UC Davis, UC Davis Health, Sacramento, California

MADELINE A. DICKS, DO
Resident Physician, Department of Rehabilitation Medicine, The University of Texas Health Science Center at San Antonio, San Antonio, Texas

DAVID F. DRAKE, MD
Assistant Professor, Department of Physical Medicine and Rehabilitation, Virginia Commonwealth University, Director, Interventional Pain Clinic, Central Virginia VA Health Care System, Richmond, Virginia

FREDA L. DREHER, MD
Private Practice, Physical Medicine and Rehabilitation and Medical Acupuncture, President, American Academy of Medical Acupuncture, Clinical Preceptor, Helms Medical Institute, The Acus Foundation

JONATHAN DROESSLER, MD
Department of Physical Medicine and Rehabilitation, VA Greater Los Angeles Health Care System, Los Angeles, California

BLESSEN C. EAPEN, MD
Chief, Physical Medicine and Rehabilitation Service, VA Greater Los Angeles Healthcare System, Associate Clinical Professor, Department of Medicine, Division of Physical Medicine and Rehabilitation, David Geffen School of Medicine at UCLA, Health Sciences Associate Clinical Professor, University of California, Los Angeles, Los Angeles, California

KRISTIN ENEBERG-BOLDON, PT, DPT
Physical Medicine and Rehabilitation Services Manager, Department of Physical Medicine and Rehabilitation Services, Greater Los Angeles VA Health Care System, Los Angeles, California

ELIZABETH P. FRATES, MD
Clinical Assistant Professor (Part Time), Physical Medicine and Rehabilitation, Harvard Medical School, Boston, Massachusetts; Spaulding Rehabilitation Hospital, Charlestown, Massachusetts

RAOUF S. GHARBO, DO
Affiliate Faculty, Department of Physical Medicine and Rehabilitation, Virginia
Commonwealth University, Williamsburg, Virginia

JARED M. GOLLIE, PhD
Health Scientist, Washington DC VA Medical Center, Department of Health, Human
Function, and Rehabilitation Sciences, School of Medicine and Health Sciences, The
George Washington University, Washington, DC; Department of Rehabilitation Science,
School of Health and Human Services, George Mason University, Fairfax, Virginia

NATHAN HINKELDEY, DC, DACRB
VA Central Iowa Health Care System, Des Moines, Iowa; Adjunct Faculty of Palmer
College of Chiropractic, Davenport, Iowa

TIMOTHY HUDSON, MD, MHA
Medical Director, Veterans Integrative Pain Center, Physical Medicine and Rehabilitation
Service, Central Virginia Veterans Healthcare System, Assistant Professor, Department of
Physical Medicine and Rehabilitation, Virginia Commonwealth University, Richmond,
Virginia

KELLY JOYCE, MSPT
Physical Therapist, Pain University Instructor, Department of Physical Medicine and
Rehabilitation Services, Tomah VA Medical Center, Tomah, Wisconsin

JAMAL KHAN, DO
Minneapolis VA Health Care System, Department of Rehabilitation Medicine,
Minneapolis, Minnesota

HEATHER L. MALECKI, PT, DPT
Washington DC VA Medical Center, Washington, DC

RASHMI S. MULLUR, MD
Associate Professor of Clinical Medicine, David Geffen School of Medicine at UCLA,
Education Lead, UCLA Integrative Medicine Collaborative, UCLA Health, Los Angeles,
California

DUDLEY K. NORMAN, EdD
Integrative Health Nurse Practitioner, Central Virginia VA Health Care System, McGuire
VA Medical Center, Richmond, Virginia

CASEY OKAMOTO, DC
Minneapolis VA Health Care System, Department of Rehabilitation Medicine,
Minneapolis, Minnesota

DAVID J. PARK, MD
Physical Medicine and Rehabilitation Resident, Tufts Medical Center, Boston,
Massachusetts

EDWARD M. PHILLIPS, MD
Assistant Professor, Physical Medicine and Rehabilitation, Harvard Medical School,
Boston, Massachusetts; Whole Health Medical Director, VA Boston Healthcare System,
West Roxbury, Massachusetts

MELISSA E. PHUPHANICH, MD, MS
Department of Physical Medicine and Rehabilitation, VA Greater Los Angeles Health Care
System, Los Angeles, California

JESSICA PIECZYNSKI, PhD
Clinical Psychologist, Greater Los Angeles VA Healthcare System, Los Angeles, California

WHITNEY PIERCE, PsyD, RN, BCB
Clinical Psychologist, VA St. Louis Healthcare System, St Louis, Missouri

HILARY PUSHKIN, BA
Department of Physical Medicine and Rehabilitation, Virginia Commonwealth University School of Medicine, Richmond, Virginia

BRADLEY SCHAACK, DPT
Physical Therapist, Pain University Instructor, Department of Physical Medicine and Rehabilitation Services, Tomah VA Medical Center, Tomah, Wisconsin

JOEL SCHOLTEN, MD
Director, Physical Medicine and Rehabilitation, Department of Veterans Affairs, Veterans Health Administration, Physical Medicine and Rehabilitation Program Office, Washington, DC

J. GREG SERPA, PhD
Clinical Psychologist, Greater Los Angeles VA Healthcare System, UCLA Department of Psychology, Los Angeles, California

DANA SHENG, MD
Resident Physician, Department of Physical Medicine and Rehabilitation, UC Davis, UC Davis Health, Sacramento, California

ALYSSA NEPH SPECIALE, MD
Assistant Professor, Department of Physical Medicine and Rehabilitation, UC Davis, UC Davis Health, Sacramento, California

BRANDEE L. WAITE, MD
Professor and Section Chief of Sports Medicine, Department of Physical Medicine and Rehabilitation, UC Davis School of Medicine, UC Davis Sports Medicine, Sacramento, California

JOSEPH WALKER III, MD
Assistant Professor, Department of Orthopedics, University of Connecticut, Farmington, Connecticut

Contents

Foreword: There is Room for Improvement   xiii

Santos F. Martinez

Preface: Integrative Medicine and Rehabilitation: Toward a New Beginning   xv

David X. Cifu and Blessen C. Eapen

Lifestyle Medicine   515

Edward M. Phillips, Elizabeth P. Frates, and David J. Park

Lifestyle medicine is a growing field of medicine that addresses key health behaviors, which are the root causes of most premature death, chronic disease, and health care costs. Coaching patients with evidence-based behavior change strategies can help them to make lasting habits in key areas, such as physical activity, healthy eating, improved sleep, cessation of tobacco, forming and maintaining relationships, and stress management. Similarities in philosophy between lifestyle medicine and physical medicine and rehabilitation make them complementary and synergistic in treating the whole patient in their social context.

Functional Medicine: A View from Physical Medicine and Rehabilitation   527

Timothy Hudson

Using the functional medicine rubric in physical medicine and rehabilitation (PM&R), a physiatrist can capitalize on addressing the root causes and downstream effects in patients with chronic diseases. Similar to the International Classification of Function model in rehabilitation, the functional medicine model uses biopsychosocial understanding with a systems biology approach to find fulcrum points to create the biggest impact on health care. Given the position of rehabilitation medicine with the type and location of patients, both functional medicine and PM&R would benefit from a mutual partnership.

Pain Neuroscience Education as the Foundation of Interdisciplinary Pain Treatment   541

Kristin Eneberg-Boldon, Bradley Schaack, and Kelly Joyce

Pain neuroscience education (PNE) can be applied as the foundational core of an interdisciplinary biopsychosocial approach to persistent pain. This article outlines a noninvasive, nonpharmaceutical, and collaborative approach to providing comprehensive pain care, applying evidence-based biopsychosocial treatment strategies within the framework of PNE. Through consistent messaging across all interdisciplinary team members, persistent pain patients can sustain a deeper level of understanding and empowerment, with goals of sustainable improvement and self-management. The application of adult learning theory by patient educators also is discussed.

Whole Medical Systems the Rehabilitation Setting (Traditional Chinese Medicine, Ayurvedic Medicine, Homeopathy, Naturopathy)   553

David F. Drake and Dudley K. Norman

> Elements of whole medical systems (WMSs) are re-emerging in a modern, patient-centered care model that leverages the benefits of evidence-based conventional medical practice with WMSs modalities. Many of these re-emerging modalities had their origins in traditional Chinese medicine, ayurvedic medicine, homeopathy, or naturopathy. To date, research has been conducted predominantly on multimodality treatment of experimental groups, drawing conclusions without a comparative control group or using modalities that are not actually WMSs.

Mind-Body Interventions for Rehabilitation Medicine: Promoting Wellness, Healing, and Coping with Adversity   563

Jessica Pieczynski, David Cosio, Whitney Pierce, and J. Greg Serpa

> Physical medicine providers work to cure organic aspects of disease while simultaneously enhancing quality of life and well-being. Mind-body interventions are evidence-based, cost-effective approaches to serve these aims. This article enhances provider knowledge and acceptance of the most effective and prevalent mind-body modalities: meditation, guided imagery, clinical hypnosis, and biofeedback. The scientific evidence is strongest for mind-body applications for chronic pain, primary headache, cardiac rehabilitation, and cancer rehabilitation, with preliminary evidence for traumatic brain injury and cerebrovascular events. Mind-body interventions are well-tolerated by patients and should be considered part of standard care in physical medicine and rehabilitation settings.

Movement-Based Therapies in Rehabilitation   577

Melissa E. Phuphanich, Jonathan Droessler, Lisa Altman, and Blessen C. Eapen

> Movement therapy refers to a broad range of Eastern and Western mindful movement-based practices used to treat the mind, body, and spirit concurrently. Forms of movement practice are universal across human culture and exist in ancient history. Research demonstrates forms of movement therapy, such as dance, existed in the common ancestor shared by humans and chimpanzees, approximately 6 million years ago. Movement-based therapies innately promote health and wellness by encouraging proactive participation in one's own health, creating community support and accountability, and so building a foundation for successful, permanent, positive change.

Spinal Manipulation and Select Manual Therapies: Current Perspectives   593

Nathan Hinkeldey, Casey Okamoto, and Jamal Khan

> Touch is fundamental to the doctor-patient relationship. Touch can produce neuromodulatory effects that mitigate pain and put patients at ease. Touch begins with a confident handshake and continues throughout the physical examination. Touching patients where they hurt is a clear indication that a provider understands their complaint. Touch often continues as a function of treatment. This article updates evidence surrounding human touch and addresses mechanisms of action for manual therapy, the

impact of manual therapy on pain management, health care conditions for which manual therapy may be beneficial, treatment plans with dose-response evidence, and the impact of manual therapy on the health care system.

Performing Arts Medicine   609

Jovauna Currey, Dana Sheng, Alyssa Neph Speciale, Camilla Cinquini, Jorge Cuza, and Brandee L. Waite

Performing artists are a unique subset of athletes. With the highly repetitive nature of performance training, emphasis on proper technique, ergonomics, and preventive cross-training is vital, as many injuries are due to overuse or poor technique. There are novel medical concerns in performers, including ENT problems, mental health concerns and substance use risks. While music is central to performances, it is also a treatment modality to address cognitive, sensory, and motor dysfunctions in certain neurological conditions. Due to this wide array of issues, it is imperative to understand the specific needs and risks of performers to provide optimal medical care.

Autonomic Rehabilitation: Adapting to Change   633

Raouf S. Gharbo

Adaption to changes of external environment or internal health, the body-mind connection, or autonomic nervous system must be flexible and healthy. Population health studies with wearable technology and remote monitoring will lead to paradigm shifts in how to approach the physiology of emotion. Heart rate variability as a whole health biomarker could emerge as a foundation for a process beginning with objective skills of real-time modulation with focused breathing for healthier decision making and autonomic health trajectory change. Physical medicine and rehabilitation is uniquely poised to refine an autonomic rehabilitation process in an integrative manner to help individuals adapt.

Physical Activity, Exercise, Whole Health, and Integrative Health Coaching   649

Heather L. Malecki, Jared M. Gollie, and Joel Scholten

Physical activity and exercise play a significant role in the management and prevention of chronic disease. Therefore, patient-center approaches offered within medical settings are essential for the promotion of health and well-being. The Whole Health model of care incorporates all aspects of care, including prevention, treatment, conventional, and complementary approaches resulting in care for the whole person. Integrative health coaching is a tool for clinicians seeking to achieve behavior changes for improved health, particularly in the areas of physical activity and exercise. The Whole Health model of care complements the rehabilitative process, using a combination of complementary and integrative medicine for health promotion. In addition to incorporating Whole Health tools into clinical care, rehabilitative specialists may partner with integrative health coaches to achieve challenging behavior changes in the areas of physical activity, exercise, and other areas of self-care.

The Basics of Nutrition: A Primary Rehabilitation Intervention   665

David X. Cifu, William Carne, Hilary Pushkin, and Isabelle Cifu

> Nutrition, the process by which a body nourishes itself through the transformation of food into energy and body tissues, is the most important factor in health maintenance, response to injury or illness, short-term and long-term rehabilitation, and longevity. Most rehabilitation providers and the individuals they treat have limited training and knowledge on even the basics of nutrition. An appropriate diet for individuals who are either in a health maintenance or an active program of rehabilitation includes 1500 to 2500 calories per day delivered via a balanced range of foodstuffs, preferably in a whole-food, plant-based manner.

The Use of Vitamins, Supplements, Herbs, and Essential Oils in Rehabilitation   685

Nathan D. Clements, Brian Ryder Connolly, Madeline A. Dicks, and Rashmi S. Mullur

> The term, dietary supplement, refers to a broad category of products, including herbal or plant-based extracts, micronutrients, and food-based nutraceuticals. The use of supplements in clinical rehabilitation requires clear communication from patients and health care providers to understand the types of products used and their effects on health. Providers should distinguish between using micronutrient supplementation for therapeutic purposes and treatment of nutritional deficiency in patients with malnutrition syndromes. Evidence supports micronutrient and nutraceutical supplementation use to improve pain, functional status, and inflammation. There is little evidence on the use of herbal or plant-based extracts in therapeutic rehabilitation; larger studies are warranted.

Acupuncture: Evidence-Based Treatment in the Rehabilitation Setting   699

Joseph Walker III and Freda L. Dreher

> Acupuncture, originally described as part of Chinese medical practice thousands of years ago, has become increasingly popular as a form of complementary medicine. This article highlights the current evidence for and against the use of acupuncture in the treatment of various rehabilitation diagnoses. This article also describes the historical aspects and basic principles of acupuncture.

PHYSICAL MEDICINE AND REHABILITATION CLINICS OF NORTH AMERICA

FORTHCOMING ISSUES

February 2021
Dance Medicine
Kathleen L. Davenport, *Editor*

May 2021
Telerehabilitation
Blessen C. Eapen, David Cifu, *Editors*

August 2021
Polio
Darren Rosenberg, Craig Alexander
Rovito, *Editors*

RECENT ISSUES

August 2020
Spinal Cord Injury
John L. Lin, *Editor*

May 2020
**Pharmacologic Support in Pain
Management**
Steven Stanos and James R. Babington,
Editors

February 2020
Cerebral Palsy
Aloysia Leisanne Schwabe, *Editor*

SERIES OF RELATED INTEREST

Orthopedic Clinics
Clinics in Sports Medicine
Neurologic Clinics

VISIT THE CLINICS ONLINE!
Access your subscription at:
www.theclinics.com

Foreword

There is Room for Improvement

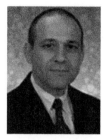

Santos F. Martinez, MD, MS
Consulting Editor

The growth of Integrative Medicine over the last 20 years has been an evolving process. Unfortunately, or possibly fortunately, traditional allopathic medicine does not have the answer for every condition or patient. It is indeed a humbling experience when confronted by a patient who is convinced that their condition has been aided more from an alternative avenue than from our algorithmic approach. In most cases, the modality is not being used as a substitute but as an adjunct to the patient's overall care. The inclusion of accepted alternative or possibly complementary disciplines into an integrative format varies depending on a clinician's disposition and the availability of evidence-based literature. The "holistic" approach to patient care is not a new concept to Physical Medicine and Rehabilitation; however, the number of ancillary modalities has outgrown most of one's knowledge base. This issue further investigates and reviews a range of specialties from more familiar topics such as Osteopathy and Acupuncture to lesser known alternatives for neuromotor retraining and mind-body exercise modalities. The article on Functional Medicine will undoubtedly spark some interest as it is instinctual that revisiting our patient history intake, dietary considerations, and being able to utilize approaches that promote overall well-being resonate with our field. Integrative and Functional Medicine departments are now gaining presence in a number of mainstream medical schools and academic institutions. This growing field, along with optimal nutritional care, is very basic for rehabilitation patients regardless of diagnosis. As patients are taking ever more responsibility for their care, they are vulnerable to the hype of media and advertising for unfound remedies. It seems like everyone has the answer or treatment option that a friend of a friend swears by. Naturally, the clinician would optimally prefer well-defined parameters, which are well researched, to offer patients the best opportunity to address their issues, and through a scientific process, the evolving standard of care becomes more inclusive, but with a scientific foundation. This malleable approach of shared decision making appears to be very satisfactory for both patients

Phys Med Rehabil Clin N Am 31 (2020) xiii–xiv
https://doi.org/10.1016/j.pmr.2020.08.006
1047-9651/20/© 2020 Published by Elsevier Inc.

pmr.theclinics.com

and physicians. I thank the guest editors' determination in bringing these lesser-known modalities for our readers consideration.

Santos F. Martinez, MD, MS
American Academy of Physical Medicine
and Rehabilitation
Campbell Clinic Orthopaedics
Department of Orthopaedics
University of Tennessee
Memphis, TN 38104, USA

E-mail address:
smartinez@campbellclinic.com

Preface

Integrative Medicine and Rehabilitation: Toward a New Beginning

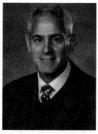 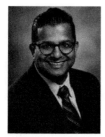

David X. Cifu, MD   Blessen C. Eapen, MD
Editors

Thoughts of "integrating" the wide ranges of health care approaches that exist across the globe have been entertained since the first contacts between peoples of different cultures tens of thousands of years ago and longer. More recently, even the concepts of "Eastern" or "Western" medicine have become moot and what began as complementary and alternative medicine has now more fully evolved into a fully patient-centric holistic model of care most appropriately labeled integrative medicine. While there exist dozens of instruction guides, book chapters, and texts highlighting some or many of the key elements of this whole-health approach to care, this easy-to-use, practical handbook represents a unique source that is both grounded in the available scientific literature and presented by real-world clinicians who are using the integrative medicine approach in their daily practice. The true art of Integrative Medicine entails applying an individualized blend of all elements of wellness and health management using learned and experiential knowledge and meeting the specific needs and wants of the individual who is receiving the care. This issue provides a broad introduction to this approach that combines a firm foundation of evidence-based information with practical, ready-to-use approaches. It may be read from cover to cover or used as a reference for specific elements of care. It is with great enthusiasm that we

Phys Med Rehabil Clin N Am 31 (2020) xv–xvi
https://doi.org/10.1016/j.pmr.2020.08.002
1047-9651/20/© 2020 Published by Elsevier Inc.

recommend taking full advantage of all the information contained in this issue and using these effective approaches to wellness.

David X. Cifu, MD
Department of Physical Medicine and Rehabilitation
Virginia Commonwealth University School of Medicine
Richmond, VA USA

U.S. Department of Veterans Affairs
Richmond, VA, USA

Long-term Impact of Military-relevant Brain Injury Consortium - Chronic Effects of
Neurotrauma Consortium (LIMBIC-CENC)
Richmond, VA, USA

Blessen C. Eapen, MD
Physical Medicine and Rehabilitation
VA Greater Los Angeles Health Care System
Los Angeles CA, USA

Department of Medicine
Division of Physical Medicine and Rehabilitation
David Geffen School of Medicine at UCLA
Los Angeles, CA USA

E-mail addresses:
dcifu@vcu.edu (D.X. Cifu)
blessen.eapen2@va.gov (B.C. Eapen)

Lifestyle Medicine

Edward M. Phillips, MD[a],*, Elizabeth P. Frates, MD[b], David J. Park, MD[c]

KEYWORDS

- Lifestyle medicine • Mind-body medicine • NCD • Health coaching

KEY POINTS

- Health behaviors are the root cause of greater than 80% of premature death, chronic disease, health care costs, and disability.
- Lifestyle medicine is a rapidly expanding field of medicine that addresses this gap with training, certification, and change in practice.
- Physical medicine and rehabilitation and lifestyle medicine are compatible fields that can learn from each other.

INTRODUCTION

"Of the 56.9 million global deaths in 2016, 40.5 million, or 71%, were due to noncommunicable diseases."[1] Heart disease, stroke, and diabetes make up a substantial portion of these deaths.[2] An estimated half of premature deaths in the United States are due to behaviors that can be modified, such as tobacco use, diet, and physical activity.[3] Chronic disability and morbidity make up approximately half the disease burden of the United States.[4] The literature has overwhelmingly suggested that modifiable behaviors and conditions, such as smoking, physical inactivity, poor diet, and excess body weight, are major contributors to noncommunicable diseases (NCD).[5–8] Ford and colleagues[9] convincingly showed that when compared with no healthy lifestyle factors, adopting 4 healthy lifestyle factors reduces the risk of developing diabetes, coronary heart disease, stroke, and cancer by nearly 80%. The fact that healthy behaviors can lead to less disease is well known and intuitive among lay people, and yet only a small fraction of the US population participates in multiple healthy behaviors,[10] which indicates that knowledge of improved behaviors alone is not sufficient to address these challenges.

[a] Physical Medicine & Rehabilitation, Harvard Medical School, Boston, MA, USA; [b] Spaulding Rehabilitation Hospital, 300 First Avenue, Charlestown, MA 02129, USA; [c] Department of Physical Medicine & Rehabilitation, Tufts Medical Center, 800 Washington Street, Boston, MA 02111, USA
* Corresponding author. VA Boston Healthcare System, 1400 VFW Parkway, West Roxbury, MA 02132.
E-mail address: ephillips1@mgh.harvard.edu

Phys Med Rehabil Clin N Am 31 (2020) 515–526
https://doi.org/10.1016/j.pmr.2020.07.006
1047-9651/20/Published by Elsevier Inc.

Lifestyle medicine (LM) is a rapidly evolving field that addresses the lifestyle-related contributors to NCD by changing health behaviors. Although physicians traditionally use medications and procedures as their main therapeutic modalities, practitioners of LM use techniques such as motivational interviewing and health coaching to engage patients in choosing and following through on their desired changes that support their reasoning for making the changes. These skills help individuals to make personalized and realistic, small goals to support improvements in diet, physical activity, sleep, stress management, avoidance of harmful substances, and social connection to treat and even reverse chronic disease.

As health care providers, we frequently try to convince patients to change their behavior in 1 way or another. Therefore, LM is applicable to all fields of medicine. The inclination of physiatry for team-based, holistic, adaptable care for our patients makes our field a natural fit for LM. Physical medicine and rehabilitation (PM&R) has significant expertise and experience to share with LM, and LM has evidence-based behavior change techniques and a whole-person perspective that aligns and enhances physiatric care.

BACKGROUND

The phrase "Lifestyle Medicine" was formalized with the publication of the first edition of the *Lifestyle Medicine* by Dr James Rippe in 1999[11] and is defined as "…the evidence based practice of helping individuals and communities with comprehensive lifestyle changes (including nutrition, physical activity, stress management, social support and environmental exposures) to help prevent, treat and even reverse the progression of chronic diseases by addressing the underlying cause."[12] LM's place in health care is bridging "the gap between health promotion, behavior change and conventional medicine."[13] The LM clinician provides direction and education while recognizing that the patient is ultimately in control of their individual choices. From a practitioner's vantage, training in LM includes a philosophic perspective that lifestyle is foundational to care, that the patient is driving the process, that core knowledge is about key health behaviors (**Fig. 1**), and the importance and active participation of the clinician in surveying and attempting to improve their own personal health behaviors and skills training in behavior change techniques and approaches (see Coaching in later discussion).

The importance of the clinician's personal health behaviors is well recognized because of its impact on the health of that individual and so that the clinician becomes a credible role model.[14] Clinicians will not readily counsel on health behaviors that they do not follow. Interestingly, even an unsuccessful attempt on the part of the clinician to adopt a new behavior will inform their efforts and improve their empathy for patients attempting meaningful lifestyle change.

CORE HEALTH BEHAVIORS
Nutrition

The standard American diet is full of fast foods, processed foods, and sweets, whereas it is almost devoid of fruits and vegetables. Data reveal that most of the US population consume less than 1 cup of fruit and less than 1.5 cups of vegetables per day, while the recommendations are to consume 1 to 2 cups of fruit and 2 to 3 cups of vegetables per day.[15] There are many controversial aspects of nutrition, but adequate consumption of fruits and vegetables is 1 area that is consistently included across the spectrum of healthy diets.[16] When reviewing diets, including low-carbohydrate, low-fat, vegan, vegetarian, low-glycemic, mixed/balanced,

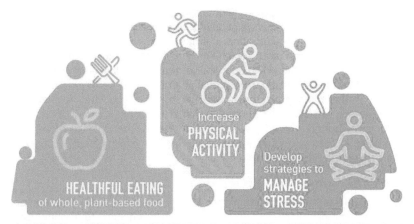

LIFESTYLE MEDICINE FOCUSES ON 6 AREAS TO IMPROVE HEALTH

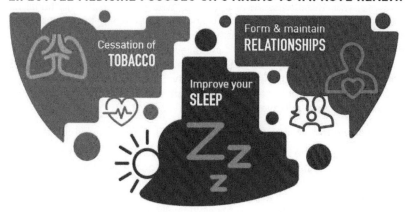

Fig. 1. Six core healthy lifestyle behaviors. (Copyright American College of Lifestyle Medicine 2019. lifestylemedicine.org.)

Mediterranean, and Paleolithic, Katz and Meller[16] conclude that all of them are potentially consistent with Michael Pollan's statement, "Eat food, not too much, mostly plants."[17]

Instead of focusing on what the patient cannot have, the LM practitioner often starts by focusing on what the patient can eat that will help their body function optimally. More often than not, people can work on consuming more plants, including vegetables, fruits, nuts, seeds, and legumes. By working with the patient to better understand the medicinal power of phytonutrients available in plants, the health care provider invites the patient to add a variety of plants to meals. The focus of nutritional counseling is on a healthy eating pattern, not a specific diet. The Harvard Healthy Plate and the Eat Lancet Plate provide a template for a healthy meal at breakfast, lunch, and dinner. The preponderance of the foods on the plates are plants.

Sleep

Although getting adequate sleep is critical to health, many people seem to pride themselves on getting by with minimal sleep. The guidelines for adults from the National

Sleep Foundation are to sleep between 7 and 9 hours per night. Routinely sleeping less than 6 hours per night puts one at risk for cancer and even death.[18] Sleep deprivation negatively impacts the immune, dermatologic, muscular, nervous, reproductive, respiratory, skeletal, and renal/urinary systems.[19] Some of the negative consequences of sleep deprivation include reducing heart rate variability and increasing risks of hypertension, myocardial infarction, and stroke. In addition, sleep deprivation is associated with an imbalance of hormones that regulate satiety, increasing ghrelin, which is the hormone that increases appetite, and decreasing leptin, which is the hormone that increases satiety. Helping patients to create a healthy bedtime routine that is conducive to sleep is key for healthy lifestyle change. The bedroom should be dark, quiet, and cool.

Physical Activity/Exercise

Physical inactivity is a global pandemic[20] and is as important as obesity and tobacco use, causing chronic disease.[21] There are myriad benefits to regular exercise, including but not limited to reduced rates of all-cause mortality, coronary heart disease, stroke, type 2 diabetes, as well as improved bone health, functional health, and improved cognition.[22–24] Despite this knowledge, attaining both the recommended 150 minutes of moderate intensity cardiovascular physical activity per week and twice weekly resistance training[22] is achieved by only 23% of US adults.[25] Lee and colleagues[21] estimated that ~30% of ischemic heart disease and ~6% to 10% of all NCDs are caused by physical inactivity. Some estimate that inactive people from the United States would gain 1.3 to 3.7 years after 50 years of age if the physical activity guidelines were achieved.[26,27]

Mind-Body/Burnout

Despite having one of the highest per capita incomes in the world, Americans are one of the most stressed populations.[28] The most common stressors among the Stress in America survey participants were work (64%) and money (60%).[29] The balance between beneficial and harmful aspects of stress must be maintained for healthy living. Chronically high levels of stress can physiologically affect the body in a multitude of ways, including contribution to the development of hypertension[30] and heart disease.[31] The presence of daily stressors has been associated with severe inflammatory skin diseases, such as psoriasis,[32] and contributes to the exacerbation of inflammatory bowel disease.[33] Furthermore, stress can lead to excess levels of cortisol, which raises blood pressure and impairs immune function.[34]

Physician burnout is a related problem that has increasingly been the focus of hospital systems. In the United States, physician burnout is prevalent in greater than 50% of practicing physicians and physicians-in-training.[35] The literature also suggests that these rates are comparable across the world.[36–38] This problem has huge implications for patient care, including lower-quality care, longer recovery times, reduced physician productivity, and increased physician turnover.[39]

LM can help reduce the negative effects of stress and help build resilience. Exercise, positive thinking, laughter, and relaxation practices, such as meditation, tai chi, and yoga, are just some of the ways that LM practitioners can help patients become more stress resilient. Mindfulness-based stress reduction is a form of meditation created by Kabat-Zinn and Hanh[40] that has promising effects in both patients with cancer and healthy individuals.[41,42] Mindfulness can be defined as a means to pay attention to particular moments with a nonjudgmental, open-minded attitude.[40,43] Another technique, called the relaxation response, was described by Benson and colleagues[44] as the ability to consciously increase blood flow to the brain and is a powerful adjunctive treatment for cardiovascular disease, headaches, insomnia, and depression.[45]

Tobacco and Substance Abuse (Including Vaping)

Modifiable behavioral risk factors, including substance use, constitute a large portion of the cause of death in the United States.[46] In 2000, the leading causes of death in the United States were tobacco (435,000 deaths; 18.1% of total US deaths), poor diet and physical inactivity (400,000 deaths; 16.6%), and alcohol consumption (85,000 deaths; 3.5%). The public health burden and financial toll on US health care from these behaviors are staggering.[46,47] These habits are difficult to break. As an example, about 80% of smokers who try to quit relapse within a month.[48]

Electronic cigarettes and other vaping devices have become more popular since their release in 2007.[49] There is increasing evidence that these products are not as harmless as initially thought, with reports of respiratory disease and deaths.[50] There is little information on the benefits of transitioning from conventional cigarettes to e-cigarettes, despite being marketed for smoking cessation. Campagna and colleagues[51] noted that smokers who partially used e-cigarettes instead of conventional cigarettes had no beneficial health benefits. Because vaping is relatively new, there are no long-term outcomes in the literature.

It takes more than just willpower for individuals to quit smoking. LM practitioners can use multiple techniques to help patients who are addicted to substances, such as motivational interviewing, listening, connecting, asking questions, being appreciative, showing compassion, exhibiting honesty, and applying the COACH approach.

Relationships/Positive Psychology

Social connection is an essential part of a healthy and happy life. Bonding with another human being starts from the day of birth when the baby connects with its mother. A sense of belonging, connection, and feeling loved is a basic human need that follows only food and shelter in Maslow's hierarchy of needs.[52] The association between social connection and health has been demonstrated for decades. One of the seminal studies,[53] a 9-year follow-up survey study, found that both men and women of all age groups who lacked social and community ties were, respectively, 2.3 and 2.8 times more likely to die than their counterparts who enjoyed extensive social connections. The American Heart Association has made loneliness a risk factor for heart disease.[54,55]

In LM, practitioners coach and counsel patients with a focus on positivity. This does not mean that people ignore problems but rather that they work to find solutions with a growth mindset, realizing every mishap or mistake is an opportunity to learn and grow.[56]

Coaching

The key to therapeutic lifestyle change is holding health coaching conversations by partnering with the patient to empower them to be an active participant in their health and to adopt healthier lifestyles. For most health care providers to embrace this type of counseling, they need to switch from the EXPERT approach to the COACH approach (**Table 1**). In the EXPERT approach, health care providers use their skills and knowledge to identify the problem and solve it. They examine the patient thoroughly, perform tests such as X rays, plan for the work-up and the treatment, explain the process to the patient and patient's family, repeat themselves for clarity, and finally, tell the patient what they need to do, including medications, procedures, and guidelines outlined by the health care provider. In this EXPERT approach, the health care provider

Table 1
Expert approach versus coach approach

EXPERT	COACH
E = Examine	C = Curiosity
X = X ray	O = Openness
P = Plan	A = Appreciation
E = Explain	C = Compassion
R = Repeat	H = Honesty
T = Tell	

From Frates B, Bonnet JP, Joseph R, et al. Lifestyle Medicine Handbook: An Introduction to the Power of Healthy Habits. Monterey CA: Healthy Learning; 2019; with permission.

does most of the talking and basically directs the patient with their words and actions. In the "COACH" approach, the health care provider uses skills to empower the patient and invites the patient to partner with them on a journey to lasting behavior change. In this partnership, the health care provider and the patient are both experts: the health care provider is expert in the LM guidelines and current research, whereas the patient is expert in their own life, knowing what has worked in the past, what motivates them, what obstacles are present, what personal strengths they have used to overcome barriers in the past, and their vision. The two work together for the benefit of the patient. In order for this partnership to work, the health care provider must embrace the skills of the "COACH" approach: Being Curious, Open, Appreciative, Compassionate, and Honest.

When working on lifestyle changes, the health care provider can envision wearing a COACH approach cap. By figuratively putting on that cap, they are reminding themselves to be genuinely curious about the patient. Instead of making assumptions about the patient's habits, the health care provider asks open-ended questions in a nonjudgmental way that elicits information from the patient. There is a focus on what is going well and on the strengths of the patient. Specifically, the health care provider asks about the patient's vision for the future, motivators for change, and feelings of confidence and importance for adopting and sustaining healthy habits. To express compassion, the health care provider must be fully present and mindful during the counseling session. Eye contact and communication that are focused and not distracted help convey empathy. Reflecting what the patient has shared is another key method to let them know they have been truly heard. Motivational Interviewing basics of asking open-ended questions, using affirmations to support any positive movement, stating reflections, and summarizing the details of the conversation all express compassion and demonstrate to the patient that they are valued and understood.[57]

If the patient tries to make excuses as to why they need to smoke or cannot exercise, the health care provider must be honest and share the dangers of smoking and sedentary behavior. However, in the COACH approach, the health care provider would not launch into a lecture on these topics. Instead, they would ask if the patient knew how smoking impacted the body and would personalize the message to that particular patient. For example, a middle-aged man who smoked and also had peripheral vascular disease might be interested to know how smoking affects all the blood vessels in his body, including those in his heart, which could cause a heart attack, and his penis, which could cause erectile dysfunction. A sedentary postmenopausal woman might want to know about how inactivity impairs bone density. Before sharing information on these topics, the health care provider asks, "Would you like to know how smoking can impact erectile dysfunction?" or "Would you like to know how lack of exercise impacts bone density after menopause?" By asking permission, the patient feels they are in charge and enjoys a sense of autonomy, which is a key part of sustained motivation for change. Coaching a patient to change is different than forcing, demanding, and telling them to change. Coaching conversations are a give-and-take between the health care provider and the patient. In these conversations, the patient does most of the talking. In the end, they co-create SMART goals (Specific, Measurable, Action oriented, Realistic, and Time-sensitive) that are important to the patient, providing enough of a challenge to be interesting but not overwhelming. Rechecking on prior goals establishes accountability and supports the therapeutic lifestyle change process. It is a process and a journey for the patient and provider. By partnering together and prioritizing healthy lifestyle habits, the patient is better equipped to adopt and sustain behavior change.

PHYSICAL MEDICINE AND REHABILITATION AND LIFESTYLE MEDICINE

LM is a field of medical practice, rather than a new specialty, that will ideally evolve the clinical interaction and impact every patient, and every specialty at every clinical visit. Physiatrists are well suited to become not only effective LM practitioners but also energetic proponents of LM based on expertise, experience, perspective, and flexibility. With the increase of lifestyle-related NCD, "[i]t seems a natural transition to apply the knowledge and skill toward emphasizing wellness and fitness in able bodied persons as well as persons with disabilities."[58]

Indeed, LM may well be the next iteration of PM&R. "The specialty of physiatry is entering into an unprecedented period with a unique opportunity; few other medical specialties are as well qualified to address the problems of obesity and inactivity."[59] "The opportunity to prescribe health and exercise regimens for those not yet experiencing—but at risk of falling ill to-the effects of obesity and its—comorbidities. Both Weinstein[58] and Laskowski[59] find tremendous potential in such a role, precisely because that role is yet unclaimed."[60]

Physiatry is focused on function more so than on specific diseases or the pathology and treatment of discrete organs or systems. This approach is consistent with the focus of LM on the root cause of health behaviors rather than on the resulting diseases, such as in the management of type 2 diabetes, heart disease, and hypertension.

What Lifestyle Medicine Can Learn from Physiatry

In order to effectively and compassionately guide patients with complex rehabilitation issues, for example, stroke, amputation, and spinal cord injury, physiatrists are trained in and demonstrate superior communication skills, patience, and compassion to address the chronic issues of disability, which intersect with patients' families, vocations, and communities. These skills and a creative, positive approach to complex, chronic issues should be shared with other health professionals who are adopting LM into their practices. Indeed, without addressing the patient in their full social context, health behavior change will not be sustainable.

For an LM intervention to be successful, the relatively short interaction between the health professional and patient must ignite a change of attitude and a flexibility on the patient's part to experiment and try to adopt improved health behaviors. Physiatrists similarly make recommendations to help patients function optimally with physical challenges whether it is a sports injury curtailing participation or a more severe physical disability. LM can learn from physiatry the sense of humility and partnership with patients as they seeks to support their patients by not just prescribing medications and balancing laboratory values.

The support necessary to help individuals adopt and sustain improved health behaviors goes beyond the efforts of an individual physician. Rather, an LM team with support from aligned health professionals, such as nurses, therapists, psychologists, health coaches, registered dietitians, and exercise physiologists, is more likely to provide the support for successful health behavior change. By physiatrist's training and experience running rehabilitation teams treating patients with complex disabilities, they are comfortable and trained to convert team leadership skills to convene and maximize the effectiveness of an LM team.

What Physiatry Can Learn from Lifestyle Medicine

Physiatrists are naturally drawn to exercise and physical activity as the cornerstone lifestyle behavior that most closely aligns with their interests, experience, and training. Indeed, an effective exercise prescription to address an outpatient's knee arthritis through cardiovascular and resistance training, most often administered by a physical therapist, can become a lifestyle prescription when the therapeutic exercise becomes a habit and enables the patient to continuously expand their physical activity levels. However, to become effective LM practitioners, physiatrists would need to learn the rudiments of other key lifestyle behaviors, including nutrition, sleep, stress modification, substance use elimination or moderation, and social connection.

Physiatrists as Leaders of Lifestyle Medicine

Physiatrists have demonstrated early leadership in the emerging field of LM. This article's lead author (E.P.) founded the Institute of Lifestyle Medicine within Spaulding Rehabilitation Hospital at Harvard Medical School in 2007. Dr Phillips was named to the American College of Lifestyle Medicine Board of Advisors in 2009 and as a Founding Board Member of the American Board of Lifestyle Medicine in 2016. His colleague at Spaulding Rehabilitation Hospital and secondary author of this article (E.F.) inaugurated the first Lifestyle Medicine Interest Group at an American medical school in 2009,[61] which has been emulated in dozens of medical schools across the country.[62] Dr Frates has served on the board of the American College of Lifestyle Medicine and is a preeminent LM educator,[63] teaching a 12-week college curriculum at the Harvard Extension School since 2014. Dr Michael Fredericson created the first LM undergraduate course at a US college, Stanford University, in 2014[64] and is currently the director of the LM program within the Stanford Center on Longevity.

LM is taking hold across the United States through the rapidly growing American College of Lifestyle Medicine[62] and through certification from the American Board of Lifestyle Medicine.[65] Physicians from all medical specialties and clinicians from a wide variety of health professions are building the infrastructure to deliver LM in multiple settings, including hospitals, private offices, medical clinics, and so forth. The LM community is joined in a concerted effort to incorporate principles and practices of LM into health professional education at all levels from preprofessional through continuing medical education, culminating in board certification. PM&R residency training is an important opportunity to incorporate LM principles and practice so that future physiatrists are best equipped to help patients adopt and sustain improved health behaviors.

SUMMARY

LM is a rapidly evolving field of medicine that crosses specialties and numerous health professions that focus on the root cause for most causes of premature death, chronic disease, and health care costs. LM addresses key health behaviors: increased physical activity, healthy eating, improved sleep, cessation of tobacco, forming and maintaining relationships, and stress management. LM uses evidence-based behavioral change strategies and practices presented as health coaching to help patients adopt and sustain improved behaviors. The philosophy and practice of LM are closely aligned with PM&R and can be readily adopted by physiatrists because of their communication skills, team-based care, the focus on treating the whole person in their social context, and their focus on pragmatic issues of function that are of importance to patients. It is a natural fit.

CLINICS CARE POINTS

- Adequate sleep for adults is 7 to 9 hours per night as per the National Sleep Foundation.
- Mindfulness is a means to pay attention to particular moments with a nonjudgmental, open-minded attitude.
- Physical Activity Guidelines for Americans call for adults to accumulate 150 minutes of moderate intensity physical activity per week and twice weekly resistance training.
- Social connection is an essential part of healthy and happy life. The American Heart Association has made loneliness a risk factor for heart disease.
- Collaborating and co-creating LM goals is more effective and rewarding than threatening and demanding change from patients.
- A healthy diet features a variety of plants, such as vegetables, fruits, nuts, seeds, and legumes.

DISCLOSURE

The authors have nothing to disclose.

REFERENCES

1. World Health Organization (WHO). Global Health Observatory (GHO) data – non communicable diseases. Available at: https://www.who.int/gho/ncd/mortality_morbidity/ncd_total/en/. Accessed March 27, 2020.
2. National Research Council. Measuring the risks and causes of premature death: summary of a Workshop. Washington, D.C.: National Academies Press; 2015. Available at: http://www.nap.edu/catalog/21656. Accessed January 27, 2020.
3. Population Reference Bureau. Up to half of U.S. premature deaths are preventable; behavioral factors key. 2015. Available at: https://www.prb.org/us-premature-deaths/. Accessed March 14, 2020.
4. Murray CJL. The state of US health, 1990-2010: burden of diseases, injuries, and risk factors. JAMA 2013;310(6):591.
5. Department of Health and Human Services, Centers for Disease Control and Prevention, National Center for Chronic Disease Prevention and Health Promotion, Office on Smoking and Health. The health consequences of smoking: a report of the surgeon general. Washington, DC: US Government Printing Office; 2004.
6. US Department of Health and Human Services. Physical activity and health: a report of the surgeon general. Atlanta (GA): US Dept of Health and Human Services, Centers for Disease Control and Prevention, National Center for Chronic Disease Prevention and Health Promotion; 1996.

7. Franz MJ, Bantle JP, Beebe CA, et al. Evidence-based nutrition principles and recommendations for the treatment and prevention of diabetes and related complications. Diabetes Care 2002;25(1):51.

8. Lichtenstein AH, Appel LJ, Brands M, et al. Diet and lifestyle recommendations revision 2006: a scientific statement from the American Heart Association nutrition committee. Circulation 2006;114(1):82–96.

9. Ford ES, Bergmann MM, Kröger J, et al. Healthy living is the best revenge: findings from the European prospective investigation into cancer and nutrition–POTSDAM study. Arch Intern Med 2009;169(15):1355–62.

10. Ford ES, Ford MA, Will JC, et al. Achieving a healthy lifestyle among United States adults: a long way to go. Ethn Dis 2001;11(2):224–31.

11. Rippe JM. Lifestyle medicine. Malden (MA): Blackwell Science; 1999.

12. Sagner M, Katz D, Egger G, et al. Lifestyle medicine potential for reversing a world of chronic disease epidemics: from cell to community. Int J Clin Pract 2014;68:1289–92.

13. Rippe JM. Definition of lifestyle medicine. In: Rippe JM, editor. Lifestyle medicine. 3rd edition. Boca Raton (FL): CRC Press; 2019. p. 961–76.

14. Abramson S, Stein J, Schaufele M, et al. Personal exercise habits and counseling practices of primary care physicians: a national survey. Clin J Sport Med 2000; 10:40–8.

15. Moore LV, Thompson FE. Adults meeting fruit and vegetable intake recommendations — United States, 2013. MMWR Morb Mortal Wkly Rep 2015;64(26):709–28.

16. Katz DL, Meller S. Can we say what diet is best for health? Annu Rev Public Health 2014;35(1):83–103.

17. Pollan M. Defense of food: an eater's manifesto. 1st ediiton. New York: Penguin Press; 2008.

18. Sleeping less than 6 hours may raise risk of cancer, even death. 2019. Available at: www.heart.org; https://www.heart.org/en/news/2019/10/02/sleeping-less-than-6-hours-may-raise-risk-of-cancer-even-death. Accessed March 22, 2020.

19. Frates EP. Sleep matters. In: Frates EP, editor. Lifestyle medicine handbook. Monterey (CA): Healthy Learning; 2019. p. 242–72.

20. Kohl HW, Craig CL, Lambert EV, et al. The pandemic of physical inactivity: global action for public health. Lancet 2012;380(9838):294–305.

21. Lee I-M, Shiroma EJ, Lobelo F, et al. Effect of physical inactivity on major noncommunicable diseases worldwide: an analysis of burden of disease and life expectancy. Lancet 2012;380(9838):219–29.

22. Physical Activity Guidelines Advisory Committee. 2018 physical activity guidelines advisory committee scientific report. Washington, DC: U.S. Department of Health and Human Services; 2018. p. 779.

23. Warburton DE, Charlesworth S, Ivey A, et al. A systematic review of the evidence for Canada's Physical Activity Guidelines for Adults. Int J Behav Nutr Phys Act 2010;7(1):39.

24. WHO. Global recommendations on physical activity for health. Geneva (Switzerland): World Health Organization; 2010.

25. Exercise or Physical Activity. Centers for Disease Control and Prevention. 2017. Available at: https://www.cdc.gov/nchs/fastats/exercise.htm. Accessed March 26, 2020.

26. Franco OH, de Laet C, Peeters A, et al. Effects of physical activity on life expectancy with cardiovascular disease. Arch Intern Med 2005;165(20):2355–60.

27. Paffenbarger RS, Hyde RT, Wing AL, et al. Physical activity, all-cause mortality, and longevity of college alumni. N Engl J Med 1986;314(10):605–13.

28. Clifton J. Gallup Global Emotions Report 2019. Washington, DC: Gallup Inc; 2019. Available at: https://www.gallup.com/analytics/248909/gallup-2019-global-emotions-report-pdf.aspx. Accessed February 3, 2020.
29. Stress in America$_{TM}$ 2019. Washington, DC: American Psychological Association; 2019. p. 9.
30. Spruill TM. Chronic psychosocial stress and hypertension. Curr Hypertens Rep 2010;12(1):10–6.
31. Rozanski A, Bairey CN, Krantz DS, et al. Mental stress and the induction of silent myocardial ischemia in patients with coronary artery disease. N Engl J Med 1988; 318(16):1005–12.
32. Evers AWM, Verhoeven EWM, Kraaimaat FW, et al. How stress gets under the skin: cortisol and stress reactivity in psoriasis: stress reactivity in psoriasis. Br J Dermatol 2010;163(5):986–91.
33. Triantafillidis JK, Merikas E, Gikas A. Psychological factors and stress in inflammatory bowel disease. Expert Rev Gastroenterol Hepatol 2013;7(3):225–38.
34. Pariante CM, Lightman SL. The HPA axis in major depression: classical theories and new developments. Trends Neurosci 2008;31(9):464–8.
35. Shanafelt TD, West CP, Sinsky C, et al. Changes in burnout and satisfaction with work-life integration in physicians and the general US working population between 2011 and 2017. Mayo Clin Proc 2019;94(9):1681–94.
36. Elit L, Trim K, Mand-Bains IH, et al. Job satisfaction, stress, and burnout among Canadian gynecologic oncologists. Gynecol Oncol 2004;94(1):134–9.
37. Goehring C, Gallacchi MB, Künzi B, et al. Psychosocial and professional characteristics of burnout in Swiss primary care practitioners: a cross-sectional survey. Swiss Med Wkly 2005;135:101–8.
38. Klein J, Grosse Frie K, Blum K, et al. Burnout and perceived quality of care among German clinicians in surgery. Int J Qual Health Care 2010;22(6):525–30.
39. West CP, Dyrbye LN, Shanafelt TD. Physician burnout: contributors, consequences and solutions. J Intern Med 2018;283(6):516–29.
40. Kabat-Zinn J, Hanh TN. Full catastrophe living: using the wisdom of your body and mind to face stress, pain, and illness. New York: Random House Publishing Group; 2009.
41. Rush SE, Sharma M. Mindfulness-based stress reduction as a stress management intervention for cancer care: a systematic review. J Evid Based Complementary Altern Med 2017;22(2):348–60.
42. Sharma M, Rush SE. Mindfulness-based stress reduction as a stress management intervention for healthy individuals: a systematic review. J Evid Based Complementary Altern Med 2014;19(4):271–86.
43. Reibel DK, Greeson JM, Brainard GC, et al. Mindfulness-based stress reduction and health-related quality of life in a heterogeneous patient population. Gen Hosp Psychiatry 2001;23(4):183–92.
44. Benson H, Beary JF, Carol MP. The relaxation response. Psychiatry 1974;37(1): 37–46.
45. Jacobs GD. Clinical applications of the relaxation response and mind–body interventions. J Altern Complement Med 2001;7(6):93–101.
46. Whiteford HA, Degenhardt L, Rehm J, et al. Global burden of disease attributable to mental and substance use disorders: findings from the Global Burden of Disease Study 2010. Lancet 2013;382(9904):1575–86.
47. Rehm J, Mathers C, Popova S, et al. Global burden of disease and injury and economic cost attributable to alcohol use and alcohol-use disorders. Lancet 2009;373(9682):2223–33.

48. Hughes JR, Keely J, Naud S. Shape of the relapse curve and long-term abstinence among untreated smokers. Addiction 2004;99(1):29–38.

49. Sood AK, Kesic MJ, Hernandez ML. Electronic cigarettes: one size does not fit all. J Allergy Clin Immunol 2018;141(6):1973–82.

50. Outbreak of lung injury associated with the use of E-cigarette, or vaping, products. Atlanta (GA): Centers for Disease Control and Prevention; 2020. Available at: https://www.cdc.gov/tobacco/basic_information/e-cigarettes/severe-lung-disease.html. Accessed March 22, 2020.

51. Campagna D, Cibella F, Caponnetto P, et al. Changes in breathomics from a 1-year randomized smoking cessation trial of electronic cigarettes. Eur J Clin Invest 2016;46(8):698–706.

52. Maslow AH. Motivation and personality. New York: Harper & Brothers; 1954.

53. Berkman LF, Syme SL. Social networks, host resistance, and mortality: a nine-year follow-up study of alameda County residents. Am J Epidemiol 1979; 109(2):186–204.

54. Caspi A, Harrington H, Moffitt TE, et al. Socially isolated children 20 years later: risk of cardiovascular disease. Arch Pediatr Adolesc Med 2006;160(8):805–11.

55. Valtorta NK, Kanaan M, Gilbody S, et al. Loneliness and social isolation as risk factors for coronary heart disease and stroke: systematic review and meta-analysis of longitudinal observational studies. Heart 2016;102(13):1009–16.

56. Dweck CS. Mindset: the new psychology of success. New York: Ballantine Books; 2006. Available at: https://books.google.com/books?id=fdjqz0TPL2wC.

57. Miller WR, Rollnick S. Motivational interviewing: helping people change. 3rd edition. New York: Guilford Press; 2013. p. xii, 482.

58. Weinstein SM. Maintaining health, wellness, and fitness: a new niche for physiatry? PM R 2009;1(9):793–4.

59. Laskowski ER. Action on obesity and fitness: the physiatrist's role. PM R. 2009; 1(9):795–7.

60. Petriceks AH, Hales HA, Srivastava S. Physical medicine and rehabilitation: trends in graduate medical education and subspecialization amid changing demographics. Am J Phys Med Rehabil 2019;98(10):931–6.

61. Pojednic R, Frates E. A parallel curriculum in lifestyle medicine. Clin Teach 2017; 14(1):27–31.

62. American College of Lifestyle Medicine. 2019. Available at: https://lifestylemedicine.org/. Accessed March 15, 2020.

63. Frates EP. Lifestyle medicine handbook. 1st edition. Monterey (CA): Healthy Learning; 2018.

64. Zhou J, Bortz W, Fredericson M. Moving toward a better balance: Stanford School of Medicine's lifestyle medicine course is spearheading the promotion of health and wellness in medicine. Am J Lifestyle Med 2017;11(1):36–8.

65. American board of lifestyle medicine – certification for lifestyle medicine. Available at: https://ablm.co/. Accessed March 15, 2020.

Functional Medicine
A View from Physical Medicine and Rehabilitation

Timothy Hudson, MD, MHA[a,b,*]

KEYWORDS

- Functional medicine • Systems biology • Biopsychosocial model • Rehabilitation
- Neuroinflammation • Chronic pain

KEY POINTS

- Functional medicine involves the use of a thorough, personalized discovery of antecedents, mediators, and triggers to an individual's health condition.
- Functional medicine looks at symptoms through a systems biology lens to see what upstream effects coming from antecedents, triggers, or mediators may be contributing to the current presentation.
- Functional medicine leverages small changes that will carry large effect on clinical scenarios.
- Functional medicine and physical medicine and rehabilitation have several similarities and differences that provide ground for an excellent partnership.

INTRODUCTION

US health care is plagued with a growing set of problems. First, obesity and metabolic disease are epidemics linked to excess sugar consumption that is killing our society.[1] Second, Americans seeking treatment for 1 or more chronic conditions make up 60% of the population but are using 90% of health care expenditures.[2] Furthermore, the cost of care is directly related to the number of chronic conditions diagnosed.[2] Among the leading causes of death and disability are heart disease, strokes, cancer, diabetes, obesity, Alzheimer disease, and tooth decay, with prevailing origins from lifestyle risk factors such as tobacco use, poor nutrition, sedentary activity, and excessive alcohol use.[3] Lifestyle stresses contribute to these as well,[4] thus lifestyle choices are driving chronic disease.

---

[a] Veterans Integrative Pain Center, Physical Medicine and Rehabilitation Service, Central Virginia Veterans Healthcare System, Richmond, VA, USA; [b] Department of Physical Medicine and Rehabilitation, Virginia Commonwealth University, Richmond, VA, USA
* Rehabilitation Medicine Service (117), 120 Broad Rock Boulevard, Hunter Holmes McGuire VAMC, Richmond, VA 23249.
E-mail address: timothy.hudson2@va.gov

Phys Med Rehabil Clin N Am 31 (2020) 527–540
https://doi.org/10.1016/j.pmr.2020.07.011
1047-9651/20/Published by Elsevier Inc.
pmr.theclinics.com

Functional medicine (FM) is a chronic care model that centers around personalized approaches to metabolic conditions. Consequently, the Center for Functional Medicine at the Cleveland Clinic studied management of chronic care and found a statistically significant improvement of health-related quality of life in comparison with matched controls using FM.[5] In the study, a cohort of 1595 participants were followed over the course of 12 months, compared with 5657 matched patients, at a family health center. Those in the FM group were found to have had a significant improvement in their PROMIS Global Physical Health scores compared with the family health center patients both at 6 months and at 1 year. The sustained benefit is suggestive of a better model of health care, but the research is a preliminary. At its core, the research challenges the basic assumptions of modern clinical care by looking deeper into the causes for conditions in each patient.

FM accomplishes its paradigm shift through personalized approaches to patient care, linking specific details in the individual's history and their status to their biology. FM focuses on treatment geared toward getting the biggest intended impact on the physiology from small efforts. Although these treatments can include pharmacology or procedures, it often starts with considering lifestyle options for the patient. Considering the patient population in physiatry, the FM model represents a synergistic opportunity for rehabilitation clinicians to develop a more in-depth systems-based understanding of the patient's case while capitalizing on ideas that they are already using. Individuals with traumatic brain injury, spinal cord injury, arthritis, or neuromuscular dysfunction are ideal patients for the FM model for a variety of reasons. There are also many ways those in FM can also benefit from mutual involvement between the fields of medicine. Indeed, rehabilitation medicine can provide even more depth to FM practice and opportunities for a uniquely appropriate patient population.

BACKGROUND

Before World War II, the contemporary industrialized model of modern medical thought developed as the need for creating scientific precision with new pharmaceuticals, such as penicillin, became important. After the usefulness of antibiotics and analgesics become vital in the life-saving treatment of acute disease, medical thought evolved into the pursuit of more evidence-based medicine (EBM), which became a driving force for current medical visits, therapies, and even algorithms for payment. EBM centers around the rapid identification of organ specific diagnoses leading to pharmacocentric or procedural-centric treatments. Although this is straightforward in acute organ dysfunction, any clinician can recognize the variability in outcomes in chronic disease owing to socioeconomic disparities (eg, genetic, ethnic, or gender differences) and individual levels of understanding and compliance. These variable outcomes demonstrate the complexity in humanity, and although an alternative view is necessary, such a change to the norm is challenging within this EBM-driven system.[6]

To find predictability in the unknown complexity of chronic care, the FM model emerged to address the growing chronic care conundrum. FM was intended to be a holistic view for all clinicians from any specialty and licensure to evaluate individuals in a personal, systems-based way. Drawing from EBM, systems biology, integrative medicine, chronic care models, personalized medicine models, and prospective health care models, FM considers the many different approaches to the chronic problems within chronic care, attempting to collate the necessary elements to achieve better results (**Table 1**).[7] By evaluating the literature and applying known physiologic concepts, it conceptualizes many of the common treatment approaches into a

Table 1	
Models that influenced functional medicine	
Evidence-based medicine	Systems biology
Chronic care model	Integrative medicine
Personalized medicine model	Prospective health care model

Data from Jones DS, Hofmann L, Quinn S. *21st Century Medicine: A New Model for Medical Education and Practice.* Gig Harbor, WA: The Institute for Functional Medicine;2009.

personalized, systems biology-based method. As the contemporary, industrial-driven, medicine model excels at acute-care evaluations and treatments, so an FM model excels at examining the root causes for chronic conditions through science and intuitive application of individual physiology.

One way of understanding the unique approach of FM is to visualize medical reasoning in as a tree (**Fig. 1**). At the base, the roots are a combination of modifiable lifestyle factors, genetic predisposition, experiences, values, and beliefs of the patient overlaid with the mental, spiritual, and emotional health of the patient. The trunk is shaped by the roots and consists of medical history and defining events in a person's life. These combine with a mixture of physiologic processes termed system biology that drive our interconnected functions such as assimilation, biotransformation/elimination, structural integrity, energy, physiologic/cellular communication, immunity, and physiologic/cellular transportation (**Table 2**). The way that the body expresses this as diseases is seen on the leaves of the tree through a person's signs and symptoms, and these are categorized in contemporary medicine terms as the well-known bastions of organ function: cardiology, neurology, immunology, gastroenterology, and so forth. Yet, analogies such as this rarely translate fully in practice.

To thoroughly consider the complexities of chronic care, clinicians need to take a different approach to the clinical visit. The foundation of the FM visit is to encourage a healing partnership and the therapeutic encounter with the individual, through active listening leading the patient to share their story in detail.[7] As the encounter progresses, which may need to be iterative over many visits, a historical chronology detailing the major themes of health and illness merge, highlighting the antecedents to the current conditions, triggers of illness, and the mediators that perpetuate symptoms within the individual's own scenario. When considered through the lens of systems biology certain opportunities can become clear as "points of leverage" to modify an individual's metabolic, epigenetic, or overall function. In turn, this method results in going upstream with signs and symptoms, allowing an individual to see farther reaching impacts of their own efforts, while making skillful pharmaceutical choices and procedural options more efficacious.

EVALUATION

A defining feature of the FM approach is to use personal medicine to flesh out clues to altered function. For the average clinician, this is an enigma, given that EBM seems to discount individuality through averages. The response of FM is to look at the individual's antecedents, triggers, and mediators (ATMs; **Table 3**).[7] Antecedents are the genetic, epigenetic, congenital and formative events that can impact an individual's health and well-being. Triggers are events in an individual's life that caused any change to the systems that create homeostasis, such as antibiotics on gut microbiota, adverse childhood events, extreme psychological or physical trauma. Mediators are ongoing aspects of an individual's lifestyle or environment that also impact health

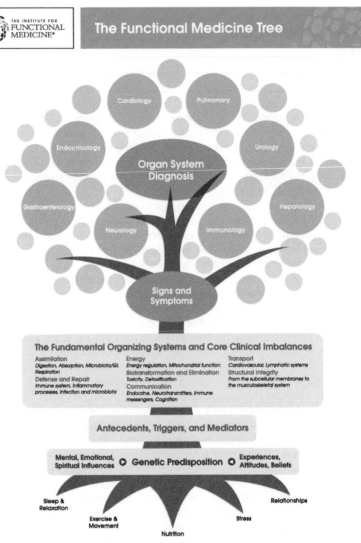

Fig. 1. Functional medicine tree. (*Courtesy of* the Institute for Functional Medicine, Federal Way, WA.)

and well-being, such as ongoing stressors, poor diet, excessive exercise, or other homeostatic disrupting activities. These tend to be forgotten in the shortened clinical visits of EBM, but they can reasonably be the cause of individualized psychological and physiologic responses to treatment recommendations.

The concept of using ATMs is not a novel idea but found in decades-old literature. A fundamental theory that points to the true complexity in medical care is the biopsychosocial (BPS) model.[8,9] Created by George Engle to describe the suffering of persons in the universe of expanding evidence-based and technical approaches

Table 2	
The systems biology matrix of functional medicine	
Assimilation	Defense and repair
Energy	Biotransformation and elimination
Transport	Communication
Structural integrity	

Data from Jones DS, Quinn S. Reversing the Chronic Disease Trend: Six Steps to Better Wellness. Federal Way, WA: The Institute for Functional Medicine;2017.

that can feel cold under the biomedical model, the BPS model was truly an innovation. The view of BPS demonstrates that causality in illness is not strictly linear; different causes can be circular and complex, forcing one to consider more than just apparent physiologic dysfunction. This can result in what is known as structural causality, or a hierarchy of causes, that can guide clinicians to recognition of the physiologic or psychological drivers of disease in individuals, recognizing many physiologic conditions are impacted by psychological states.[9]

Beyond the connections that move the provider from sympathy to empathy, the BPS model has further included the addition of the diathesis-stress model.[9] This model incorporates the genetic vulnerabilities of each individual, coupled with their external or internal stresses; when these reach an individual threshold, they may exacerbate metabolic or hormonal abnormalities. With the biopsychosocial–diathesis-stress (BPSDS) model, clinicians can see more clearly the importance of a team built to include mental professionals, physical therapists, physicians, physician extenders, and dietitians. Considering the genetic background of an individual in context of their biopsychosocial stresses helps more completely view the causes variations in common presentation and treatment response. This is the purpose of collecting the ATMs.

Specifically, in chronic pain conditions in which the effects of pain are felt emotionally and socially, deepened knowledge of the individual's experience can cross several domains. This can go beyond the physician, and advances in understanding pain current literature recommends that treatment be sought not just from one clinician, but in an interdisciplinary format.[10] In addition, clinicians must find the details of what pain means to individuals and how badly it can impact their quality of life.[9] An example of incorporating the BPSDS into action is the Departments of Defense and Veterans Health Administration collaboration on a substitute pain scale, the Defense and Veterans Pain Rating Scale (DVPRS; see **Box 1**),[11] which forgoes the traditional "How bad is your pain?" for "How does pain affect your activity, mood, sleep, and stress?"

The role of BPSDS in brain injury rehabilitation goes further than recognizing the psychosocial impacts. Research shows that outcomes with mild traumatic brain injuries (TBIs) are worsened with impaired biopsychosocial status.[12] In addition, those

Table 3		
Examples of antecedents, triggers, and mediators		
Antecedents	**Triggers**	**Mediators**
Family history	Physical trauma	Lifestyle choices
Genetic information	Psychological/moral trauma	Psychosocial stressors
Congenital effects	Acute health conditions	Chronic disease
Maternal/birth history	Major life events	Medications

> **Box 1**
> **Defense and Veterans Pain Rating Scale (DVPRS)**
>
> In the last 24 hours, on a scale of 0 to 10, 10 being the worst:
> - How has pain interfered with your usual activity?
> - How has pain interfered with your sleep?
> - How has pain affected your mood?
> - How has pain contributed to your stress?
>
> *Data from* Nassif TH, Hull A, Holliday SB, Sullivan P, Sandbrink F. Concurrent Validity of the Defense and Veterans Pain Rating Scale in VA Outpatients. Pain Med. 2015;16(11):2152-2161.

with premorbid mental health issues demonstrate more post-concussive symptoms after a year of recovery.[13] This carries further with preinjury histories of substance abuse and psychiatric disorders predicting employment status and independent living status following more significant brain injury. Although there are clear biologic impacts from brain injury on neuronal function, psychosocial impacts of brain injury may provide a better understanding to the changes seen in personality, and conversely impacting overall biopsychosocial function. Thus, the ATMs have a predictive value in neurotrauma, the role of the BPSDS is becoming more essential for individual treatment.

APPLICATION

As the ATMs paint the details and specifics of the individual's condition, the principles of systems biology (SB) provide color to the overall picture. SB is a view connecting the networks of genetics and metabolism to the greater networks function of the organism.[14,15] Rather than examine only individual proteins or genes in isolation, SB considers the behavior of these among multiple systems using computational models that range from molecular networks to social networks.[16] FM adapts this viewpoint to create a web of interconnecting physiologic processes that are required for our bodies to work appropriately. FM has created a matrix of these (see **Table 3**), such as intracellular and extracellular communication, energetics, structural integrity, bioelimination, immune function/defense, transportation, and assimilation.[7] The SB of these categories challenges the provider to look from the genetic up through the social impacts, and it allows the provider to create a web of connections, helping to identify specific points of abnormality.

To reflect on the approach to SB in rehabilitation, it would be illustrative a look into common pathways in chronic pain and brain injury. The role and impact of neuroinflammation is being increasingly appreciated in common brain disorders like stroke and brain injury, and also in chronic pain, spinal cord injury, and others.[17,18] SB has been working to elucidate many of the biochemical pathways in neurotrauma to elaborate on the proteomics of the neuroinflammation.[19] The 2 most relevant advances in understanding neuroinflammation have to do with the role of the microglia[20] and the loss of the dogma of immune privilege through discovery of the Dural lymphatic network.[21] In context to brain injury and chronic pain, neuroinflammation then is an important co-factor in a patient's management, one that would be seen in FM as a possible treatment fulcrum.

On neuronal level, microglia has been shown to be more involved in our daily living than previously known.[22] The macrophage-derivative origin of the cell explains some of its vital functions within the brain, particularly as a neural innate immune responder.[18] Roles such as initial inflammation, debris and pathogen management, and cleanup are regulated through this cell, alternating its own morphology.[23] Amazingly, microglia influence such broad brain functions as learning, emotion, and cognition. Its darker side can be seen in various ways after trauma, infection, inflammation, and auto-immune processes, but it can be guided through neurofeedback, nutrition, supplements, exercise and pharmacology.[24] Neuroinflammation requires certain microglial morphologic changes, and so these 2-faced cells become centers of attention in chronic neurologic conditions.

In addition to recent discoveries on microglial function, lymphatic function in the brain has more fully been elucidated through the understanding of glymphatic circulation and Dural lymphatic drainage.[21] Just as the microglial work in acting as the primary housekeeping cell has become more understood, their role has as both driving and following immune changes is become clearer in drawing in immune cells through the blood brain barrier.[18,25] Following this, T-helper differentiation helps explain a series of complex events that can lead to chronic states of inflammation or autoimmunity. These T cells, depending on their own morphology, can increase the inflammation, lessen it, or convert it to an acquired immune response.[26] Dural lymphatic access to the cervical lymph nodes encourages B-cell activation, risking autoantibodies in significant, prolonged inflammation as tissue debris is collected and presented.[27] This is the spectrum of severity in immune dysfunction within neuroinflammation.

Notably, neuroinflammation is not isolated within the central nervous system. A change in vagal outflow following brain injury and in neuroinflammation as a part of an immune reflex response suppresses gastrointestinal function, parasympathetic influence on the heart, and complicates immune regulation.[28,29] Increasingly there is recognition that this impacts other systems as well. Particularly, the vagal depression causing gastrointestinal dysfunction leads to intestinal inflammation and change in the gut microbiota.[30] Individually or together, brain inflammation and gut inflammation can cause system release of cytokines and chemokines, generating a milieu prone to metabolic dysfunction.[31]

As surmised from the BPSDS model, neuroinflammation does not incur in isolation from previous antecedents or mediators. Antecedents to neuroinflammation and chronic pain can be genetic, for example, genetic variations in HTE2C, Catechol-O-Methyltransferase (COMT), interleukin-6, interleukin 1β, and μ-opioid receptors (OPRM1) can impact pain perception, exacerbation to stresses, and the overall pain management plan. Similarly, severity, recovery and ongoing neuroinflammation in TBI has been linked to several polymorphisms in inflammatory cytokines, ApoE, brain derived neurotrophic growth factor (BDNF), and serotonin receptors.[32] Unfortunately, testing for these is not done frequently, likely due to cost or privacy concerns.

Similarly, mediators will be cumulative to body inflammation and can also hypothalamic function, changing vagal tone, and allows for increased neuroinflammation. So, the impact of common conditions, such as insulin resistance or obesity, that can cause hypothalamic function can further explain some the variation in post injury outcome.[33] Similarly, gut dysfunction and microbiota causing inflammation can also have a significant role on neuroinflammation.[34] The ATMs become a critical point of individuality that can drive neuroinflammation in addition to direct pathology.

Ominously, in its various degrees, central nervous system (CNS) trauma such as brain injury and stroke have resultant neuroinflammation with debris removal, immune reaction and self-antigen presentation.[27] As noted, neuroinflammation is also a cause of acute severe secondary injury to brain tissue following acquired brain injury, making it a target for neuropreservation.[35] Unfortunately, chronic neuroinflammation can persist for years following such an intercranial injury,[36] and there appears to be a feedback loop in which neuroinflammation can also lead to gastrointestinal dysfunction and body inflammation, and these can lead to worsened neuroinflammation.[37] This puts an exclamation on the role of current comorbidities causing inflammatory disorders can exacerbate that dysfunction in spontaneous CNS dysfunction.

Arguably, a sequela of neuroinflammation seen in chronic pain is central sensitization.[38] Chronic pain can begin with a peripheral noxious stimulus that can lead to peripheral sensitization, and central sensitization follows. However, neuroinflammation can also lead to central sensitization.[38] Central sensitization can be driven from neuroinflammation through actions of microglia and astrocytes releasing chrome inflammatory cytokine and chemokines in the spinal cord and brain. Peripheral sensitization can also cause long-term potentiation of the spinal cord modulating the receptors and cytokines release within the cerebrospinal fluid, impacting distant locations.[39] Another example of a feedback system, various external and internal conditions can either prime or drive the CNS for neuroinflammation, which can cause chronic pain sensitization with or without the peripheral stimulus.

THERAPEUTIC OPTIONS

Treatment of the interconnected network of SB is very complex and requires appreciating the ATMs to place context around a plan. Even then, a provider can feel overwhelmed looking at where to begin. A simple way to proceed into FM treatment is to consider the concept that if one applies enough pressure upstream then a large downstream effect can result.[7] This concept of finding "points of leverage" can begin with examining how modifiable lifestyle factors can impact the downstream effects, or from the previous analogy, how the roots can impact the leaves on the FM tree. Ultimately, this can be applied to pharmacologic, procedural or advanced therapeutics; however, the conservative treatments often have the least adverse effect for the biggest gain.

Paradoxically, a check-in with a patient in FM starts with a check-in with one's self, a step back. This opens the attention of the provider to be aware of any nonverbal communications by gathering self-intentions before gathering information from the individual.[7] Echoing this recommended ritual from FM, it was suggested that providers should calibrate themselves with mindfulness and self-awareness.[9] It is also suggested that providers work to create trust with the patient, cultivate curiosity in the patient's condition, recognize bias within the research and within themselves, educate their own emotions, and use informed intuition for nonlinear problems.[9] These suggestions are likely to be hollow in a technical, biomedical model, but they ring true considering FM approaches to patient care.

Beginning with an individual with health concerns, the clinician works to gather the relevant ATMs, attempting to understand the complexity in chronic care, while communicating the severity and prognosis of a pathology. The lifestyle-dependent expression of epigenetic traits can cast a light onto the interconnectedness of systems and the variation from individual to individual. In addition to the mediators or triggers previously mentioned, antecedents (or diathesis) can open the personalized differences in symptoms, prognosis or treatment. Genetic testing can help describe differences in prognostic or treatment expectations. Further investigation needs to be done into the proteomics of the genetic variations in rehabilitation conditions, but they can impact the history and severity of neuroinflammation and contribute to the depth or complexity of chronic diseases.

As treatment planning starts, it makes sense to initially recommend the most common approach within physiatry: exercise and activity. Just as other areas of the treatment plan, exercise needs to be understood in relation to its biochemical effects: the type, length and intensity of exercise.[40] BDNF produced by exercise in traumatic brain injury recovery can be helpful in reducing neural inflammation and improving neurologic recovery, and even lactate and β-hydroxybuterate may be neuroprotective.[41] In addition, the frequency of firing of neurons will reduce the impact of microglial activation, and the presentation of tissue antigen to T cells. However, these inflammation markers can exacerbate chronic pain syndromes,[38] though most often they are seen as beneficial.[42] In cases of exercise hyperalgesia, using modulation therapy such as acupuncture can reduce the impact of serotonin in the dorsal root ganglia before engaging clients in significance exercise therapies.[43]

Impacting parasympathetic function through Vagal nerve modulation is a fulcrum to provide heavy lifting. The Vagal nerve function plays a role in neuroinflammation including the ability to modulate the inflammatory response, but it can be modified by a number of conditions and actions. Vagal activity is decreased in chronic pain patients as seen through Heart Rate Variability (HRV) analysis, and treatment with biofeedback focused on HRV seems to improve outcome with these patients.[44] Additionally, HRV can be used in TBI to correlate the social and emotional functions of the patient vacating a possible role for HRV biofeedback,[45] though a large-scale trial has not been tested. Alternatively, electric simulation of the Vagal nerve (tVNS) has been shown to be effective in chronic pain treatments with patients.[46] The use of tVNS has also been shown to be effective in rodent models of brain injury at reducing neuroinflammation and early observational results are positive.[47] Using the inflammatory reflex of the Vagal nerve through either biofeedback or tVNS are expanded methods of treating the neuroinflammation present in complex patients.

Another downstream dysfunction of neuroinflammation is sleep. Sleep disturbances are common in both chronic pain and in brain injury, and in either, it can be multifactorial.[48] Importantly, the impact of sleep on brain injuries bidirectional related to the changes in hormonal regulation and is also related to impairments during the neuro-rehabilitation process.[49] These underidentified effects can be persistent in long-standing following brain injury.[50] Beyond traditional sleep studies and noninvasive ventilation support, supplementation of melatonin does seem to help this population,[51] whereas cognitive behavioral therapy can be used successfully to treat chronic pain related sleep disturbances.[52]

One of the last basic recommendations to consider is the effect of diet on the overall epigenetic and metabolic function of patients because of nutrition. This is evident from the effect of overconsumption of sugar on metabolic syndrome.[1] FM considers the biochemical and cellular impact on the various systems previously mentioned. By initiating a thorough history of dietary intake, a provider can assess if there is a tendency to eat foods that cause gut inflammation or systemic inflammation, or avoiding the helpful phytonutrients, polyunsaturated fats, or antioxidants.[53] Despite growing research that nutrition forms the basics of health and disease, clinicians are still poorly educated on strategies of dietary interventions.[54] An example of a unique intervention is using the ketogenic diet in neurodegenerative diseases, which has shown benefit in ischemic conditions and traumatic brain injury.[55] There is also evidence that a diet heavy in antioxidant foods, otherwise known as an anti-inflammatory diet, can improve chronic pain syndromes.[56] Fasting and plant-based options also show promise in improving outcomes.[57,58] Outside of strict nutrition, supplements such as resveratrol,[59] omega 3 fatty acids,[60] or N-acetylcysteine[61] may provide needed support in TBI patients, and the use of vitamin D,[62] polyunsaturated fatty acids[63] and turmeric[64] can be of benefit in chronic pain syndrome, among plenty of other emerging evidence.

SUMMARY

Rehabilitation medicine sees many of the chronic diseases that are the progeny of metabolic dysfunction, or metabolic dysfunction produced through trauma. It's well recognized that treating metabolic function impacts future disability, thus, pertinent evaluation of evident ATMs allows an opportunity to reconsider the complex care of rehabilitation patients. Through personalized SB a rehabilitation physician can attune themselves to the various prevailing factors that will influence the course of chronic illness. Using leverage points, an individualized treatment plan incorporating different systems and team members will create a patient-centered and efficacious health care plan.

These concepts are not entirely new to physical medicine and rehabilitation (PM&R), because they have been seen in rehabilitation-based research and models. As noted, there are several explorations in the literature into what amounts to the SB of chronic neurologic disease at the levels of genetics, cellular function, organ physiology, and treatments. Similarly, through the lens of the BPS model, the World Health Organization published the International Classification of Functioning, Disability, and Health (ICF) Model of Functioning and Disability, which considers patient and environmental factors, as well as body structures/functions, activities and participation in evaluating overall function or health condition.[65] Interestingly, this is a close approximation of the ATMs and the SB approach. The differences largely center around the external functioning of the body in its environment within the ICF model versus the internal functioning of the body by SB.

There is, of course, another shared philosophy between FM and PM&R. The interdisciplinary team is the prototypic example of the physiatric approach to chronic problems by using multiple team members input with the physician facilitation Organizations like the Institute for Functional Medicine also promote this interdisciplinary team approach and function with an diverse core of teaching faculty who help a variety of learners from various clinical backgrounds to apply FM principles within the scope of their practice.[7] Both FM and PM&R endorse value to the variety of treatments providers.

However, one point of leverage in the current curriculum of FM taught with the matrix concept of SB is the paucity of musculoskeletal application for the structural integrity portion of the matrix. Such work as the ICF Model, the Feldenkrais technique and the inpatient rehabilitation process would help enlighten providers within the FM curriculum on the interplay between neuromuscular function and the other systems. Furthermore, the impact of loss of function on the factories of metabolism is evident with those with physical disabilities. Similarly, the biochemistry of activities of daily living, the role of exercise on blood transportation, the interdependent role of muscle cellular function and effects on bone metabolism are important considerations in daily practice.

There are advantages to having a relationship between FM and PM&R, as the approaches, individuals they serve, and locations are well aligned. As mentioned, the interdisciplinary team and ICF models of rehabilitation fit well with the personal, SB model of FM. Interestingly, inpatient rehabilitation also offers a unique platform for trying many of the intensive lifestyle changes and may represent a positive opportunity for change for many patients, including using FM on previously "functional" diagnoses.

CLINICS CARE POINTS

- The use of FM is beneficial in chronic disease management.
- Many complex rehabilitation cases will be more thoroughly managed by attentive clinicians collecting ATMs; avoiding only a linear medical approach.
- Accepted approaches for chronic pain and TBI, such as exercise prescription and sleep management, need to be thoughtfully considered rather than applied blindly.
- Vagal nerve stimulation and nutritional management are further methods of improving symptoms in chronic pain and TBI.

DISCLOSURE

Nothing to Disclose.

REFERENCES

1. Bentley AR, DJ, Fouts HN. U.S. obesity as delayed effect of excess sugar. Econ Hum Biol 2020;36.
2. Buttorff CR, T, Bauman M. Multiple chronic conditions in the United States. Santa Monica (CA): RAND Corporation; 2017.
3. Health and Economic Costs of Chronic Diseases. Centers for Disease Control and Prevention. 2020. Available at: https://www.cdc.gov/chronicdisease/about/costs/index.htm. Accessed April 9, 2020.
4. Sapolsky RM. Why zebras don't get ulcers. 3rd edition. New York: Owl Book/Henry Holt and Co.; 2004.
5. Beidelschies M, Alejandro-Rodriguez M, Ji X, et al. Association of the functional medicine model of care with patient-reported health-related quality-of-life outcomes. JAMA Netw Open 2019;2(10):e1914017.
6. Jones DS, Hofmann L, Quinn S. 21st Century medicine: a new model for medical education and practice. Gig Harbor (WA): The Institute for Functional Medicine; 2009.
7. Jones DS, Quinn S. Reversing the chronic disease trend: six steps to better wellness. Federal Way (WA): The Institute for Functional Medicine; 2017.
8. Wade DT, Halligan PW. The biopsychosocial model of illness: a model whose time has come. Clin Rehabil 2017;31(8):995–1004.
9. Borrell-Carrio F, Suchman AL, Epstein RM. The biopsychosocial model 25 years later: principles, practice, and scientific inquiry. Ann Fam Med 2004;2(6):576–82.
10. Bevers K, Watts L, Kishino N, et al. Touch Medical Media, Ltd: The Biopsychosocial Model of the Assessment, Prevention, and Treatment of Chronic Pain. US neurology 2016;12(2):98–104.
11. Nassif TH, Hull A, Holliday SB, et al. Concurrent validity of the defense and veterans pain rating scale in VA outpatients. Pain Med 2015;16(11):2152–61.
12. Waljas M, Lange RT, Hakulinen U, et al. Biopsychosocial outcome after uncomplicated mild traumatic brain injury. J neurotrauma 2014;31(1):108–24.
13. Waljas M, Iverson GL, Lange RT, et al. A prospective biopsychosocial study of the persistent post-concussion symptoms following mild traumatic brain injury. J neurotrauma 2015;32(8):534–47.
14. Ideker T, Galitski T, Hood L. A new approach to decoding life: systems biology. Annu Rev Genom Hum Genet 2001;2:343–72.
15. Yu C, Kobeissy F. Systems biology applications to decipher mechanisms and novel biomarkers in CNS trauma. In: Kobeissy FH, editor. Brain neurotrauma:

molecular, neuropsychological, and rehabilitation aspects. Seattle: Institute for Systems Biology; 2015.

16. What is systems biology. Institute for Systems Biology. 2020. Available at: https://isbscience.org/about/what-is-systems-biology/. Accessed April 8, 2020.

17. Lyman M, Lloyd DG, Ji X, et al. Neuroinflammation: the role and consequences. Neurosci Res 2014;79:1–12.

18. Simon DW, McGeachy MJ, Bayir H, et al. The far-reaching scope of neuroinflammation after traumatic brain injury. Nat Rev Neurol 2017;13(3):171–91.

19. Le Thuc O, Blondeau N, Nahon JL, et al. The complex contribution of chemokines to neuroinflammation: switching from beneficial to detrimental effects. Ann N Y Acad Sci 2015;1351:127–40.

20. Hong S, Dissing-Olesen L, Stevens B. New insights on the role of microglia in synaptic pruning in health and disease. Curr Opin Neurobiol 2016;36:128–34.

21. Louveau A, Herz J, Alme MN, et al. CNS lymphatic drainage and neuroinflammation are regulated by meningeal lymphatic vasculature. Nat Neurosci 2018;21(10):1380–91.

22. Jackson Nakazawa D. The angel and the assassin. New York: Ballantine Books; 2020.

23. Perry VH, Nicoll JA, Holmes C. Microglia in neurodegenerative disease. Nat Rev Neurol 2010;6(4):193–201.

24. Chowen JA, Garcia-Segura LM. Microglia, neurodegeneration and loss of neuroendocrine control. Prog Neurobiol 2020;184:101720.

25. Javidi E, Magnus T. Autoimmunity after ischemic stroke and brain injury. Front Immunol 2019;10:686.

26. Kempuraj D, Thangavel R, Selvakumar GP, et al. Brain and peripheral atypical inflammatory mediators potentiate neuroinflammation and neurodegeneration. Front Cell Neurosci 2017;11:216.

27. Engelhardt B, Carare RO, Bechmann I, et al. Vascular, glial, and lymphatic immune gateways of the central nervous system. Acta Neuropathol 2016;132(3):317–38.

28. Andersson U, Tracey KJ. Neural reflexes in inflammation and immunity. J Exp Med 2012;209(6):1057–68.

29. Kox M, Pompe JC, Pickkers P, et al. Increased vagal tone accounts for the observed immune paralysis in patients with traumatic brain injury. Neurology 2008;70(6):480–5.

30. Sundman MH, Chen NK, Subbian V, et al. The bidirectional gut-brain-microbiota axis as a potential nexus between traumatic brain injury, inflammation, and disease. Brain Behav Immun 2017;66:31–44.

31. Rea K, Dinan TG, Cryan JF. The microbiome: A key regulator of stress and neuroinflammation. Neurobiol Stress 2016;4:23–33.

32. Krishnamurthy K, Laskowitz DT. Cellular and Molecular Mechanisms of Secondary Neuronal Injury following Traumatic Brain Injury. In Laskowitz D and Grant G, editors. Translational Research in Traumatic Brain Injury: Frontiers in Neuroscience. p. 134-71.

33. Han C, Rice MW, Cai D. Neuroinflammatory and autonomic mechanisms in diabetes and hypertension. Am J Physiol Endocrinol Metab 2016;311(1):E32–41.

34. Singh V, Roth S, Llovera G, et al. Microbiota dysbiosis controls the neuroinflammatory response after stroke. J Neurosci 2016;36(28):7428–40.

35. Kumar A, Loane DJ. Neuroinflammation after traumatic brain injury: opportunities for therapeutic intervention. Brain Behav Immun 2012;26(8):1191–201.

36. Lozano D, Gonzales-Portillo GS, Acosta S, et al. Neuroinflammatory responses to traumatic brain injury: etiology, clinical consequences, and therapeutic opportunities. Neuropsychiatr Dis Treat 2015;11:97–106.

37. Hoogland ICM, Westhoff D, Engelen-Lee JY, et al. Microglial activation after systemic stimulation with lipopolysaccharide and Escherichia coli. Front Cell Neurosci 2018;12:110.

38. Ji RR, Nackley A, Huh Y, et al. Neuroinflammation and central sensitization in chronic and widespread pain. Anesthesiology 2018;129(2):343–66.

39. Kuner R, Flor H. Structural plasticity and reorganisation in chronic pain. Nat Rev Neurosci 2017;18(2):113.

40. Moghetti P, Bacchi E, Brangani C, et al. Metabolic effects of exercise. Front Horm Res 2016;47:44–57.

41. Stephan JS, Sleiman SF. Exercise factors as potential mediators of cognitive rehabilitation following traumatic brain injury. Curr Opin Neurol 2019;32(6):808–14.

42. Rice D, Nijs J, Kosek E, et al. Exercise-induced hypoalgesia in pain-free and chronic pain populations: state of the art and future directions. J Pain 2019;20(11):1249–66.

43. Lin L, Skakavac N, Lin X, et al. Acupuncture-induced analgesia: the role of microglial inhibition. Cell Transplant 2016;25:621–8.

44. Berry ME, Chapple IT, Ginsberg JP, et al. Non-pharmacological intervention for chronic pain in veterans: a pilot study of heart rate variability biofeedback. Glob Adv Health Med 2014;3(2):28–33.

45. Francis HM, Fisher A, Rushby JA, et al. Reduced heart rate variability in chronic severe traumatic brain injury: Association with impaired emotional and social functioning, and potential for treatment using biofeedback. Neuropsychol Rehabil 2016;26(1):103–25.

46. Chakravarthy K, Chaudhry H, Williams K, et al. Review of the uses of vagal nerve stimulation in chronic pain management. Curr Pain Headache Rep 2015;19(12):54.

47. Hakon J, Moghiseh M, Poulsen I. Transcutaneous Vagus Nerve Stimulation in Patients With Severe Traumatic Brain Injury: A Feasibility Trial. Neuromodulation 2020;23(6):859–64.

48. Burgess HJ, Burns JW, Buvanendran A, et al. Associations between sleep disturbance and chronic pain intensity and function: a test of direct and indirect pathways. Clin J Pain 2019;35(7):569–76.

49. Wolfe LF, Sahni AS, Attarian H. Sleep disorders in traumatic brain injury. NeuroRehabilitation 2018;43(3):257–66.

50. Ouellet MC, Beaulieu-Bonneau S, Morin CM. Sleep-wake disturbances after traumatic brain injury. Lancet Neurol 2015;14(7):746–57.

51. Grima NA, Rajaratnam SMW, Mansfield D, et al. Efficacy of melatonin for sleep disturbance following traumatic brain injury: a randomised controlled trial. BMC Med 2018;16(1):8.

52. Koffel E, McCurry SM, Smith MT, et al. Improving pain and sleep in middle-aged and older adults: the promise of behavioral sleep interventions. Pain 2019;160(3):529–34.

53. Totsch SK, Quinn TL, Strath LJ, et al. The impact of the standard American diet in rats: effects on behavior, physiology and recovery from inflammatory injury. Scand J Pain 2017;17:316–24.

54. Cresci G, Beidelschies M, Tebo J, et al. Educating future physicians in nutritional science and practice: the time is now. J Am Coll Nutr 2019;38(5):387–94.

55. Gasior M, Rogawski MA, Hartman AL. Neuroprotective and disease-modifying effects of the ketogenic diet. Behav Pharmacol 2006;17(5–6):431–9.
56. Rondanelli M, Faliva MA, Miccono A, et al. Food pyramid for subjects with chronic pain: foods and dietary constituents as anti-inflammatory and antioxidant agents. Nutr Res Rev 2018;31(1):131–51.
57. Towery P, Guffey JS, Doerflein C, et al. Chronic musculoskeletal pain and function improve with a plant-based diet. Complement Ther Med 2018;40:64–9.
58. Brain K, Burrows TL, Rollo ME, et al. A systematic review and meta-analysis of nutrition interventions for chronic noncancer pain. J Hum Nutr Diet 2019;32(2): 198–225.
59. Zhang X, Wu Q, Zhang Q, et al. Resveratrol attenuates early brain injury after experimental subarachnoid hemorrhage via inhibition of NLRP3 inflammasome activation. Front Neurosci 2017;11:611.
60. Chen X, Chen C, Fan S, et al. Omega-3 polyunsaturated fatty acid attenuates the inflammatory response by modulating microglia polarization through SIRT1-mediated deacetylation of the HMGB1/NF-κB pathway following experimental traumatic brain injury. J Neuroinflammation 2018;15(1):116.
61. Bhatti J, Nascimento B, Akhtar U, et al. Systematic review of human and animal studies examining the efficacy and safety of N-Acetylcysteine (NAC) and N-Acetylcysteine Amide (NACA) in traumatic brain injury: impact on neurofunctional outcome and biomarkers of oxidative stress and inflammation. Front Neurol 2018;8:744.
62. Guida F, Boccella S, Belardo C, et al. Altered gut microbiota and endocannabinoid system tone in vitamin D deficiency-mediated chronic pain. Brain Behav Immun 2020;85:128–41.
63. Prego-Dominguez J, Hadrya F, Takkouche B. Polyunsaturated fatty acids and chronic pain: a systematic review and meta-analysis. Pain Physician 2016; 19(8):521–35.
64. Daily JW, Yang M, Park S. Efficacy of turmeric extracts and curcumin for alleviating the symptoms of joint arthritis: a systematic review and meta-analysis of randomized clinical trials. J Med Food 2016;19(8):717–29.
65. Steiner WA, Ryser L, Huber E, et al. Use of the ICF model as a clinical problem-solving tool in physical therapy and rehabilitation medicine. Phys Ther 2002; 82(11):1098–107.

Pain Neuroscience Education as the Foundation of Interdisciplinary Pain Treatment

Kristin Eneberg-Boldon, PT, DPT[a], Bradley Schaack, DPT[b],*,
Kelly Joyce, MSPT[b],*

KEYWORDS

- Pain neuroscience education • Persistent pain • Biopsychosocial factors
- Adult learning theory

KEY POINTS

- Complexity of persistent pain calls for a collaborative team-based approach, using pain neuroscience education at its core.
- Treatment approaches should be individualized and reflect findings of the comprehensive biopsychosocial evaluation.
- Using a common approach and consistent messaging across all pain, clinicians can lead to improved understanding of pain and functional outcomes.
- Development of the patient-clinician therapeutic alliance influences outcomes.

INTRODUCTION

Each year in the United States, an estimated 100 million adults with persistent pain diagnoses carry the burden of health care costs, totaling up to $635 billion annually.[1] Every pain patient has a diverse variety of influencing factors having an impact on function, pain, and overall health. The complexity of pain care options should be met with a clear navigational strategy that fosters efficient, direct pathways to the most appropriate treatment plan that is specific to an individual's unique pain condition. Not only the perspective of patient well-being and provision of high-quality care but also the financial aspect of pain treatment must be considered. Whereas many patients and clinicians desire a quick remedy to pain, evidence indicates that interdisciplinary, biopsychosocial interventions provide longer-lasting improvement for patients with persistent pain. Due to the nature of the health care system and training of health care providers, this type of care often is not accessed until long into the chronic phase

[a] Physical Medicine and Rehabilitation Services (117A), Greater Los Angeles VA health Care System, 11301 Wilshire Blvd, Los Angeles, CA 90073, USA; [b] Physical Medicine and Rehabilitation Services (117A), Tomah VA Medical Center, 500 East Veterans Street, Tomah, WI 54660, USA
* Corresponding authors.
E-mail addresses: Bradley.Schaack@va.gov (B.S.); Kelly.Joyce@va.gov (K.J.)

of pain, if at all. Investigators have recognized the lack of comprehensive pain education training for primary care providers in medical school as well as limited training in comprehensive pain assessment and management strategies as contributing factors.[2,3] Lack of a thorough understanding of persistent pain can lead to a trial-and-error approach by inexperienced clinicians across many professions, including the ordering of unnecessary tests and treatments in the absence of a comprehensive musculoskeletal pain evaluation.

PAIN NEUROSCIENCE EDUCATION

From a patient perspective, unnecessary tests or treatments lead to increasing financial burden and stress from the increasing fears of why pain persists long after tissues have healed.[2] These are just 2 factors that have an impact on the pain cycle.[2] By understanding pain and the contributing biopsychosocial factors connected to persistent pain, as knowledgeable health care clinicians, physical medicine and rehabilitation professionals can be leaders in helping patients navigate through multiple health care options and consumer-driven products, using the most current evidence related to pain neuroscience education (PNE)[3] as a foundational core for navigating pain treatment. PNE provides a central understanding of how pain works and conveys common messages that can be understood by patients and reinforced by all health care professions (**Box 1**). From this perspective, current PNE techniques can be considered as a part of the therapeutic treatment plan. The importance of teaching patients to understand their individual pain condition can lead to an improved quality of life and increase in functional gains.[3] A higher level of compliance and relevant behavior changes, such as empowered decision making and independence in self-treatment techniques over time, also may exist when clinicians target treatment approaches with a more efficient and effective plan of care. Compliance with treatment ultimately can help patients escape their pain cycle.[2] A combination of increasing mobility, activity, and exercise with psychology-based approaches, such as cognitive behavior therapy, motivational interviewing, and mindfulness techniques, along with PNE has shown an effective method for controlling pain, reducing fear, and improving function.[3,4]

EVALUATION WITH EDUCATION

A comprehensive musculoskeletal evaluation is indicated for patients with persistent pain to assure no underlying disease or neurologic diagnoses exist and to guide

---

Box 1
Common pain neuroscience terms

- Nociception
  Nervous system response to harmful or potentially harmful stimuli

- Peripheral sensitization
  Increased sensitivity to afferent nerve stimuli, such as with swelling after acute injury

- Central sensitization
  Increased responsiveness of nociceptors in the central nervous system resulting in hypersensitivity or an increased pain response

- Neuroplasticity
  Changes in the nervous system brought about by physical and cognitive activity

Data from Refs.[3,4,9–12]

treatment decisions based on objective strengths, limitations, and goals. Bio-psychosocial factors and patient preferences are important to consider as treatment planning and therapeutic alliance-building begin. During the initial evaluation, by intro-ducing concepts of PNE, choosing language carefully to reduce fear regarding their persistent pain condition, a strong therapeutic alliance can be created.[3,4] Allowing pa-tients to tell their pain story instead of simply using a checklist or intake form may seem less efficient; however, it actually may lead to more directly relevant information than an intake form. A significant amount of information can and should be gathered from the comprehensive evaluation:

- Medical history, including biopsychosocial factors
- Comprehensive pain interview
  - Frequency, intensity, and duration
  - Continuous versus intermittent
  - Pain treatment history
  - Pain triggers
  - Pain patterns
  - Actions that increase or decrease pain
  - Comorbidities having an impact on pain
  - Fatigue level
  - Coping skills
  - Level of pain catastrophizing
  - Level of pain understanding
  - Patient treatment preferences
  - Patient goals and expectations
- Vital signs, red flags, and neurologic screening
- Range of motion
- Joint mobility, as indicated
- Strength
- Coordination
- Functional outcome measures
- Activity or exercise tolerance

TREATMENT CONSIDERATIONS

Once underlying disease and influential comorbid conditions have been ruled out, the question of which of many potential treatments to prescribe arises. Societal influences encourage the desire for quick fixes for chronic and persistent conditions, leading to high patient expectations. Medication, surgeries, or 1-time procedures often are the hope of the patient but often not a realistic care plan. As research evolves, it becomes more apparent that, for persistent pain, changes in physical activity and psychosocial and lifestyle behaviors have promising results.[5,6] Lowering stress, increasing exercise, and insuring a healthy diet often are included in the multimodal treatment plan for many different conditions, including persistent pain conditions.[5,6] The challenge lies is in motivating patients to create long-term lifestyle changes. Physical, social, and cognitive habits are hard to break and belief patterns are difficult to change.[7,8] Although recommendations for changes commonly are provided, implementing long-term change in patients can be challenging.

By offering comprehensive PNE as a primary focus early in the treatment plan, a strong foundation is provided to create a more intentional approach to multimodal pain care, with a more engaged and knowledgeable patient. To ensure learning by the adult patient with persistent pain, evidence found in educational sciences provides guidance. Many health care providers place less emphasis on patient education, simply by providing a brochure, handout, or Internet link. This may be due to time constraints, reimbursement concerns, or simply not having learned effective patient education skills. Patient education typically occurs at nearly every appointment in some form; however, many clinicians may lack formal understanding or the ability to effectively apply adult learning theory in patient care. How clinicians communicate and teach patients can influence the amount and quality of information that a patient retains and ultimately have an impact on the decisions patients make about their treatment. Level of retention can modify the level of compliance with the pain treatment plan. Whether pain education, medication management, home exercise program instruction, or stress management techniques, effective clinicians must understand principles of adult learning theory as it applies to patient education.

Andragogy, developed by Malcolm Knowles in 1988, is the theory that adult learners desire an understanding of why something should be done a certain way and how something works.[7] When adults understand "the why," it establishes a greater level of intrinsic motivation.[8] Explaining to a patient how pain works and its relationship to the nervous system is an example of andragogy. When developing instructional material, the clinician turned teacher should understand what the patient wants to know as well as what is needed to know. Assessing a patient's readiness to learn and motivations to learn can assist in directing treatment planning. Comprehending a patient's pain experience also helps in building a stronger therapeutic alliance. Experiential learning theory[8] describes a scenario where the patient experience provides the framework for applying PNE. The initial pain onset and patterns of pain, as well as the experiences from health care treatments and non–health care influences, are important to identify. Clinicians must have respect for the learner and their pain experience in order to create an environment suitable for learning and ensure time is carved out for discussion, reflection, and questions.

Across the spectrum of biopsychosocial therapeutic treatment options (**Fig. 1**), the application of pain education offers a strong foundation for all therapeutic options for which to connect. PNE teaches patients why they have persistent pain and helps to reframe their beliefs about pain and their abilities.[4] The therapeutic effect of the education focuses on reducing the heightened sensitivity of the nervous system.[3,9] When reflecting on the pain cycle (see **Box 1**), treatment should address the reduction of fear, increasing movement, and applying cognitive behavior changes.[3,10] Patients become self-managers of their pain by understanding and controlling the variety of

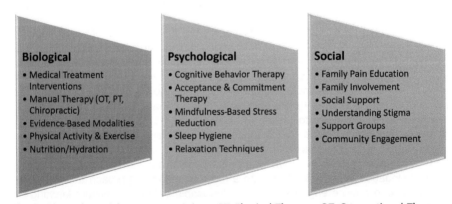

Fig. 1. Biopsychosocial treatment options. PT, Physical Therapy; OT, Occupational Therapy.

influencing factors and understanding that intentional, sensible treatment approaches can lead to long-term gains. Evidence shows that patients who have a deeper understanding of modern pain science have reduced, pain, dysfunction, and kinesiophobia while increasing movement and improving function.[11–13] Adults learn best when they understand why something happens and how something works.[7] Not only does this apply to patients but also to clinicians. Staying current in modern pain neuroscience advances is required in order to provide accurate patent education. As members of a pain team, it is everyone's role to present potential treatment options and help patients choose long-term strategies that achieve lasting results instead of a trial-and-error approach. Altering a patient's beliefs requires uniform messaging, recurring interaction, and pain coaching to make a sustainable difference. It is advised that consistent messaging and treatment choices focus on decreasing the sensitivity of the nervous system.

TREATMENT: PRESCRIBING MOVEMENT

Although PNE has been beneficial for patients with chronic pain, evidence shows that combining PNE with safe, progressive exercise increases function and reduces fear.[13] The comprehensive evaluation, including biopsychosocial factors, guides a physical therapist in prescribing the most appropriate exercise for each patient based on individual clinical needs and personal preferences. In some situations, manual therapy techniques may be required prior to or in conjunction with therapeutic exercise, when indicated to improve joint mobility. Many forms of exercise have shown to benefit patients with persistent pain (**Fig. 2**). The consistent factor in research is that movement plays a significant role and should be part of the treatment plan, beginning at an appropriate intensity, frequency, and duration to avoid flare-up of pain. Therapeutic movement and exercise have an important role in the treatment of persistent pain.[6] In the same manner that each patient's pain experience is different from others' experiences, each patient also has an exercise preference for type, style, and mode of exercise. When prescribing exercise, discussion between an informed clinician and their patient should include the following considerations:

- What is the current level of mobility and activity?
- Is there a preference for independent, personal instruction or group exercise?
- Is there a preference for activity in home, rehabilitation clinic, or community?
- Is there a preference for virtual or in-person exercise?

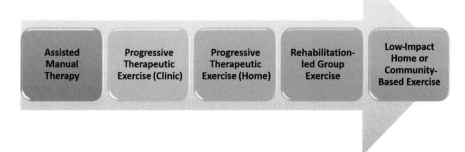

Fig. 2. Movement continuum.

- Is there a preference for structured classes or a general increase of activity, such as gardening or walking?
- Based on biopsychosocial factors, should activity focus on flexibility, strength, motion, balance, socialization, aerobic exercise, or a combination?
- Which medical comorbidities must be taken into consideration when prescribing exercise?
- How frequently is the patient able and willing to commit to exercise?

Movement and exercise goals for patients begin with improving functional deficits, leading to gains in independence with compliance and progression. Physical therapists identify a patient's preferred, sustainable activity that promotes better health. Although an inexperienced clinician or local gym may advocate for a specific type of exercise based on internal biases or current trends, an experienced clinician prescribing exercise understands that long-term success occurs when patient preferences help guide the decision, along with insuring an appropriate frequency, intensity, and duration. Pending no negative effects, an exercise prescription that combines, flexibility, strengthening, balance, and endurance that a patient can tolerate, self-modify, and progress through is the long-term goal of an exercise prescription. When prescribing exercise, there are several specific considerations that must be made:

1. Throughout a progressive exercise continuum, it is recommended to reinforce pain neuroscience concepts while experiencing the exercise. Repeating key points applied to different experiences leads to a deeper understanding of how the brain responds to movement. This teaches the patient that pain can be controlled through awareness of movement, while justifying the benefits of the exercise.[13,14]
2. Fear-avoidance behaviors often limit follow-through on recommended exercise prescription. Adequate time must be taken in initial and subsequent visits to build trust and allow patients to experience the motion, reinforce their ability to control the exercise intensity, and stay safe in a supportive setting to reduce or eliminate fear-avoidance behaviors.[15]
3. Activity pacing recommendations can be a fine balance. If too little pacing is incorporated, the risk of increased fear or pain may occur. If too many pacing limits are incorporated, the risk of no improvement and boredom may occur, leading to noncompliance. In early stages, rather than prescribing exercise to perform independently, it is recommended to ensure an effective communication feedback loop between therapist and patient, until the patient's awareness of the association between exercise and pain has been mastered.

THERAPEUTIC MODALITIES AND COMPLEMENTARY AND INTEGRATED HEALTH IN PAIN REHABILITATION

When considering the application of modalities, such as therapeutic dry needling, electrical stimulation, biofeedback, acupuncture, or other modalities, all clinicians must critically assess the reason for their intended application in relation to how pain works and weigh the evidence behind why the modality is considered. A review of individual modalities is not the intent of this article; however, when considering the introduction of modalities, some questions to consider for any modality include the following:

- Is there evidence supporting the use of the selected modality for the specific condition?
- What physiologic or cognitive responses are expected from the modality?

- What other treatment approaches complement the modality?
- Is the time spent providing a modality the best use of clinical and patient time compared with other treatment approaches?
- Will the use of the modality allow the patient to progress faster compared with no modality being used?
- How might the modality fit within a PNE framework? That is, would it help calm the sensitivity of the nervous system by initiating relaxation or mindfulness?
- Would it inspire or inhibit the progression toward long-term goals of independent self-care?
- Prior to delivering the modality, can the clinician explain and the patient understand how it relates to other pain neuroscience messaging?

PSYCHOSOCIAL TREATMENT OPTIONS

Rehabilitation clinicians receive education and training that focus on the ability to see and treat the whole person beyond the diagnosis. When it comes to applying PNE as a foundation for treating the whole person, clinicians must realize the benefit and perspective that mental health professionals also bring to the interdisciplinary pain team. Although techniques for coaching, motivational interviewing, and cognitive behavior techniques are used frequently among rehabilitation professionals, by incorporating pain psychologists into the team, more directed mental health expertise for the complex, persistent pain patient deepens the strength of the pain team. Evidence supports the use of treatments, such as mindfulness-based stress reduction, acceptance and commitment therapy,[15] and cognitive behavior therapy. Because mental health diagnoses and stressors can influence pain, individual mental health treatment to address psychosocial factors, such as relationships, addiction, anxiety, and depression, can be an effective contribution to a multimodal team. Whereas PNE alone has been shown to lead to some improvement, by adding both prescribed progression of movement by a physical therapist and cognitive behavior treatment approaches, evidence has shown greater gains in function.[16,17] Therapeutic alliance is another factor that must be considered when treating patients with persistent pain.[18] Patient adherence to clinical recommendations often is poor, which can lead to ineffective results or a false perception regarding the therapeutic benefits of therapy, exercise, or other professional interventions. The incorporation of good communication skills can lead to improved compliance, with potential for improved function and self-motivation.[19–21]

NUTRITIONAL CONSIDERATIONS

Clinical dietitians bring value to the multimodal pain to not only encourage healthy eating strategies but also individually address a variety of comorbidities that may be either a result of chronic pain or a contributing factor to chronic pain. The dietitian who treats pain also should understand and deliver consistent pain neuroscience messaging regarding the sensitivity of the nervous system as it relates to pain and nutrition.[22] Although general introductory nutritional advice can be provided relevant to healthy eating by many professions or accessed via the Internet, the advanced understanding by a clinical dietitian brings a deeper level of individualization in relation to patient comorbidities and advanced nutritional recommendations in the same way that a physical therapist prescribes individualized exercise and that psychologists or occupational therapists with a mental health focus address cognitive and psychosocial factors. By developing a pain team that includes these core clinicians and ensuring all members deliver consistent messaging related to PNE, the patient with complex persistent pain can receive a direct, comprehensive, and integrated treatment plan. For conditions that developed over an extended period, the ability to break down habitual behaviors and replace with healthy biopsychosocial behaviors also takes time.

MULTIMEDIA CONSIDERATIONS

Through the advancement of technology, persistent pain has reached a new era as multimedia strategies to deliver pain education begin to be implemented and clinically based visits are expanded to adding creative methods of supporting the pain patient from a motivational and coaching perspective using telehealth, streaming rehabilitation exercise, Internet-based education, and mobile applications for pain, stress management, nutrition and water intake, and other supportive features. Technology should not replace the individualized expertise that health care clinicians can provide; however, their use to supplement, motivate, and transition the patient to independence has significant potential for contributing to sustainable long-term gains, when applied with appropriate health-focused intention.

CASE STUDY

The patient is a 55-year-old female Air Force veteran who presented to outpatient physical therapy with complaints of low back pain and bilateral lower extremity paresthesia. Although the patient reported previous ongoing low back pain, she described a motor vehicle accident and subsequent flare of symptoms 17 years ago. After the accident, patient reported trialing many nonsurgical options with minimal success. Ultimately, patient underwent an L3-5 fusion with limited postsurgical follow-up for physical therapy.

At the time of the physical therapy evaluation, the patient reported difficulty with prolonged walking for more than 30 minutes, standing for more than 20 minutes, and general housework. She reported utilizing over-the-counter anti-inflammatories and a generalized home stretching program with moderate relief. The patient's goals for treatment included improvement in ongoing pain and increased tolerance with activities of daily life.

Key elements of objective evaluation
- Transfers/mobility: independent transfers with no ambulation unsteadiness
- Active trunk range of motion: gross flexion and extension measurements were limited by lumbar pain to 80° and 20°, respectively.
- Manual muscle test: 5/5 for all lower extremity motions
- Neurologic screen: patellar reflex (2+ bilateral), Achilles reflex (not elicited bilateral)

Treatment strategies
- PNE highlighted multiple concepts, including nervous system sensitivity and its role in a person's pain experience, the brain being the driver of a person's pain, the role of nontissue influences, and the importance of exercise pacing principles in relation to desensitizing the nervous system. These concepts were implemented via a workbook format. Homework required reading and reflection activities, which were provided as part of every treatment session.
- Disbursed transcutaneous electrical nerve stimulation unit as self-management option with education regarding its role in helping desensitize the nervous system
- Trigger point dry needling to affected area
- Myofascial soft tissue mobilization techniques to the lumbar spine

- Prior lumbar radiograph reviewed with patient, in relation to fear-avoidance thoughts (negative for hardware misalignment)
- Joint mobilization of the pelvis and lumbar spine
- Progressive home exercise program focused on full-body, functional movement
- Consistent, progressive cardiovascular exercise (stationary bike) daily
- Nutritional Changes per Registered Dietitian Recommendation
- Stopped smoking
- Daily meditation exercise as directed by psychologist
- Individualized mental health appointments focused on treatment of stress management, fear-avoidance behaviors, and cognitive behavior approaches
- Private, weekly yoga sessions patient pursued independently, following recommendation by physical therapist

Outcome

- Thirteen treatments spanning 5 months, with decreasing frequency per month
- Patient reported constant low back pain being resolved and decreased intensity of intermittent flare ups.
- Walking—patient reported walking up to 45 minutes with no increase in low back pain.
- Standing—patient reported being able to stand for 45 minutes with no increase in low back pain.
- Patient reported no increase in low back pain during or after completing all needed household activities.

Clinics care points

- This case reinforces the benefit of a multimodal approach when treating persistent pain, using an interdisciplinary approach to address not only mobility but also mental health, nutrition, and other identified areas of need.
- With persistent pain clients, the clinician's focus was less on tissue damage and more on improving the patient's function and overall mobility.
- This case presents a situation where fear was an integral part of the veteran's pain persisting beyond normal healing periods. Once the fear of reinjury was addressed and lessened, the veteran saw immediate gains in exercise tolerance. As exercise tolerance increased and stress levels decreased, pain lessened and function improved.
- The importance of noting the benefit of normalizing a pain flare allows the patient to realize that during recovery, mild or moderate flares in pain are normal and that increasing pain does not directly suggest further tissue damage.
- In most persistent pain cases, the complexity of the education provided, the level of understanding needed, and the need for activity pacing may require a lengthier treatment course. In the grand perspective, 5 months and 13 visits to improve a 17-year persistent pain condition and change health behaviors is a reasonable duration; when a patient is steadily progressive, change is the expectation versus expecting an immediate resolution in 1 or 2 treatments.
- Patient motivation and the clinician's ability to influence self-motivation played an integral part in the overall treatment success of this patient with persistent pain.
- This case represents the importance of education in combination with movement, manual therapy, mental health nutrition, and complementary strategies, with progression to independent self-care. Using techniques together may allow for central nervous system changes and subsequent decreased nervous system sensitivity in a patient with persistent pain.

SUMMARY

Due to the numerous factors that contribute to pain, 1 standardized treatment plan or intervention does not benefit most patients with persistent pain. Collaborative teamwork, among physiatrists, physical and occupational therapists, psychologists, registered dietitians, and other health care professionals who have a deep and comprehensive understanding of persistent pain conditions, offers an individualized, functionally focused approach to treating pain.

Following a comprehensive musculoskeletal-psychosocial evaluation, an individualized treatment plan combines appropriate levels of progressive mobility and exercise, nutrition, and cognitive-based treatment strategies, with consistent PNE strategies implemented throughout the course of treatment. As self-care strategies and independence develop and the understanding of PNE principles strengthens, the incorporation of complementary and integrated self-care treatment options or community-based exercise groups that promote safe movement or decreasing the sensitivity of the nervous system can be a good tool for the transition to an independence. Adult learning theory teaches including the patient as a student, with the goal of patient becoming independent in all necessary knowledge and applied learning upon discharge. Applying this patient education tool early and regularly into the chain of health care appointments also may help prevent persistent pain. To effectively unlearn or reverse the biopsychosocial factors that contributed to the persistent state, understanding the why reinforces patient effort and action.[8] Long-term treatment success is built within a therapeutic alliance between patient and clinicians by listening, ensuring good communication, and building trust.

ACKNOWLEDGMENTS

Wesley Kurszewski, DPT, for sharing his expertise, passion of treating patients with persistent pain, and mentoring clinicians through the years.

DISCLOSURE

The authors have nothing to disclose.

REFERENCES

1. Relieving Pain in America: a blueprint for transforming prevention, care, education, and research. Mil Med 2016;181(5):397–9.
2. Stones C, Cole F. Breaking the cycle: extending the persistent pain cycle diagram using an affective pictorial metaphor. Health Commun 2014;29(1):32–40.
3. Louw A, Nijs J, Puentedura EJ. A clinical perspective on a pain neuroscience education approach to manual therapy. J Man Manip Ther 2017;25(3):160–8.
4. Brumagne S, Diers M, Dannels L, et al. Neuroplasticity of Sensorimotor Control in Low Back Pain. J Orthop Sports Phys Ther 2019;49(6):402–14.
5. Davin S, Lapin B, Mijatovic D, et al. Comparative effectiveness of an interdisciplinary pain program for chronic low back pain, compared to physical therapy alone. Spine (Phila Pa 1976) 2019;44(24):1715–22.
6. Seers K. Review: intensive multidisciplinary biopsychosocial rehabilitation reduces pain and improves function in chronic low back pain. Evid Based Nurs 2002;5:116.
7. Franco MS. Instructional strategies and adult learning theories: an autoethnographic study about teaching research methods in a doctoral program. Education 2019;139(3):178–85.

8. Breese U, French R. Adult learning theory and patient education for low back pain. J Allied Health 2012;41(4):198–203.

9. Graven-Nielsen T, Arendt-Nielsen L. Peripheral and central sensitization in musculoskeletal pain disorders: an experimental approach. Curr Rheumatol Rep 2002;4(4):313–21.

10. Woolf CJ, Latremoliere A. Central Sensitization: A generator of pain hypersensitivity by central neural plasticity. J Pain 2009;10(9):895–926.

11. Meeus M, Nijs J. Central Sensitization: a biopyschosocial explanation for chronic widespread pain in patients with fibromyalgia and chronic fatigue syndrome. Clin Rheumatol 2007;26:465–73.

12. Loeser JD, Treede RD. The Kyoto protocol of IASP basic pain terminology. Pain 2008;137:473–7.

13. Puljak L, Arienti C. Can Physical Activity and Exercise Alleviate Chronic Pain in Adults? Am J Phys Med Rehabil 2019;98(6):526–7.

14. Kawada T. Exercise therapy for low back pain. Am J Phys Med Rehabil 2018; 97:10.

15. Casey M-B, Cotter N, Kelly C, et al. Exercise and acceptance and commitment therapy for chronic pain: a case series with one-year follow-up. Musculoskeletal Care 2020;18:64–73.

16. Markfelder T, Pauli P. Fear of pain and pain intensity: Meta-analysis and systematic review. Psychol Bull 2020;146(5):411–50.

17. Daniel HC, Narewska J, Serpell M, et al. Comparison of psychological and physical function in neuropathic pain and nociceptive pain: Implications for cognitive behavioral pain management programs. Eur J Pain 2008;12:731–41.

18. Miciak M, Mayan M, Brown C, et al. A framework for establishing connections in physiotherapy practice. Physiother Theor Pract 2019;35(1):40–56.

19. Lonsdale C, Hall AM, Murray A, et al. Communication skills training for practitioners to increase patient adherence to home-based rehabilitation for chronic low back pain: results of a cluster randomized controlled trial. Arch Phys Med Rehabil 2017;98(9):1732–43.

20. Diener I, Kargela LA. Listening is therapy: Patient interviewing from a pain science perspective. Physiother Theor Pract 2016;32(5):356–67.

21. Taccolini Manzoni AC, Bastos de Oliveira NT, Nunes Cabral CM, et al. The role of the therapeutic alliance on pain relief in musculoskeletal rehabilitation: A systematic review. Physiother Theor Pract 2018;34(12):901–15.

22. Brain K, Burrows TL, Rollo ME, et al. A systematic review and meta-analysis of nutrition interventions for chronic noncancer pain. J Hum Nutr Diet 2019;32(2): 198–225.

Whole Medical Systems the Rehabilitation Setting (Traditional Chinese Medicine, Ayurvedic Medicine, Homeopathy, Naturopathy)

David F. Drake, MD[a,b,*], Dudley K. Norman, EdD[c]

KEYWORDS

- Ayurveda • Complementary • Conventional • Homeopathy • Integrative
- Naturopathy • Traditional Chinese medicine

KEY POINTS

- Traditional Chinese medicine, ayurveda, homeopathy, and naturopathy are re-emerging as approaches integrated into contemporary medical practice.
- Research of whole medical systems, although experiencing a renaissance, continues to be methodologically weak.
- Whole medical systems treatments and conventional treatments all carry inherent risks, which the clinician and patient should consider in a balanced, informed, manner.
- Recently emerging integrative medical group visits can be an effective practice that is complementary to conventional medical practice.

More than 30% of American adults utilize health care approaches that are not considered mainstream. Mainstream approaches to health care most often are referred to as *conventional*, non-mainstream practices as *alternative approaches*, and the combination of mainstream and non-mainstream approaches as *complementary*. Integrative medicine (IM) brings together conventional, alternative, and complementary approaches into a holistic approach to health and wellness.[1] These IM approaches range from as broad in scope as the field of nutrition or movement therapy to as specific as acupuncture or massage. Many elements of IM, for example, mindfulness and meditation, increasingly are applied to myriad ailments. The IM trends emerging today

[a] Department of Physical Medicine and Rehabilitation, Virginia Commonwealth University, Richmond, VA, USA; [b] Interventional Pain Clinic, Central Virginia VA Health Care System, Richmond, VA, USA; [c] Central Virginia VA Health Care System, McGuire VA Medical Center, 1201 Broad Rock Boulevard #117, Richmond, VA 23249, USA
* Corresponding author. 14530 Sailview Ct, Midlothian, VA 23112.
E-mail address: David.Drake4@va.gov

Phys Med Rehabil Clin N Am 31 (2020) 553–561
https://doi.org/10.1016/j.pmr.2020.07.009
1047-9651/20/Published by Elsevier Inc.

represent a renaissance of millennial-old practices and their efficacy increasingly is supported by scientific evidence.

Many non-mainstream approaches to health care had their origins in ancient practices of whole medical systems (WMSs), in particular, traditional Chinese medicine (TCM) and ayurveda. Naturopathy and homeopathy have roots in ancient practices but have re-emerged and been formalized through modern educational systems over the past century. *The Merck Manual* defines WMSs as "complete systems that include philosophy and explanation of disease diagnosis, and therapy."[2] WMSs include TCM, ayurveda, homeopathy, and naturopathy, which each represent unique philosophic foundations, yet they commonly utilize overlapping techniques of diagnosis and treatment. Even though WMSs developed from within variant cultural histories, and most systems borrowed techniques from each other, all relied on the perspective that treatment of identifiable diseases or illnesses was dependent on treating the body and mind as a whole rather than focusing on the disease, illness, or symptoms, thus the name WMSs. This holistic care, although new to conventional Western medicine, is evolving standards of practice that are transforming modern medical systems (eg, allopathic medicine and osteopathic medicine).

Recent trends have moved away from alternative approaches and toward integrative therapies. Rather than offering historically WMSs modalities as stand-alone treatments or as multimodality treatments from one WMSs philosophic basis, evidence-based modalities now are integrated with conventional practices, providing options to patients and providers alike. Thus, contemporary medicine can be seen as borrowing singular and multimodality approaches from the historical WMSs paradigms into an emerging, modern, IM approach. Unfortunately, the evolving integration of WMSs approaches has not kept pace with modern research methodologies. Much of the available research reported still relies on (1) testing of multiple simultaneous treatments; (2) absence of control groups; (3) failure to blind subjects, assessors, or both; and (3) only rare comparison to conventional treatments or to no treatment. That said, studying WMSs by its very nature includes multiple, uncontrolled variables, so applying conventional medical research techniques is problematic. A sampling of these overlapping practices is discussed, with focus on those most emphasized in contemporary integrative practice, particularly in rehabilitative medicine. Example modalities, although overlapping, are representative mindfulness, movement, nutritional, and biomechanical.

TRADITIONAL CHINESE MEDICINE

TCM found its origins in China thousands of years ago.[3] TCM holds that pathology results from a disruption in the flow of natural body energy, referred to as *qi*. Diseases may arise from this disruption as well as from an imbalance in homeostasis, referred to in TCM as *yin and yang*, or from similar disturbances in the 5 elements: wood, fire, metal, earth, and water. TCM treatments involve re-establishing the proper flow of qi and improving the balance between yin and yang. Many colleges and universities in North America offer master's-level education in TCM. Many, but not all, states and provinces offer licensing to practice TCM, in particularly acupuncture.

A systematic review and meta-analysis[4] of TCM for neck pain and low back pain, in 2015, that included 75 randomized controlled trials (RCTs) examining more than 11,000 participants, found acupuncture, acupressure, and cupping to be efficacious for chronic neck pain and chronic low back pain; gua sha, tai chi, qigong, and Chinese manipulation showed modest changes but definite conclusions could not be drawn; and tui na, moxibustion, and herbal medicine were not studied (**Table 1**). Although

Table 1
Systematic review and meta-analysis of traditional Chinese medicine–defined key healing practices

Acupuncture	Acupuncture is a therapeutic method of penetrating needles into specific acupoints on the human body, guided by the theory of energy channels called meridians and the associated acupoints of traditional Chinese medicine.
Acupressure	Acupressure uses the application of fingers and pressure to stimulate specific acupoints on the human body, focusing on the balance of yin and yang.
Cupping	Cupping is a technique to induce local congestion and blood stasis for healing. Cups are made in different sizes and come in bamboo, plastic, glass, or porcelain. The treatment consists of creating a vacuum inside a cup and placing the cup over the selected area to include moving the cup with suction along tissue planes. TCM holds that the resulting suction effect invigorates blood and qi flow.
Gua sha	Gua sha is a technique of using a tool to massage the surface of the body at targeted locations, often over fascial planes. After gua sha, ecchymosis and petechia are evident at the local skin site, which are called *sha*. Traditionally, it is believed that poisons in the inner body were extracted in the shape of the sha. Gua sha is a technique used for pain relief, muscular tension, and spasms.
Qigong	Qigong refers to a mind and body training method that focuses on breathing adjustment and physical activity modulation. Qigong has varied forms of expression, some of which are based on imitating animal movements.
Tai chi	Tai chi is a combination of Chinese theoretic thinking and martial arts, guiding methodology, and traditional Chinese medicine. Tai chi is a high-level expression of the human body and has multiple functions, which include taking care of one's temperament, building one's body, and the art of attack and defense.
Chinese herbal medicine	Herbal therapies generally are formula-based, and single herbs rarely are used. Every medicinal substance has its strengths and its shortcomings, and each ingredient in the formula should be balanced carefully in quality and quantity.
Chinese manipulation	Chinese manipulation can be classified into 3 approaches: rotation, traction, or a combination. Chinese manipulation disciplines share the same principles to reconstruct the balance of the musculoskeletal system through relaxing the muscles and rectifying abnormalities in the relationships between joints. Chinese manipulation is based on meridians and acupoints.
Moxibustion	Moxibustion treats diseases by means of the heat generated by burning an herbal preparation, usually containing mugwort.
Tui na	Tui na has 2 components: soft tissue manipulation and spinal manipulation. The soft tissue techniques, which are analogous to massage, include stroking, kneading, and drumming. In contrast, the spinal manipulations consist of manual operation procedures without thrust.

Data from Yuan Q, Guo T, Liu L, et al. Traditional Chinese medicine for neck pain and low back pain: a systematic review and meta-analysis. PLoS ONE. 2015; 10(2):e0117146.

this review reported on 75 RCTs, the investigators advised caution about interpretation of the reported results because they found that most studies showed low strength of evidence, a few demonstrated moderate evidence, and none revealed a high level of evidence. The poor quality of results was attributed to (1) failure to include a blinded control group, (2) small sample sizes, and (3) inconsistency of results between trials.

Looking at the levels of evidence for specific types of TCM in this comprehensive review,[4] 13 studies compared acupuncture to sham acupuncture and 4 studies compared acupuncture to no treatment; all demonstrated some level of efficacy. Two other studies on pain that compared acupuncture to a conventional therapy, the transcutaneous electrical nerve stimulation unit, showed no difference. On the other hand, 6 studies compared acupuncture to usual care for pain and found results in favor of acupuncture. Acupressure was found favorable for pain care compared with physical therapy or with no care. Cupping was found favorable for pain care compared with both standard medical care and with heating pad application, but there was no significant difference found between cupping and progressive muscle relaxation.

Tai chi has received extensive research, with more than 500 trials and 120 systematic reviews published on the health benefits of tai chi in the past half-century. Based on their review of more than 200 studies of the benefits of tai chi, Huston and McFarlane drew several conclusions.[5] They found that tai chi showed benefits of improved balance and aerobic capacity for patients with poor fitness, increased lower limb strength, decreased incidences of falls, improved chronic obstructive pulmonary disease, and improved cognitive capacity in older adults. They also found that studies demonstrated improvements from tai chi in depression, cardiac rehabilitation, stroke rehabilitation, and dementia. They also noted that studies reported no benefit for quality of life in cancer patients, fibromyalgia, hypertension, and osteoporosis. This review also highlighted the limitations were noted for these studies. Many of the studies were small and methodologically weak and lacked blinding of participants. On the other hand, in addition to systematic reviews and meta-analyses, there were some RCTs; thus, providers should have some confidence in recommending tai chi as an evidenced-based practice.

AYURVEDA

Ayurvedic medicine has its roots in India and evolved over several thousand years.[3] The philosophy of ayurveda focuses on treating the whole body by integrating body, mind, and spirit. Illness is thought to represent an imbalance between these 3 dimensions. The objective of balancing the body, mind, and spirit is thought to prevent illness and promote wellness. According to ayurvedic medicine, everything, from a thought to a person to a tree, is composed of 5 building blocks or elements: space, air, fire, water, and earth. To create health and well-being, ayurveda focuses on harmonizing the 5 elements in both the mind, the body, and the spirit.[6] There are several colleges and universities in the United States offering degree programs in ayurveda. Graduates may be eligible for board certification as Holistic Nutritionists by the National Association of Nutrition Professionals.

Ayurveda therapies include herbs, diet, meditation, yoga, oil massage, and steam heat treatments. Ayurvedic medicine uses techniques and products to cleanse the body and restore balance. Some of the products used to cleanse the body have been documented as producing drug interactions.[7] Aloe vera has been shown to potentiate conventional medicines used to lower blood glucose and also cardiac glycosides and antiarrhythmic drugs. Bala, which contains ephedrine, is known to interact with caffeine and monoamine oxidase inhibitors, elevating blood pressure and reducing effectiveness of β-blockers. Cayenne has potential for decreasing absorption of aspirin, increasing absorption of ciprofloxacin and theophylline, and altering absorption of cefalexin and digoxin. Turmeric and curcumin can affect the absorption of β-blockers, midazolam, and tallinolol. *Stockley's Herbal Medicines Interactions*[8] offers an in-depth review of ayurvedic herb interactions with conventional medications.

A systematic review and meta-analysis of 33 studies that was published in 2015 was aimed at measuring the effect of ayurvedic interventions on pain, physical function, and global improvement in populations with osteoarthritis.[6] They included 12 different ayurvedic formulas and 3 nonpharmaceutical interventions and revealed evidence of effectiveness for several ayurvedic interventions; however, the preponderance of the published reports lacked rigorous methodology, adequate sample sizes, adequate randomization, intention-to-treat methodology, and blinding of outcome assessors. One study[9] examined the practice of obtaining supplements via the Internet and found that 193 of 230 ayurvedic medications sold on the Internet had unacceptable levels of mercury, lead, or arsenic in a significant portion of products. Of the products researched, 21.7% were manufactured in the United States and 40.6% of in India. The US Food and Drug Administration regulates herbal product labeling and promotional materials distributed at the point of sales, whereas the US Federal Trade Commission regulates product claims made by herb manufacturers and distributers. Safety concerns led to changes in federal regulations on labeling herbal supplements effective January 1, 2020, and the American Herbal Products Association has updated its labeling guidance to comply with these regulatory changes.[10]

HOMEOPATHY

Homeopathy has its origins in Germany in the nineteenth century. Homeopathic practitioners select various treatments for illnesses according to the total picture of the patient, including lifestyle, symptoms, emotional states, and mental states.[3] The objective of homeopathic treatments is to stimulate the body's defense mechanisms to prevent or to treat diseases. Homeopathic treatments often involve using very small doses of remedies that are used in larger dosage in conventional medicine. Many colleges and universities in the United States offer training programs in homeopathy and, although specific certifications examinations are available, homeopathy usually is practiced as a complementary modality by practitioners licensed in a conventional health care field.[3] Two systematic analyses, one by the Australian Government[11] and one by the US government,[12] determined that there are no research studies supporting the beneficial use of homeopathic remedies in the treatment of illness.[11] A 2019 National Center for Complementary and Integrative Health (NCCIH)[12] concurred and noted, "there's little evidence to support homeopathy as an effective treatment for any specific health condition." Furthermore, the NCCIH emphasized that some products labeled as homeopathic may contain substantial amounts of active ingredients and could cause side effects and drug interactions.

NATUROPATHY

Naturopathic medicine focuses on maintaining health rather than treating disease.[3] A key tenet is to do no harm by selecting therapies intended to minimize side effects rather than to suppress symptoms. Naturopaths seek to promote the healing power of nature. Practitioners seek to treat the cause of illness or disease rather than the symptoms. The causes generally are thought to emerge from a combination of the physical, mental, emotional, genetic, environment, and social factors. Symptoms are viewed as indications of the body attempting to fight disease, adapt to it, or recover from it. Naturopathic practitioners are teachers to their patients, attempting to promote healthy ways of living and the importance of patients taking responsibility for their own health. Many colleges and universities offer degrees in naturopathic medicine, and in North America some states and provinces license graduates to practice naturopathic medicine. Naturopathic medicine utilizes practices such as the following[13]: dietary and lifestyle changes, stress reduction, herbs and other dietary supplements, manipulative therapies, exercise therapy, guided detoxification, psychotherapy, and counseling.

A systematic review of naturopathic medicine, published in 2019,[14] included 33 studies evaluating the effectiveness of naturopathic medical care where 2 or more naturopathic modalities were provided by naturopathic clinicians and sample size exceeded 5 subjects. Naturopathic multimodality therapies were shown to be effective in the treatment of cardiovascular disease, musculoskeletal pain, type 2 diabetes mellitus, polycystic ovary syndrome, depression, anxiety, and other chronic complex conditions. A 2016 study from India[15] examined 104 participants with hypertension who were enrolled into an integrated naturopathic hospital for 3 months and then had 3-months' follow-up; 79 of the subjects achieved target blood pressure control (<140/90) and 66 of these patients achieved this with an antihypertensive medication dose reduction of greater than 50%. Eight of these patients were able to completely eliminate antihypertensive medications. Another 2016 study from India[16] looked at 101 participants with type 2 diabetes mellitus who were admitted to an integrative naturopathic hospital. Mean glycemic control at the 30-day follow-up represented a reduction of 39 mg/mL in fasting blood sugar, 39 mg/dL in postprandial blood sugar, and a reduction of 1.2% hemoglobin A_{1c} (HbA_{1c}) in patients with baseline HbA_{1c} of greater than or equal to 7%. A 2012 report from Germany[17] studied 221 participants with musculoskeletal pain who received 2 weeks of inpatient naturopathic care. At 1-year follow-up, analysis demonstrated a statistically significant decrease in back pain. A 2009 Canadian study[18] of 85 participants with rotator cuff tendinitis compared a set naturopathic treatment protocol to a standardized placebo exercise routine. The naturopathic treatment decreased a Shoulder Pain and Disability Index by 54.5% compared with a control group decrease of only 18%. The State of the Evidence for Whole Systems, Multi-modality Naturopathic Medicine: A Systematic Scoping Review[14] reported on 33 naturopathic, multimodality research studies and concluded there is a need for real-world trials in which complex naturopathic treatments are compared with usual care. Although further controlled research is needed, these diverse studies support the emerging preventive approach to a wide range of acute and chronic conditions.

FUTURE DIRECTIONS IN RESEARCH

WMSs research accelerated in 1990 when the US Congress appropriated funds to stimulate the National Institutes of Health (NIH)[19] to evaluate traditional, complementary, and IM practices. Although the initial goals of Congress were to implement and measure implications of value-based care, 4 themes emerged as the focus of the NIH evaluations progressed: (1) complex, behaviorally focused interventions; (2) patient-centered outcomes; (3) team-based care; and (4) resilience and well-being. The ongoing convergence of conventional, nonconventional, alternative, complementary, and integrative services is clearly having an impact on health care, including moving health settings toward shared medical group services.[18]

Over the past 3 decades, a new health care paradigm, whole health (WH),[20] has emerged and gaining momentum and support. This WH movement is an integrative health model that integrates the best of ancient wisdom and modern medicine.

More importantly, the WH movement has embraced a major shift toward empowering patients to take charge of their life and health. This model, the WH paradigm, encompasses the meditative approaches taken from TCM; the mind-body balance of ayurveda; the lifestyle balance of homeopathy; and naturopathic emphasis on patient education and responsibility for self. Conventional Western medicine historically has taken a paternalistic view of care, making the patient a passive recipient. Whereas WH educates and empowers patients to make choices and to take responsibility for improving their health and wellness, health care providers, in this new paradigm, guide patients in making self-care and lifestyle choices to improve their health and well-being in alignment with the conventional medical care available to them. Improved health and a higher sense of well-being are achieved through synergy between the patient's conventional, evidence-based medical services and the guided, self-selected, self-care and lifestyle modifications.[21] Many of these patient choices have their origins in the ancient practices, which have, of late, garnered a degree of supportive scientific evidence and which no longer are dependent on the active involvement of a health care provider. This is resulting in a multidimensional benefit, enhancing patient experience, improving provider satisfaction, bettering population health, and lowering per capita costs. These results mirror the major goals of the 1990 Congress, in implementing and measuring the implications of value-based care.[19]

A 2019 RCT examined the effectiveness of IM group visits (IMGVs) compared with primary care provider (PCP) visits in patients with chronic pain and depression[22] and found no difference in pain or depression at any point in time; however, the IMGV participants did demonstrate a reduction in pain medication and in emergency department visits. The participants had no worsening of pain reports despite this significant reduction in medication usage. Thus, for pain care, IMGV clinics are particularly valuable in balancing of the costs and availability of PCP services and the costs of emergency department visits and medications. This study also reported a high variability of attendance to both IMGV and PCP visits, indicating that some patients may be good candidates for either service while other patients may be good candidates for only one of the services and not the other. Therefore, in designing an effective IGMVs program, attention must be paid toward differentiating patients who are most compliant with the services offered.

The multimodal approach to research that is necessary to fully understand and study WMSs can be challenging to traditional researchers and clinicians who are more confident in research that isolates a single, active experimental treatment. That is, researches often find greater comfort with research that compares a control population with double blinded results and analysis. On the other hand, WMSs research most often uses patient-reported outcomes rather than traditional biomarkers.[19] Importantly, WMSs modalities, particularly when used in combination, carry risks of injury, harm from toxic chemicals, medication interactions, and opportunity costs that can be difficult to fully appreciate and study. On the other hand, even with these inherent risks, most WMs modalities actually carry lower overall risks than the conventional therapies that otherwise would be used. Imagine the dissonance created for the clinician who is considering acupuncture for pain versus injection, surgery, or narcotic medications.[23] This dissonance may often be colored by a clinician's own philosophic preferences between the 2 paradigms rather than by the actual risk profiles. As with any type of health care delivered, all potential risks should be disclosed and balanced with potential benefits; however, there are few RCTs available to quantify these comparisons. A final research challenge seen with WMSs is that its reliance on healthy lifestyle changes can make it difficult to fully study, because many individuals already may be practicing some of these healthy behaviors and, therefore, already experiencing some of the benefits.

CLINICS CARE POINTS

- Acupuncture, acupressure, and cupping have been found effective for chronic neck pain and chronic low back pain.
- Tai chi has shown benefits for improving balance and aerobic capacity; increased lower limb strength; decreased incidents of falls; improved chronic obstructive pulmonary disease; improved cognitive capacity; improved depression; cardiac and stroke rehabilitation; and decreased dementia. Tai chi has not been demonstrated, however, to improve quality of life in fibromyalgia, hypertension, or osteoporosis.
- Some evidence exists for the use of ayurvedic interventions for osteoarthritis. Ayurvedic herbal remedies should be used cautiously and should be researched in sources, such as *Stockley's Herbal Medicines Interactions*, prior to use. Many ayurvedic supplements sold on the Internet have been found to contain toxic levels of heavy metals.
- Naturopathic, multimodality therapies that often are utilized along with yoga (originally an ayurvedic intervention), have shown effectiveness in the treatment of cardiovascular disease, musculoskeletal pain, type 2 diabetes mellitus, polycystic ovarian syndrome, depression, and anxiety.
- Some patients respond better to IM group interventions compared with other patients who respond better to PCP visits. Costs and compliance rates, therefore, must be considered.
- Risks and benefits of contemporary versus WMSs approaches must be disclosed and be considered by both the patient and provider in a balanced, fully informed manner.

DISCLOSURE

The authors have nothing to disclose.

REFERENCES

1. Complementary, Alternative, or Integrative Health: What's in a Name. Available at: https://nccih.nih.gov/health/integrative-health. Accessed March 18, 2020. Microsoft edge.
2. Merck Manual. Types of Complementary and Alternative Medicine, Whole Medical Systems. Available at: https://www.merckmanuals.com/home/special-subjects/integrative,-complementary,-and-alternative-medicine/types-of-complementary-and-alternative-medicine. Accessed March 17, 2020. Microsoft Edge.
3. The National Psoriasis Foundation. Whole Medical Systems. Available at: https://www.psoriasis.org/about-psoriasis/treatments/alternative/whole-systems. Accessed March 17, 2020. Microsoft Edge.
4. Traditional Chinese medicine for neck pain and low back pain: a systematic review and meta-analysis. PLoS One 2015. https://doi.org/10.1371/journal.pone.0117146.
5. Huston P, McFarlane B. Health Benefits of Tai Chi. Available at: https://www.cfp.ca/node/23428.full.print. Accessed March 20, 2020. Microsoft Edge.
6. Christian S, Pinders L, Michalsen A, et al. Ayurvedic intervention for osteoarthritis: a systematic review and meta-analysis. Rheumatol Int 2015;35:211–32.

7. Ayurvedic Herbs – Drug Interactions. Available at: https://saiayurvediccollege.com/ayurvedic-herb-drug-interactions/. Accessed April 1, 2020. Microsoft Edge.
8. Williamson E, Driver D, Baxter K, editors. Stockley's herbal medicines interactions. London: RPS-Pharmaceutical Press; 2009. updated 2020.
9. Lead. Mercury, and Arsenic in US- and Indian-Manufactured Ayurvedic Medications Sold Via the Internet. Available at: https://www.ncbi.nim.nih.gov/pmc/articles/PMC2755247/. Accessed March 26, 2020. Microsoft Edge.
10. American Herbal Products Association: AHPA Guidance Documents. Available at: https://www.ahpa.org/Resources/TechnicalGuidance/AHPAGuidanceDocuments.aspx. Accessed March 2t, 2020. Microsoft Edge.
11. Australian Government. Evidence on The Effectiveness of Homeopathy for Treating Health Conditions. Available at: https://chopra.com/articles/bacis-principles-of-ayurvedis-medicine. Accessed March 23, 2020. Microsoft Edge.
12. National Center for Complementary and Integrative Health, Homeopathy. Available at: https://nccih.nih.gov/health/homeopathy#hed4. Accessed March 23, 2020. Microsoft Edge.
13. National Center for Complementary and Integrative Health. Naturopathy. Available at: https://nccih.nih.gov/health/naturopathy. Accessed March 21, 2020. Microsoft Edge.
14. The State of the Evidence for Whole Systems, Multi-modality Naturopathic Medicine: A Systematic Scoping Review. Available at: https://www.ncbi.nih.gov/pmc/articles/PMC6389764. Accessed March 18, 2020. Microsoft Edge.
15. Edla S, Kumar A, Srinivas B. Integrated naturopathy and yoga reduces blood pressure and the need for medications among a cohort of hypertensive patients in south india: a three- month follow-up study. Adv Integr Med 2016;3:90–7.
16. Barry S, Kumar A, Raju M. Is Adjunctive naturopathy associated with improved glycemic control and a reduction in need for medications among type 2 diabetic patients? a prospective cohort study from India. BMC Complement Altern Med 2016;16:290.
17. Stange R, Hackermier U, Franzen G. 1-year sustaining efficacy of multi-dimensional therapy for inpatients with different conditions of chronic musculoskeletal pain. BMC Complement Altern Med 2012;12(Supp 1):p228.
18. Szczurko O, Cooley K, Mills E. Naturopathic treatment of rotator cuff tendonitis among canadian postal workers: a randomized controlled trial. Arthritis Rheumatol 2009;61:1037–45.
19. Convergent Points for Conventional Medicine and Whole Systems Research: A User's guide. Available at: https://www.lieberpub.com/doi/10.1089/acm.2018.0515. Accessed March 18, 2020. Microsoft Edge.
20. What is Whole Health. Available at: https://tami-brady.com/what-is-whole-health. Accessed March 18, 2020. Microsoft Edge.
21. Promoting the Whole Health Model, From Science to Practice. Available at: https://www.mentalhealth.va.gov/suicide_prevention/docs/Literature_Review_FSTP_Whole_Health_Final_508_8-19-2019.pdf. Accessed March 18, 2020. Microsoft Edge.
22. Effectiveness of Integrative Medicine Group Visits in Chronic Pain and Depressive Symptoms: A Randomized Controlled Trial. Available at: https://doi.org/10.1371/journal.pone.0225540. Accessed March 18, 2020. Microsoft Edge.
23. Acupuncture Treatment is Safe. Available at: https://www.webmd.com/balance/news/20010904/acupuncture-treatment-is-dafe#2. Accessed March 27, 2020. Microsoft Edge.

Mind-Body Interventions for Rehabilitation Medicine

Promoting Wellness, Healing, and Coping with Adversity

Jessica Pieczynski, PhD[a],*, David Cosio, PhD, ABPP[b], Whitney Pierce, PsyD, RN, BCB[c], J. Greg Serpa, PhD[d]

KEYWORDS

- Meditation • Mindfulness • Mind-body techniques • Biofeedback • Guided imagery
- Hypnosis

KEY POINTS

- Meditation, guided imagery, clinical hypnosis, and biofeedback are cost-effective evidenced-based approaches used in physical medicine and rehabilitation settings that are well-tolerated by patients.
- There is good evidence for their applications for chronic pain, primary headache, cardiac rehabilitation, cancer rehabilitation, and preliminary evidence for traumatic brain injury and cerebrovascular events.
- Outcomes are strongest for mental health and quality-of-life indicators and are often less robust for disease-specific physiologic indicators (eg, acute pain).
- High-quality, longitudinal designs across diverse patient populations are still needed to fully understand the benefits and limitations for rehabilitation medicine populations.

A cure, traditionally the resolution of a medical condition, may be out of reach for many patients presenting in rehabilitation settings with debilitating injuries or conditions. For example, with chronic pain an overreliance on pharmacotherapy for management has resulted in the opioid epidemic without meeting the 3 key treatment goals of effective pain relief, improved quality of life, and improved functional capacity.[1] Interdisciplinary providers in physical medicine attempt to cure organic aspects of disease when possible while simultaneously providing healing approaches to enhance quality of

[a] Greater Los Angeles VA Healthcare System, 11301 Wilshire Boulevard, Los Angeles, CA 90073, USA; [b] Jesse Brown VA Medical Center, 820 South Damen Avenue, Chicago, IL 60612, USA; [c] VA St. Louis Healthcare System, 915 North Grand Boulevard, St Louis, MO 63106, USA; [d] Greater Los Angeles VA Healthcare System, UCLA Department of Psychology, 11301 Wilshire Boulevard, Los Angeles, CA 90073, USA
* Corresponding author.
E-mail address: Jessica.Pieczynski@va.gov

Phys Med Rehabil Clin N Am 31 (2020) 563–575
https://doi.org/10.1016/j.pmr.2020.07.008
1047-9651/20/© 2020 Elsevier Inc. All rights reserved.

life and well-being. Healing entails reducing anxiety and stress related to their physical ailment, and retaining a sense of personal integrity and agency despite facing an ongoing, disabling organic illness.[2] Mind-body interventions (MBI) are evidence-based, cost-effective approaches that serve these aims.[3] Although it has been more than 20 years since the National Institutes of Health determined the evidence is *strong* for the effectiveness of relaxation approaches in the treatment of chronic pain, implementation of mind-body approaches in rehabilitation medicine has not kept pace with the science.[4] Barriers to implementation have included provider and patient knowledge and acceptance of these approaches, the influence of health insurance reimbursements on access, and state regulation/scope of practice variability.[5] In this review, the aim was to increase provider knowledge and acceptance of some of the most effective and popular mind-body modalities that are used by providers in rehabilitation settings: meditation, guided imagery, clinical hypnosis, and biofeedback training. Often times, clinicians and patients alike have difficulty differentiating these interventions, so our primary objective is to help providers understand their unique offerings and to evaluate the current state of the literature of these mind-body modalities for rehabilitation populations.

MEDITATION

Meditation is one of the most commonly used complementary and integrative health (CIH) approaches. According to the annual National Health Interview Survey, the use of meditation has increased more than threefold from 4.1% in 2012 to 14.2% in 2017 among adults aged 18 and older.[6] The practice of meditation originated in the ancient Vedic times of India and appears in many religious traditions, from Judaism to Christianity.[7] The mind-body practice encompasses a variety of styles designed to focus attention to enhance well-being. In the past 40 years meditation has been applied in a secular manner to a variety of integrative modalities, and it is these secular versions that have become widely researched and popularized in health care settings. Secular meditation techniques are often categorized by researchers into 2 forms: those that emphasize use of a mantra, such as transcendental meditation (TM) and mantrum repetition, and those that emphasize "mindfulness," such as mindfulness-based stress reduction (MBSR) and mindfulness-based cognitive therapy (MBCT). There is also a more recent body of research exploring the effects of compassion meditation. While some might consider these categorizations overly reductionistic,[8] we will use this framework for ease of organizing the literature.

Mantra-Based Meditation

Mantra-based meditation techniques practiced in the United States primarily consist of TM, a program established by Maharishi Mahesh Yogi in the 1950s. A mantra is given to or chosen by each patient and is used as a vehicle to "transcend" mental activity.[8,9] Benefits derived from completion of a TM program have included reduced frequency of pain symptoms, headaches and backaches, pain during pregnancy and childbirth, and medical care utilization for pain-related conditions such as chest and abdominal pain,[7,10,11] TM has also demonstrated benefits for cardiac rehabilitation.[12] Although these outcomes are promising, sample sizes in TM research are typically small and highly controlled studies are lacking. In addition, over the past couple of decades TM has appeared less prevalent within the literature as mindfulness meditation gained popularity among researchers and clinical practitioners.

Mindfulness Meditation

Mindfulness meditation is the most widely studied variation of meditation. Mindfulness meditation is derived from Vipassana, or insight meditation from the Theravada tradition of Buddhism. Mindfulness has been described as self-regulating attention toward the present moment and adopting a stance marked by curiosity, openness, and acceptance.[13] In this form of meditation, participants are instructed to become aware of thoughts, feelings, and sensations and to observe them in a nonjudgmental way. It is based on the philosophy that full and nonjudgmental experience of the present moment creates positive outcomes for health, even in the midst of chronic illness.[14] MBIs include MBSR and its adaptation, MBCT for depression. MBSR was developed in the 1970s for patients with chronic pain and other complex medical conditions, and involves guided sitting meditation, mindful movement, and psycho-education.[15] Other interventions that incorporate mindfulness include dialectical behavioral therapy (DBT) and acceptance and commitment therapy (ACT), but these approaches do not use mindfulness meditation as the primary mechanism of therapeutic change.[16]

One of the most well-researched areas on the application of MBIs for rehabilitation populations is that for pain. Those that emphasize cultivating acceptance, nonattachment, and social engagement may be most effective in decreasing pain and psychological symptoms.[17] A meta-analysis examining the impact of mindfulness meditation on primary headache found mindfulness meditation reduces pain intensity and headache frequency, suggesting that clinicians can consider mindfulness meditation as a viable CIH approach for primary headache.[18] A review of studies examining the effects of MBIs for cancer-related pain found that they reduced pain severity, anxiety, stress, depression, and increased quality of life.[19] Comprehensive reviews on mindfulness for chronic back pain, fibromyalgia, and musculoskeletal pain show small positive effects for pain and have found improvements in pain, pain acceptance, quality of life, and functional status.[20,21] Researchers determined that although mindfulness meditation interventions show significant improvements for chronic pain, depression, and quality of life, the magnitude of effect is stronger for depression and mental health–related quality of life outcomes than for self-reported pain. Of studies that reported on change in analgesic use, however, results have been mixed. Adverse events are rare and not classified as serious[22] and there is some evidence to show that as many as 88% of patients continue to practice 4 months post-MBI, suggesting that MBIs are a feasible long-term self-management strategy for pain.[23]

Following a cerebrovascular event, people may derive benefits from MBIs. One study found MBSR may be a promising nonpharmacological treatment for mental fatigue after a stroke or traumatic brain injury (TBI),[24] whereas another 2-week MBI for poststroke spasticity showed statistically significant improvements in spasticity in both the elbow and wrist, improvements in quality-of-life measures for energy, personality, and enhanced work and productivity.[25] However, further methodologically robust trials are required to accurately assess clinical utility.

In a randomized controlled trial exploring the impact of MBSR on cardiac rehabilitation, 3-month results revealed that participants exhibited greater improvements in depression, anxiety, and cardiovascular risk factors (blood pressure, biomarkers, lipids, HbA1c, C-reactive protein), with an attenuation of treatment effects at 9 months, suggesting that MBSR is a safe and well-received secondary prevention strategy for cardiac rehabilitation.[26]

Compassion Meditation

Although most physical psychosocial interventions are intended to alleviate or reduce negative states, in the past decade, there has been growing interest in creating interventions to cultivate or enhance positive states such as compassion to promote well-being and reduce suffering.[27] Self-compassion is taking a stance of compassion directed to oneself, although the field continues to explore differences between self-directed and other-directed compassion. Neff[28] has proposed 3 interacting components of self-compassion, including mindfulness, self-kindness (being caring toward oneself instead of judgmental about perceived or actual shortcomings), and common humanity (an awareness that accepting flaws or struggles actually connects one to the human condition). A meta-analysis of 14 studies demonstrated a significant, inverse relationship between self-compassion and psychopathology,[29] indicating compassion is an important variable for resilience. Compassion-based interventions (CBIs) include Cognitively-Based Compassion Therapy (CBCT).[30] Compassion Cultivation Training (CCT),[31] Compassion-Focused Therapy (CFT),[32] and Mindful Self-Compassion (MSC).[33] A recent meta-analysis of 27 studies found compassion interventions improved 11 diverse psychosocial outcomes, such as depression, self-criticism, and anxiety.[34] Biomarker studies also suggest compassion interventions can positively influence modulation of stress and inflammation.[35]

Although the impact of these interventions in the rehabilitation healing space has not yet fully been explored, recent studies on CBIs show promise. Among cancer survivors who completed a CBCT group, participation led to greater improvements in depression, avoidance of intrusive thoughts, functional impairment associated with fear of recurrence, mindfulness, and vitality/fatigue compared with controls.[30] In addition, completion of a compassion-focused therapy intervention was associated with significant reductions in measures of self-criticism, anxiety, and depression for those with acquired brain injury.[36] Self-compassion has also been studied in the chronic pain literature, but to date there have not been studies on formalized interventions.[37] Although rehabilitation-specific research is lacking, CBIs offer a promising approach for healing in rehabilitation medicine and will undoubtedly proliferate the scientific literature in the near future.

GUIDED IMAGERY

Guided imagery (GI) is a therapeutic technique that uses inwardly focused visualization and imaginative content to evoke sensory perceptions for improving mental and/or physical well-being. A facilitator uses descriptive language intended to assist the patient in using their imagination to create sensory images that decrease unpleasant symptoms, such as pain or agitation. This often involves going to a place in their mind (eg, beach or forest) and using several or all the senses in the mind of the listener, including vision (eg, trees, grass, sun, people, or animals), smell (eg, ocean, pine, or flowers), sounds (eg, birds, sticks cracking, or waves), touch (eg, cool breeze, warm sun, or water), and taste (eg, salty air, sweet berries, or cool water). The facilitator may precede the GI with diaphragmatic breathing. The length is tailored to the patient's preference and energy level. Often times, GI sessions can use an audiotaped script or a live guide. Interventions, such as virtual reality or mirror therapy, rely on external sensory input and are thus excluded from this category and this review.[38] There is some evidence to suggest a practice akin to GI was used as far back as the twelfth to ninth centuries BC to 600 AD in ancient Greek civilization. However, it was Hanscarl Leuner, a German psychiatrist, who first developed guided affective imagery in the 1940s and the research soon followed.

GI interventions have been used for a variety of rehabilitation populations, including arthritis, cancer, cardiac surgery, critical illness/intensive care unit (ICU) patients, fibromyalgia, headaches, musculoskeletal pain, and stroke. Findings from systematic reviews suggest there is evidence of a positive effect for arthritis[39] and secondary outcomes of anxiety and depression in cancer.[40] There is also evidence of a potential positive effect for diagnosis-related outcomes for cancer,[41] cardiac surgery,[42] critical illness/ICU,[39] and motor imagery for stroke.[43] There is unclear or insufficient evidence for headaches[44] and musculoskeletal pain.[45] There is no evidence of a positive effect for fibromyalgia, but potential positive effects on secondary outcomes including psychological distress and coping with pain.[46]

CLINICAL HYPNOSIS

Clinical hypnosis is a procedure involving cognitive processes, like imagination, in which a patient is guided by a health professional to respond to suggestions for changes in perceptions, sensations, thoughts, feelings, and behaviors,[47] which is intended to invoke heightened focus and suggestibility.[48] Hypnosis involves learning how to use your mind and thoughts to manage emotional distress, unpleasant physical symptoms, and certain habits or behaviors. Sometimes, people are also trained in self-hypnosis where they learn to guide themselves through a hypnotic procedure or may be provided audio recordings of the sessions to help assist with home practice. There are many myths, misconceptions, and misinformation about hypnosis. Thus, clinical hypnosis should only be conducted by trained health care professionals, such as licensed psychologists or master's level clinicians. At its most basic, hypnosis treatment consists of 4 stages, including an induction (to focus attention), then some deepening (to deepen relaxation of the body), followed by suggestions (to change the experience), and ends with a debriefing. Most people describe hypnosis as a pleasant experience, feel focused and absorbed in the experience, more alert, relaxed and comfortable, and peaceful. Certain cases are discouraged to pursue clinical hypnosis, including anyone with severe psychological disorders that have gone untreated, persons under the influence of recreational drugs or alcohol, and anyone who is delusional or hallucinatory at the time of treatment. It is important to note that some patients may object to hypnosis due to their religious beliefs, cultural beliefs, or other factors.

Clinical hypnosis has a long history of being used as a therapeutic tool. During ancient times, the treatment of physical ailments was shrouded by mystical practices. Egyptians used "dream temples" and the Greeks used sleep temples called "hypnos." Evidence of the practice of hypnosis can be found in the Bible and Hindu Vedas dating back to 1500 BC. The practice resurfaced in the late eighteenth century with Mesmer's use of the imagination and magnet baths, and Braid finally introduced the term "hypnosis" in 1795 to describe the treatment process. In the beginning of the nineteenth century, hypnosis was being used as anesthesia until chloroform started being used in 1831. In the twentieth century, clinical hypnosis re-emerged as a conventional treatment modality, being used in clinical psychotherapy by Erickson, dentistry, and medicine.[49]

Clinical hypnosis has been successful for a variety of health conditions, including obesity/weight loss, anxiety related to medical procedures, insomnia, and irritable bowel syndrome.[50–53] However, hypnosis interventions have not been as widely studied in rehabilitation populations as other CIH modalities, although there is a small body of literature examining its application to cancer and chronic (noncancer) pain. Systematic reviews suggest there is evidence of a positive effect for cancer anxiety[54] and breast cancer care.[55] However, there is mixed evidence for pain.[56] For chronic pain management, clinical hypnosis has been found to be generally more effective than nonpharmacological interventions, such as physical therapy and pain education.[57–60] There is growing evidence to suggest that hypnosis has greater influence on the effects of pain in that it reduces stress, relieves anxiety, improves sleep, improves mood, and reduces need for opioids. Similar to the literature on meditation, the effects on the direct sensation of pain are limited.[61,62] The final mind-body modality to consider in the current examination is biofeedback training.

BIOFEEDBACK TRAINING

Biofeedback training is a form of applied psychophysiology that enables individuals to learn how to change physiologic activity for the purposes of improving health and performance. It draws on the learning principles of operant conditioning to enable self-regulation of physiologic responses that were once thought beyond voluntary control.[63] During training sessions, electronic devices with precise sensors measure physiologic signals (eg, heart function, breathing, muscle activation, and electroencephalographic brain waves) and provide visual, auditory, or vibrotactile feedback to a patient and their provider. Real-time physiologic feedback enhances the patient's ability to process and interpret somatosensory information and learn new strategies to achieve the desired psychophysiological change. It is the presence of a knowledgeable training provider that can offer guidance in skills such as breathing, relaxation, GI, mindful awareness, and cognitive reappraisal that distinguishes true biofeedback training from the widely available technology that provides basic metrics such as activity, sleep, and heart rate.[64] With proper feedback and training, the patient will internalize the learning process and become capable of sustaining changes without the continued use of an external device. Modern biofeedback training has its roots in the psychophysiology laboratories that developed in university settings during the 1950s and 1960s. Since that time, rapid advancements in technology and growing interest in alternative and complementary health interventions have fueled a renewed interest in the field of biofeedback training.

Surface electromyography (EMG) biofeedback offers the opportunity to increase awareness of dysfunctional muscle use patterns, and training can be used to facilitate relaxation practice and strengthening exercises. For example, EMG biofeedback has been shown to reduce knee pain, improve quadriceps strength, and increase functional rehabilitation performance for patients with osteoarthritis, juvenile rheumatoid arthritis, and following arthroscopic meniscectomy surgery.[65–67] There is also good evidence for the efficacy of EMG biofeedback training for chronic back pain as a recent meta-analysis concluded that training as a standalone or adjunctive treatment can lead to improvements on ratings of pain intensity, disability, cognitive coping, and measures of muscle tension.[68] EMG biofeedback-assisted therapy has also been found to be comparable to cognitive therapy and superior to a wait-list control in the treatment of low back pain.[69] When used as an adjunct to traditional medical and physical therapy treatments, EMG biofeedback may shorten duration and cost of treatment, while increasing skill for muscle self-regulation and decreasing dysfunctional use patterns that may create additional sources of reinjury and pain.[70]

There is strong evidence for treatment of tension and migraine headaches with biofeedback training, with many studies demonstrating superiority of biofeedback training to control and relaxation alone treatment groups.[71,72] A meta-analysis that included 55 studies showed that blood volume, pulse, temperature, and EMG biofeedback were all more effective than control conditions for decreasing frequency of migraine headaches, with stable improvement lasting for an average of 17 months.[73]

Similarly, a meta-analysis of 53 studies showed biofeedback training for treatment for tension-type headache was more effective than headache monitoring, placebo, and standalone relaxation therapies. Improvements proved stable over an average follow-up phase of 15 months.[74] When compared with medication, one randomized controlled trial found biofeedback training and propranolol prescription to have comparable short-term outcomes; however, biofeedback training demonstrated significantly better long-term prophylactic effect compared with propranolol for migraine at 1-year posttreatment.[75]

Although there is relatively little research for using biofeedback training as an adjunct to cancer treatments, the physiologic and psychological symptoms that accompany a cancer diagnosis and treatment would appear to be a relatively good fit for biofeedback training.[76,77] Findings from a study of EMG biofeedback-assisted relaxation treatment showed beneficial effects of reduced subjective pain scores for patients with advanced cancer.[78] Studies of electroencephalographic neurofeedback (NFB) training have also demonstrated some promising results for offering a new treatment option for the debilitating symptoms of chemotherapy-induced peripheral neuropathy (CIPN).[79,80] The findings of those studies have shown significant improvement in pain, numbness, cancer symptom interference, physical functioning, general health, and fatigue compared with control groups. Posttreatment follow-up indicated sustained reduction of CIPN symptoms at 4 months.

There is also some evidence that support the use of NFB to enhance cognitive rehabilitation following stroke. A systemic review found 8 studies that showed improvements in a broad range of cognitive and psychological symptoms including memory, mood, concentration, energy, reading and speech abilities, and motivation.[81] Kober and colleagues[82] compared NFB with traditional cognitive rehabilitation and found a stronger effect on pre- and post-verbal short- and long-term memory for the NFB experimental group compared with the control group. Sensorimotor Rhythm (SMR) training protocol produced specific improvements in visuo-spatial short-term memory performance, whereas an Upper Alpha protocol improved working memory performance.[82] Those results demonstrated a potential for more effective and individualized poststroke cognitive rehabilitation treatment plans with the addition of NFB, but larger controlled studies need to be conducted before broader claims can be made.

In HRV biofeedback training, an individualized breath pace is used to induce vagal modulation that results in a respiratory sinus arrhythmia (RSA). RSA has been found to be helpful in the management of physical and psychological symptoms of stress. Research has shown that patients with ischemic heart disease have little naturally occurring HRV, and they may struggle to increase it without intensive practice and coaching.[83,84] Those findings have been attributed to a combination of disease-related decreases in cardiac capacity for demand adjustments and psychological symptoms of depression or anxiety. Related research has shown that following coronary artery bypass surgery, patients are at a greater risk for symptoms of depression. Moreover, postoperative depression is linked to greater risk for cardiac morbidity and fatal cardiac events.[85,86] However, the findings of one randomized clinical trial provided evidence that biofeedback training can significantly increase RSA and decrease depression screening scores, suggesting a potential use for postoperative risk reduction in cardiac rehabilitation programs.[87]

FUTURE DIRECTIONS

Although there is a growing body of literature exploring the benefits of MBI, some researchers have argued that these findings are based on a body of evidence that is, at best, of moderate quality. The quality of the evidence for the efficacy of mind-body modalities appears to be higher for mental health–related indicators and quality-of-life outcomes than for disease-specific physical or physiologic indicators (eg, acute pain). Just as with any line of research, inflated findings can be the result of non-randomized studies, underreporting of negative trials and moderate heterogeneity among the studies that have been conducted. Several investigators cited in this review echoed concerns of limited evidence for the efficacy of MBI due to of methodological issues, and that additional high-quality research is warranted. Given the popularity of these interventions among patients and their transdiagnostic applicability to address a variety of health-related constructs, we hope to continue to see high-quality, longitudinal designs across diverse patient populations to fully appreciate the benefits and limitations of MBI for healing and coping with adversity within physical medicine and rehabilitation settings.

SUMMARY

Whether they have been practiced for thousands of years or harness modern technological advancements, mind-body modalities represent low-risk, cost-effective adjunctive treatment options for rehabilitation medicine settings. It was important for the current review to help providers understand the unique offerings of each mind-body modality and to evaluate the current state of the literature for rehabilitation populations. As nonpharmacological and noninvasive treatments, many patients benefit from the option to incorporate MBIs into their overall treatment plan, as they are able to actively work on their healing even in the midst of potentially incurable ailments. Moreover, integration of mind-body modalities may decrease stigma for accessing mental health treatment and improve their prognosis by creating an opportunity to address psychological risk factors such as anxiety and depression that might otherwise go unaddressed and lead to deterioration of their physical health. Ultimately, the goal of every intervention reviewed in this article is to empower patients with knowledge and skills that extend beyond their primary medical treatment to increase their capacity for responses that promote health and balance in the mind and body.

CLINICS CARE POINTS

- Although mind-body modalities are widely available to the general public and continue to gain popularity in medical settings, some are more efficacious than others.
- Meditation, GI, clinical hypnosis, and biofeedback are cost-effective evidence-based approaches that are well-received with minimal side-effect profiles for most patients.
- Providers are encouraged to offer measured optimism around setting patient expectations as outcomes for mind-body modalities are strong for mental health and quality of life, yet can be less robust for disease-specific indicators.
- Although a traditional cure is often out of reach for many patients, promoting healing, wellness, and coping in the midst of adversity are not.

DISCLOSURE

The authors have nothing to disclose.

REFERENCES

1. Eriksen J, Sjogren P, Bruera E, et al. Critical issues on opioids in chronic non-cancer pain: an epidemiological study. Pain 2006;125(1–2):172–9.
2. Toombs K. Living at the boundary: healing and incurable illness. Baylor University; 2008.
3. Rogan C, Fortune DG, Prentice G. Post-traumatic growth, illness perceptions and coping in people with acquired brain injury. Neuropsychol Rehabil 2013;23(5):639–57.
4. Health UNIo. Integration of behavioral and relaxation approaches into the treatment of chronic pain and insomnia. Paper presented at: Technology assessment conference statement 1995.
5. Pollack SW, Skillman SM, Frogner BK. The health workforce delivering evidence-based non-pharmacological pain management. University of Washington: Center for Health Workforce Studies; 2020.
6. Black LI, Barnes PM, Clarke TC, Stussman BJ, Nahin RL. Use of yoga, meditation, and chiropractors among US children aged 4-17 years. US Department of Health and Human Services, Centers for Disease Control and Prevention, National Center for Health Statistics; 2018.
7. Sharma H. Meditation: process and effects. Ayu 2015;36(3):233–7.
8. Goyal M, Singh S, Sibinga EM, et al. Meditation programs for psychological stress and well-being: a systematic review and meta-analysis. JAMA Intern Med 2014;174(3):357–68.
9. Travis F, Shear J. Focused attention, open monitoring and automatic self-transcending: Categories to organize meditations from Vedic, Buddhist and Chinese traditions. Conscious Cogn 2010;19(4):1110–8.
10. Orme-Johnson DW, Schneider RH, Son YD, et al. Neuroimaging of meditation's effect on brain reactivity to pain. Neuroreport 2006;17(12):1359–63.
11. Innes KE, Selfe TK, Kandati S, et al. Effects of mantra meditation versus music listening on knee pain, function, and related outcomes in older adults with knee osteoarthritis: an exploratory randomized clinical trial (RCT). Evid Based Complement Alternat Med 2018;2018:7683897.
12. Zamarra JW, Schneider RH, Besseghini I, et al. Usefulness of the transcendental meditation program in the treatment of patients with coronary artery disease. Am J Cardiol 1996;77(10):867–70.
13. Bishop SR, Lau M, Shapiro S, et al. Mindfulness: a proposed operational definition. Clin Psychol Sci Pract 2004;11(3):230–41.
14. Williams JMG, Kabat-Zinn J. Mindfulness: diverse perspectives on its meaning, origins, and multiple applications at the intersection of science and dharma. Contemporary Buddhism 2011;12(1):1–18.
15. Kabat-Zinn J. An outpatient program in behavioral medicine for chronic pain patients based on the practice of mindfulness meditation: Theoretical considerations and preliminary results. Gen Hosp Psychiatry 1982;4(1):33–47.
16. Hempel S, Taylor SL, Marshall NJ, et al. VA evidence-based synthesis program reports. In: Evidence map of mindfulness. Washington, DC: Department of Veterans Affairs (US); 2014.
17. Adler-Neal AL, Zeidan F. Mindfulness meditation for fibromyalgia: mechanistic and clinical considerations. Curr Rheumatol Rep 2017;19(9):59.
18. Gu Q, Hou JC, Fang XM. Mindfulness meditation for primary headache pain: a meta-analysis. Chin Med J (Engl) 2018;131(7):829–38.

19. Ngamkham S, Holden JE, Smith EL. A systematic review: mindfulness intervention for cancer-related pain. Asia Pac J Oncol Nurs 2019;6(2):161–9.
20. Lee C, Crawford C, Hickey A. Active Self-Care Therapies for Pain Working Group. Mind-body therapies for the self-management of chronic pain symptoms. Pain Med 2014;15(Suppl 1):S21–39.
21. Bawa FL, Mercer SW, Atherton RJ, et al. Does mindfulness improve outcomes in patients with chronic pain? Systematic review and meta-analysis. Br J Gen Pract 2015;65(635):e387–400.
22. Hilton L, Hempel S, Ewing BA, et al. Mindfulness meditation for chronic pain: systematic review and meta-analysis. Ann Behav Med 2017;51(2):199–213.
23. Morone NE, Rollman BL, Moore CG, et al. A mind-body program for older adults with chronic low back pain: results of a pilot study. Pain Med 2009;10(8):1395–407.
24. Johansson B, Bjuhr H, Ronnback L. Mindfulness-based stress reduction (MBSR) improves long-term mental fatigue after stroke or traumatic brain injury. Brain Inj 2012;26(13–14):1621–8.
25. Wathugala M, Saldana D, Juliano JM, et al. Mindfulness meditation effects on poststroke spasticity: a feasibility study. J Evid Based Integr Med 2019;24. 2515690X19855941.
26. Nijjar PS, Connett JE, Lindquist R, et al. Randomized trial of mindfulness-based stress reduction in cardiac patients eligible for cardiac rehabilitation. Sci Rep 2019;9(1):18415.
27. Balslev AN, Evers D. Compassion in the world's religions: envisioning human solidarity, vol. 8. Münster: LIT Verlag; 2010.
28. Neff K. Self-compassion: an alternative conceptualization of a healthy attitude toward oneself. Self and Identity 2003;2(2):85–101.
29. MacBeth A, Gumley A. Exploring compassion: a meta-analysis of the association between self-compassion and psychopathology. Clin Psychol Rev 2012;32(6):545–52.
30. Dodds SE, Pace TW, Bell ML, et al. Feasibility of Cognitively-Based Compassion Training (CBCT) for breast cancer survivors: a randomized, wait list controlled pilot study. Support Care Cancer 2015;23(12):3599–608.
31. Jazaieri H, Jinpa GT, McGonigal K, et al. Enhancing compassion: a randomized controlled trial of a compassion cultivation training program. J Happiness Stud 2013;14(4):1113–26.
32. Gilbert P. Introducing compassion-focused therapy. Adv Psychiatr Treat 2009;15(3):199–208.
33. Neff KD, Germer CK. A pilot study and randomized controlled trial of the mindful self-compassion program: a pilot and randomized trial of MSC program. J Clin Psychol 2013;69(1):28–44.
34. Ferrari M, Hunt C, Harrysunker A, et al. Self-compassion interventions and psychosocial outcomes: a meta-analysis of RCTs. Mindfulness 2019;10(8):1455–73.
35. Pace TWW, Negi LT, Adame DD, et al. Effect of compassion meditation on neuroendocrine, innate immune and behavioral responses to psychosocial stress. Psychoneuroendocrinology 2009;34(1):87–98.
36. Ashworth F, Clarke A, Jones L, et al. An exploration of compassion focused therapy following acquired brain injury. Psychol Psychother 2015;88(2):143–62.
37. Purdie F, Morley S. Compassion and chronic pain. Pain 2016;157(12):2625–7.
38. Hattan J, King L, Griffiths P. The impact of foot massage and guided relaxation following cardiac surgery: a randomized controlled trial. J Adv Nurs 2002;37(2):199–207.

39. Giacobbi PR, Stabler ME, Stewart J, et al. Guided imagery for arthritis and other rheumatic diseases: a systematic review of randomized controlled trials. Pain Manag Nurs 2015;16(5):792–803.

40. Roffe L, Schmidt K, Ernst E. A systematic review of guided imagery as an adjuvant cancer therapy. Psycho Oncol 2005;14(8):607–17.

41. King K. A review of the effects of guided imagery on cancer patients with pain. Complement Health Pract Rev 2010;15(2):98–107.

42. Casida J, Lemanski SA. An evidence-based review on guided imagery utilization in adult cardiac surgery. Clin Scholars Rev 2010;3(1):22–30.

43. Li R-Q, Li Z-M, Tan J-Y, et al. Effects of motor imagery on walking function and balance in patients after stroke: A quantitative synthesis of randomized controlled trials. Complement Ther Clin Pract 2017;28:75–84.

44. Kanji N, White AR, Ernst E. Autogenic training for tension type headaches: A systematic review of controlled trials. Complement Ther Med 2006;14(2):144–50.

45. Posadzki P, Ernst E. Guided imagery for musculoskeletal pain.: a systematic review. Clin J Pain 2011;27(7):648–53.

46. Zech N, Hansen E, Bernardy K, et al. Efficacy, acceptability and safety of guided imagery/hypnosis in fibromyalgia - A systematic review and meta-analysis of randomized controlled trials. Eur J Pain 2017;21(2):217–27.

47. Association AP. Hypnosis for the relief and control of pain. 2004. Available at: https://www.apa.org/research/action/hypnosis. Accessed February 20, 2020.

48. Freeman M. Guided imagery, biofeedback, & hypnosis: a map of the evidence 2019. Podcast. Department of Veterans Affairs, Veterans Health Administration, Health Services Research and Development.

49. Bastarache RB, Bastarache RE. Hypnotherapy certification training manual from A-Z. Biddeford (ME): American School of Hypnosis; 2005.

50. Milling LS, Gover MC, Moriarty CL. The effectiveness of hypnosis as an intervention for obesity: A meta-analytic review. Psychol Conscious (Wash D C) 2018;5(1): 29–45.

51. Cheseaux N, de Saint Lager AJ, Walder B. Hypnosis before diagnostic or therapeutic medical procedures: a systematic review. Int J Clin Exp Hypn 2014;62(4): 399–424.

52. Lam T-H, Chung K-F, Yeung W-F, et al. Hypnotherapy for insomnia: A systematic review and meta-analysis of randomized controlled trials. Complement Ther Med 2015;23(5):719–32.

53. Schaefert R, Klose P, Moser G, et al. Efficacy, tolerability, and safety of hypnosis in adult irritable bowel syndrome: systematic review and meta-analysis. Psychosom Med 2014;76(5):389–98.

54. Chen P-Y, Liu Y-M, Chen M-L. The effect of hypnosis on anxiety in patients with cancer: a meta-analysis: hypnosis effect anxiety in cancer patients. Worldviews Evid Based Nurs 2017;14(3):223–36.

55. Cramer H, Lauche R, Paul A, et al. Hypnosis in breast cancer care: a systematic review of randomized controlled trials. Integr Cancer Ther 2015;14(1):5–15.

56. Bowker E, Dorstyn D. Hypnotherapy for disability-related pain: a meta-analysis. J Health Psychol 2016;21(4):526–39.

57. Huet A, Lucas-Polomeni M-M, Robert J-C, et al. Hypnosis and dental anesthesia in children: a prospective controlled study. Int J Clin Exp Hypn 2011;59(4): 424–40.

58. Jensen MP, Ehde DM, Gertz KJ, et al. Effects of self-hypnosis training and cognitive restructuring on daily pain intensity and catastrophizing in individuals with multiple sclerosis and chronic pain. Int J Clin Exp Hypn 2010;59(1):45–63.

59. Lew MW, Kravits K, Garberoglio C, et al. Use of preoperative hypnosis to reduce postoperative pain and anesthesia-related side effects. Int J Clin Exp Hypn 2011; 59(4):406–23.

60. Nusbaum F, Redouté J, Le Bars D, et al. Chronic low-back pain modulation is enhanced by hypnotic analgesic suggestion by recruiting an emotional network: a PET imaging study. Int J Clin Exp Hypn 2010;59(1):27–44.

61. Jensen MP. Hypnosis for chronic pain management: a new hope. Pain 2009; 146(3):235–7.

62. Rainville P, Carrier B, Hofbauer RK, et al. Dissociation of sensory and affective dimensions of pain using hypnotic modulation. Pain 1999;82(2):159–71.

63. Skinner BF. 'Superstition' in the pigeon. J Exp Psychol 1948;38(2):168–72.

64. Schwartz MS. Appl Psychophysiol Biofeedback 1999;24(1):43–54.

65. Eid MAM, Aly SM, El-Shamy SM. Effect of electromyographic biofeedback training on pain, quadriceps muscle strength, and functional ability in juvenile rheumatoid arthritis: Am J Phys Med Rehabil 2016;95(12):921–30.

66. Kirnap M, Calis M, Turgut AO, et al. The efficacy of EMG-biofeedback training on quadriceps muscle strength in patients after arthroscopic meniscectomy. N Z Med J 2005;118(1224):U1704.

67. Anwer S, Quddus N, Miraj M, et al. Effectiveness of electromyographic biofeedback training on quadriceps muscle strength in osteoarthritis of knee. Hong Kong Physiother J 2011;29(2):86–93.

68. Sielski R, Rief W, Glombiewski JA. Efficacy of biofeedback in chronic back pain: a meta-analysis. Int J Behav Med 2017;24(1):25–41.

69. Newton-John TRO, Spence SH, Schotte D. Cognitive-behavioural therapy versus EMG biofeedback in the treatment of chronic low back pain. Behav Res Ther 1995;33(6):691–7.

70. Sella GE. Neuropathology considerations: Clinical and SEMG/biofeedback applications. Appl Psychophysiol Biofeedback 2003;28(2):93–105.

71. Blanchard EB, Andrasik F, Evans DD, et al. Behavioral treatment of 250 chronic headache patients: a clinical replication series. Behav Ther 1985;16(3):308–27.

72. McGrady A, Wauquie A, McNei A, et al. Effect of biofeedback-assisted relaxation on migraine headache and changes in cerebral blood flow velocity in the middle cerebral artery. Headache 1994;34(7):424–8.

73. Nestoriuc Y, Martin A. Efficacy of biofeedback for migraine: a meta-analysis. Pain 2007;128(1):111–27.

74. Nestoriuc Y, Rief W, Martin A. Meta-analysis of biofeedback for tension-type headache: efficacy, specificity, and treatment moderators. J Consult Clin Psychol 2008;76(3):379–96.

75. Kaushik R, Kaushik RM, Mahajan SK, et al. Biofeedback assisted diaphragmatic breathing and systematic relaxation versus propranolol in long term prophylaxis of migraine. Complement Ther Med 2005;13(3):165–74.

76. Syrjala KL, Jensen MP, Mendoza ME, et al. Psychological and behavioral approaches to cancer pain management. J Clin Oncol 2014;32(16):1703–11.

77. Mayden KD. Mind-body therapies: evidence and implications in advanced oncology practice. J Adv Pract Oncol 2012;3(6):357–73.

78. Prinsloo S, Novy D, Driver L, et al. The long-term impact of neurofeedback on symptom burden and interference in patients with chronic chemotherapy-induced neuropathy: analysis of a randomized controlled trial. J Pain Symptom Manage 2018;55(5):1276–85.

79. Prinsloo S, Novy D, Driver L, et al. Randomized controlled trial of neurofeedback on chemotherapy-induced peripheral neuropathy: a pilot study: neurofeedback for neuropathy. Cancer 2017;123(11):1989–97.
80. Tsai P-S, Chen P-L, Lai Y-L, et al. Effects of electromyography biofeedback-assisted relaxation on pain in patients with advanced cancer in a palliative care unit: Cancer Nurs 2007;30(5):347–53.
81. Renton T, Tibbles A, Topolovec-Vranic J. Neurofeedback as a form of cognitive rehabilitation therapy following stroke: a systematic review. PLoS One 2017; 12(5):e0177290.
82. Kober SE, Schweiger D, Witte M, et al. Specific effects of EEG based neurofeedback training on memory functions in post-stroke victims. J Neuroeng Rehabil 2015;12(1):107.
83. Lang PJ, Troyer WG, Twentyman CT, et al. Differential effects of heart rate modification training on college students, older males, and patients with ischemic heart disease. Psychosom Med 1975;37(5):429–46.
84. Palomba D, Stegagno L, Zanchi C. Biofeedback-assisted heart rate modification after myocardial infarction. J Psychosom Res 1982;26(5):469–73.
85. Blumenthal JA, Lett HS, Babyak MA, et al. Depression as a risk factor for mortality after coronary artery bypass surgery. Lancet 2003;362(9384):604–9.
86. Connerney I, Shapiro PA, McLaughlin JS, et al. Relation between depression after coronary artery bypass surgery and 12-month outcome: a prospective study. Lancet 2001;358(9295):1766–71.
87. Patron E, Messerotti Benvenuti S, Favretto G, et al. Biofeedback assisted control of respiratory sinus arrhythmia as a biobehavioral intervention for depressive symptoms in patients after cardiac surgery: a preliminary study. Appl Psychophysiology Biofeedback 2013;38(1):1–9.

Movement-Based Therapies in Rehabilitation

Melissa E. Phuphanich, MD, MS[a],*, Jonathan Droessler, MD[a], Lisa Altman, MD[b,c], Blessen C. Eapen, MD[a,c]

KEYWORDS

- Movement therapy • Yoga • Pilates • Tai chi • Qigong • Feldenkrais method
- Rehabilitation

KEY POINTS

Movement-based therapies

- Decrease fear avoidance and empower individuals to take a proactive role in their own health and wellness.
- Can benefit patients of any ability; practices are customizable to the individual's needs and health.
- Are safe, cost-effective, and potent adjunct treatments used to supplement (not replace) standard care.
- Deliver patient-centered, integrative care that accounts for the physical, psychological, social, and spiritual aspects of health and illness.
- Have diverse, evidence-based benefits, including reduction in pain, stress, and debility, and improvements in range of motion, strength, balance, coordination, cardiovascular health, physical fitness, mood, and cognition.

INTRODUCTION

Movement therapy refers to a broad range of Eastern and Western mindful movement–based practices used to treat the mind, body, and spirit concurrently. Forms of movement practice are universal across human culture and exist in ancient history. Research demonstrates forms of movement therapy, such as dance, existed in the common ancestor shared by humans and chimpanzees, approximately 6 million years ago.[1] Movement-based therapies innately promote health and wellness by encouraging proactive participation in one's own health, creating community support

[a] Department of Physical Medicine and Rehabilitation, VA Greater Los Angeles Health Care System, 11301 Wilshire Boulevard (117) Los Angeles, CA 90073, USA; [b] Healthcare Transformation, VA Greater Los Angeles Health Care System, 11301 Wilshire Boulevard (117) Los Angeles, CA 90073, USA; [c] University of California Los Angeles- UCLA, Los Angeles, CA, USA
* Corresponding author. Physical Medicine and Rehabilitation Department, Veterans Administration Greater Los Angeles Healthcare System, (117), 11301 Wilshire Boulevard, Los Angeles, CA 90073.
E-mail address: mphuphanich@gmail.com

Phys Med Rehabil Clin N Am 31 (2020) 577–591
https://doi.org/10.1016/j.pmr.2020.07.002
1047-9651/20/© 2020 Elsevier Inc. All rights reserved.

and accountability, and so building a foundation for successful, permanent, positive change.

Movement therapies used in conjunction with conventional medicine allow physicians to offer comprehensive, patient-centered treatment plans. This holistic approach embodies the essence of Physical Medicine and Rehabilitation by maximizing patient function and improving quality of life (QOL) to treat the whole person, not just the disease. The combination of modern medicine with mind-body practices offers an opportunity for "a state of complete physical, mental, and social well-being and not merely the absence of disease or infirmity," the definition of health by the World Health Organization.[2]

This article described evidence supporting the concept that mindful movement is medicine. Scientific evidence supports broad benefits of movement therapy, including reduction in pain, stress, and debility, and improvements in range of motion (ROM), strength, balance, coordination, cardiovascular health, physical fitness, mood, and cognition. Compelling evidence demonstrates that movement practices promote optimal health and are integral in the prevention and treatment of many medical conditions.

YOGA
The Yoga Practice

Yoga is a practice of physical postures, breathing techniques, and sometimes meditation derived from ancient India to promote physiologic and psychological well-being. Many types of yoga have evolved and become widespread in the United States. Although all forms of yoga share a common foundation in ancient philosophy focused on mind-body connection, each style has a different emphasis (**Table 1**). Styles range from handstand practices that would challenge an Olympic athlete to Kundalini yoga, which involves only poses lying down. Consequently, it may be challenging for a patient to choose the style that best suites his or her needs.

Despite the large variety of yoga classes available, all forms are based in the fundamentals of yoga philosophy that nourish physical and mental wellness, which include the following:

1. Asana—physical poses
2. Pranayama—breathing techniques
3. Meditation
4. Advice for ethical lifestyle
5. Spiritual practice

Introduction to Yoga Research

There are many research studies highlighting the benefits of yoga on mental health and medical conditions. A bibliometric analysis on yoga as a therapeutic intervention from 1967 to 2013 reported 486 articles published in 217 different peer-reviewed journals and included 28,080 participants from 29 different countries and a vast variety of conditions.[3] Studies in almost every field of medicine examine yoga's benefits (**Table 2**).[4–9] The most studied disorders are in (1) mental health, (2) cardiovascular disease, and (3) respiratory disease.[3]

Research shows that yoga improves physical fitness and cognitive function, and yoga may serve as an effective adjunct treatment of many medical and psychiatric conditions.

The literature demonstrates that yoga is more effective than waitlist control comparisons; however, yoga cannot yet be recommended as an equivalent or superior treatment to standard-of-care physical therapy or traditional exercise.[4] All 13 Cochrane

Table 1 Commonly practiced yoga styles	
Yoga Style	**Brief Description**
Ashtanga	A rigorous style that requires exertion equivalent to a conventional gym workout. The same preset sequence of poses, referred to as a "series," is practiced each session. Classes are a supervised self-practice, in which each student moves through the same series at his or her own pace and level; the teacher supervises by providing individualized adjustments to each student.
Bikram	A fixed sequence of 26 poses taught by an instructor with verbal instruction and physical example. Bikram yoga is practiced in a mirrored room heated to 105 F. The instructor gives no individualized adjustments; students are expected to correct themselves using the mirrors. The sequence does not include any poses that significantly bear weight on the hands.
Vinyasa	An athletic continuous flow through a series of poses that synchronizes one breath per movement. The sequence of poses is choreographed by the instructor, and thus every Vinyasa class is unique.
Hatha	A slower paced practice that focuses on flowing breathwork in static postures, rather than the strenuous breath-to-movement flows more commonly found in Vinyasa or Ashtanga yoga.
Iyengar	A practice that intensely focuses on proper form and precise bodily alignment of poses. An Iyengar class may consist of only a few poses, but each pose is held for a longer duration and can be individually modified with props, such as chairs. The attention to detail and customization of poses can make this style appropriate for individuals recovering from an injury.

reviews on yoga concluded that further, large-scale, methodological robust trials are required to establish evidence for yoga as a stand-alone treatment.[6–15] Accordingly, yoga should be used as a potent therapy in addition to standard care.

Yoga for Oncologic Rehabilitation

The mind-body-spirit connection applied in yoga is particularly valuable for conditions that affect both physical and mental health, such as cancer. Oncologic patients often

Table 2 Research studies on yoga for many conditions	
Medical Field	**Conditions Studied**
Neurologic	Parkinson disease, multiple sclerosis, stroke, epilepsy, dementia, neuropathy, myelopathy, Guillain-Barre syndrome
Psychiatric	Anxiety, depression, stress, PTSD, eating disorders, sleep disturbance
Cardiovascular	Hypertension, primary prevention of cardiovascular disease, secondary prevention of coronary heart disease, hyperlipidemia
Chronic	Diabetes, COPD, asthma, HIV, obesity, osteoporosis, irritable bowel syndrome, chronic fatigue
Geriatric	Osteoarthritis, balance, falls
Oncological	Breast cancer, colorectal cancer, hematological malignancies
Chronic Pain	Low back pain, headaches, arthritis, fibromyalgia
Women's Health	Urinary incontinence, pregnancy, perinatal depression

suffer from long-term psychological distress, anxiety, depression, fatigue, and chronic pain. A recent Cochrane meta-analysis on yoga for breast cancer, the most commonly diagnosed cancer in women worldwide, includes an impressive 24 randomized control trials (RCTs) involving 2166 women. The review recommends yoga as a complementary intervention for improving health-related QOL and reducing fatigue, sleep disturbances, depression, and anxiety.[10] Furthermore, yoga may boost the immune system of oncology patients. Patients with breast cancer in a Hatha yoga program showed decreases in interleukin-6, tumor necrosis factor-alpha, interleukin-1beta cytokine from isolated peripheral blood mononuclear cells stimulated with lipopolysaccharide, and interferon-gamma, suggesting that yoga protects against stress-related immune suppression.[16]

Yoga for Mental Health

Mental health influences the effectiveness of rehabilitation treatment plans, and yoga can efficiently address these psychosocial components of care. RCTs establish that the addition of yoga to standard-of-care treatment is more effective in reducing depression symptoms than standard care alone.[10,17] Yoga enhances mood through improved regulation of the sympathetic and hypothalamic-pituitary-adrenal systems. RCTs illustrate that these changes are mediated by decreases in cortisol and autonomic measures, such as heart rate and blood pressure, and upregulation of gamma-aminobutyric acid (GABA) levels.[16] Moreover, a longitudinal study found these benefits to mood were sustained at 1 year after only an 8-week yoga intervention.[18] The strongest evidence endorses yoga for depressive symptoms. The evidence on yoga for anxiety and posttraumatic stress disorder (PTSD) is also encouraging but not definitive due to lack of large-scale RCTs with high methodological and reporting quality.[19]

Yoga for Chronic Pain

Chronic pain syndromes are particularly susceptible to exacerbation by psychosocial factors, and yoga mitigates these negative influences by decreasing fear avoidance, increasing self-efficacy, and reducing stress and sleep disturbance.[20] Quality reviews show improvements in function, QOL, and pain level for chronic pain conditions, such as knee osteoarthritis (OA), rheumatoid arthritis, neck pain, headaches, and low back pain.[4,21–24] One quality study used MRI techniques to show that yoga improves pain tolerance.[25] Yogis tolerated pain more than twice as long as individually matched controls and had more brain matter in areas uniquely correlated to pain tolerance and areas responsible for integrating nociceptive input and parasympathetic activation. This finding of use-dependent hypertrophy suggests a consistent yoga practice improves pain tolerance by teaching different ways to deal with sensory inputs and the potential emotional reactions attached to those inputs. An RCT of yoga for low back pain also highlighted yoga's impact on neuromodulation. This study demonstrated that yoga led to decreased pain scores, improved ROM, and higher levels of serotonin and brain-derived neurotrophic factor (known modulators of nociception).[26]

Yoga for Spinal Conditions

More specifically, yoga may improve pain related to spinal conditions due to its focus on postural awareness and correction and subsequent reduction in excess muscle tension. RCTs demonstrated that yoga improved cervical proprioception, ROM, QOL, and mood and reduces pain and associated disability.[21,27] Evidence also affirmed that yoga decreased headache frequency, duration, and pain intensity in patients suffering from tension or cervicogenic headaches.[23] Iyengar yoga, which emphasizes precise body alignment, may be the most appropriate style for patients with chronic spine pain who need posture training.

Yoga for Neurologic Rehabilitation

Yoga can also effectively treat debilitating neurologic conditions that are often exacerbated by stress. Studies demonstrate yoga's alleviating effect on traumatic brain injury, stroke, spinal cord injury, Parkinson disease, dementia, multiple sclerosis, epilepsy, and neuropathies. Multiple systematic reviews reproduced improvements in function and mood, using tools such as the Berg Balance Scale, 6-minute walk, Timed Up and Go, State Trait Anxiety Inventory, Geriatric Depression Scale, Stroke Impact Scale, and Unified Parkinson Disease Rating Scale.[4,5] Even patients with paretic neurologic conditions may benefit from yoga. A study revealed that Kundalini yoga, a style that practices only poses lying down, improved both aphasia and fine motor dexterity in stroke patients.[28] In addition, a case study on a man who sustained an incomplete C3-C6 spinal cord injury and underwent a 12-week Hatha yoga practice showed improvements in functional goals, balance, endurance, flexibility, posture, and muscle strength of the hip extensors, hip abductors, and knee extensors.[29] Yoga is also used to reduce seizures triggered by stress. Sahaja yoga, a simple form of meditation, reduced seizures and EEG changes in patients with epilepsy. The potent effect of meditation was attributed to stress reduction, as evidenced by changes in galvanic skin resistance and levels of blood lactate and urinary vanillylmandelic acid, which are objective indicators of stress.[30,31]

Yoga for Cardiopulmonary Rehabilitation

The holistic yoga philosophy promotes a sustainably healthy lifestyle that may be useful for cardiopulmonary rehabilitation patients. A meta-analysis of 44 RCTs found that yoga improved systolic and diastolic blood pressures, heart rate, respiratory rate, waist circumference, waist/hip ratio, cholesterol, triglycerides, hemoglobin A1c, and insulin resistance.[32] The improvements in autonomic measures were attributable to increased parasympathetic activity through upregulation of GABA. This modulation counteracts the excessive activity of the sympathetic nervous system that has been associated with hypertension.[33] Rigorous yoga styles, such as Ashtanga or Vinyasa yoga, are more suitable for cardiovascular fitness, as no reductions in blood pressure were appreciated with Kundalini yoga interventions, which only uses poses lying down.[34]

Yoga Therapy in Summary

Yoga is a powerful adjunct tool for health promotion and maintenance and can be used to minimize pharmacologic treatments; alleviate chronic pain; and supplement neurologic, cardiopulmonary, and spinal cord injury rehabilitation. The diversity of yoga styles allows this therapy to be adaptable for a broad variety of ailments and physical abilities. However, this variability also makes it inherently difficult to apply the scientific method standards traditionally used for validating treatments. Clinical trials cannot blind yoga participants, which makes this research intrinsically susceptible to bias and not amenable to the gold standard of double-blinded RCTs. Yoga is highly supported as a safe and effective remedy for a plethora of conditions but cannot yet be recommended as a stand-alone treatment until stronger evidence is established. Research urges that additional high-quality RCTs are needed to improve confidence in estimates of effect, to evaluate long-term outcomes, and to provide additional information on comparisons between yoga and other exercise.

PILATES

The Pilates Method

Pilates is low-impact exercise based on holistic movement principles including concentration, centering, control, breathing, precision, and flow (**Table 3**).[35] Its mindful approach stimulates awareness of body structure, muscle recruitment, body alignment during movement, and posture awareness and control and stabilizes the core muscles during dynamic movement.[36] Pilates uses isokinetic exercises with resistance to strengthen deep muscle groups. In contrast to yoga, there are only 2 major forms of Pilates (**Table 4**).

Introduction to Pilates Research

Research supports Pilates ability to improve pain, function, psychological health, and kinesiophobia in people with disability.[37,38] Systematic reviews have investigated the effectiveness of Pilates on health outcomes related to body compositions, low back pain, breast cancer rehabilitation, physical fitness and fall prevention in seniors, and pelvic floor muscle function.[36,39] However, the benefits of Pilates are considerably less established in the literature when compared with the thousands of research articles examining yoga.

Pilates for Low Back Pain

Of the limited Pilates research, the strongest evidence suggests that Pilates effectively treats low back pain. This style of exercise builds lumbar stability and incorporates posture training and thus may alleviate low back pain using the same strategies as conventional evidence-based physical therapy programs. Pilates activates deep abdominal muscles for core strengthening and focuses on precise body alignment and awareness, resulting in a physique that mediates low back pain. The resultant physical changes identified in studies include increased rectus abdominis strength, elimination of muscular asymmetries in transversus abdominis and obliques, improved isolation of transversus abdominis, improved spinal stability with limb loading, improved hamstring flexibility, and improved abdominal muscular endurance.[40] The design of the Pilates method is highly compatible to the treatment of low back pain disorders. These exercises use a recruitment pattern of the abdominal muscles that may be particularly efficacious. A study examining activation of the

Table 3
Key principles of the Pilates method

Pilates Principle	Brief Description
Concentration	Focusing full attention of proper execution of Pilates exercises
Centering	Activation of deep trunk musculature such as the transverse abdominals, obliques, diaphragm, multifidus, and pelvic floor muscles. These muscles stabilize the lumbosacral spine and pelvis
Control	Performing movements and postures with careful muscular recruitment and control
Precision	Focuses on the bodily alignment and emphasizes proper technique of the Pilates movements
Breathing	Exercises are synchronized to a breathing rhythm, which stabilizes and strengthens deep abdominal muscles
Flow	Smoothness of movements with graceful transitions

Table 4 Types of Pilates	
Pilates Styles	**Brief Description**
Mat Pilates	Only equipment required is a mat and only bodyweight is used for resistance. Mat Pilates provides a foundation for learning muscle control
Reformer Pilates	Requires special equipment with springs that provide adjustable resistance. Reformer Pilates requires familiarity with a reformer machine but has the benefit of added resistance to improve strength

transversus abdominis, a primary contributor to spine stability, found Pilates practitioners performed significantly better on transversus abdominis isolation and lumbopelvic stability testing compared with the group that trained with standard abdominal crunches.[41] Another RCT compared Pilates against aerobic exercise and proposed that Pilates is a more effective treatment of low back pain and disability because the exercises are targeted to the muscles of pelvis and trunk.[42] Research also identified higher patient satisfaction and compliance with Pilates programs compared with traditional back school.[40]

Pilates Therapy in Summary

Although the Pilates method was established over a hundred years ago, there is a paucity of scientific experiment examining its health effects. The existing studies, along with established biomechanical theory, suggest Pilates is an effective treatment of low back disorders; however, the current evidence is not strong enough to be conclusive.[43] Consequently, Pilates is recommended as a powerful supplement (not replacement) to traditional physical therapy programs for low back pain.

TAI CHI
The Tai Chi Practice

Tai chi is a Chinese, meditative, martial arts practice designed to gently strengthen and relax the body and mind. It is a system featuring coordinated movements, meditation, and purposeful breathing that is believed to help unlock the body's Qi (**Table 5**).[44] Qi is the energy source that is believed to flow throughout every person's

Table 5 Key characteristics of tai chi	
Tai Chi Characteristic	**Brief Description**
Circular	All movements flow in a circular path, promoting dynamic stretching and balance
Relax	Deep breathing facilitates relaxation throughout entirety of the practice. Overexertion is avoided
Calm	Calmness in movement and mind, meaning no excessive movements and the mind is clear of superfluous thoughts
Continuous	Smooth transitions with one movement flowing to the next
Intent	Mind is present and fully focused on moving with purpose
Energy	Movements are biomechanically efficient, using the least amount of effort to execute

body and accounts for physical, mental, and spiritual health. When Qi becomes "unbalanced or blocked," pain and sickness result.[45] Tai chi is the process by which each person's Qi can be restored, generating improved functional capacity, balance, stress reduction, and enhancement of peacefulness, healing, and life-expectancy.[46]

Introduction to Tai Chi Research

Ancient tai chi is known for its complex, choreographed movement patterns that can take years to master. Given its accessibility to a wide age range, low cost, and theoretic benefit to functional ability and general health, a standardized and simplified form of tai chi was sought. In 2003, an expert panel on tai chi agreed that a simplified, standardized practice could be used for the general population.[46] There are now more than 500 trials and 120 systematic reviews over the past 45 years on the health benefits of tai chi.[44]

Tai Chi for Fall Prevention

The strongest evidence supports tai chi for fall prevention. Many strategies have been investigated, including various exercise modalities, vitamin supplementation, medication reconciliation, and vision screening or cataract surgery.[47] A Cochrane review on tai chi exercise and falls found high-certainty evidence that tai chi reduces the number of falls in elderly by 20% compared with controls.[48] In addition, a systematic review comparing the most common approaches to prevent falls found that tai chi is the most cost-effective fall prevention strategy.[47] Similarly, there is strong evidence that tai chi improves balance and reduces falls in patients with Parkinson disease.[44,49,50] Meta-analyses also suggest a possible role for tai chi in stroke rehabilitation to improve balance and gait and prevent falls.[44,51,52] Further, studies indicate tai chi may reduce fractures, a common consequence of falls, by improving bone mineral density in osteoporosis. A clinical trial demonstrated statistically significant improvements after 9 months, with participation in at least 75% of classes, suggesting results may depend on length and compliance with intervention.[44] These promising results are attributed to tai chi's ability to reduce the fear of falling and improve lower extremity strength, aerobic capacity, flexibility, and static and dynamic balance.[44,53,54]

Tai Chi for Chronic Pain

Tai chi's integrative approach is recommended in current guidelines for reducing chronic general musculoskeletal pain and associated disability.[55] Tai chi significantly reduces pain in patients with OA and is recommended by American College of Rheumatology for knee and hip OA.[56] Tai chi may also improve pain and QOL for patients with fibromyalgia. An RCT on fibromyalgia revealed that tai chi was superior to aerobic exercise, the current first-line exercise treatment.[44,57] This advantage could be attributed to the biopsychosocial care tai chi offers over conventional aerobic exercise.

Tai Chi Therapy in Summary

The highest quality evidence supports tai chi for fall prevention in community dwelling elderly and patients with Parkinson disease. These results are especially important given that tai chi has minimal adverse events and has the potential to reduce health care costs.[44] Research suggests the benefits of tai chi may apply to a wider range of conditions, including depression, anxiety, posttraumatic stress disorder, sleep disturbance, schizophrenia, rheumatoid arthritis, spinal cord injury, traumatic brain injury, and immune disorders.[44,58] However, there is a lack of conclusive evidence broadening the utility of tai chi due to small study size and methodological heterogeneity. Improvements must be made in standardizing tai chi class type, length of treatment, and assessing the long-term effects.[44]

QIGONG
The Qigong Practice

Qigong is another "moving" mindfulness practice that originated from traditional Chinese medicine.[58] Similar to tai chi, qigong uses the "mind" (or concentration) to coordinate breathing and smooth movements that promote the circulation of Qi.[46] There are several forms of qigong performed standing, sitting, or lying down with little to no movement. The forms make qigong adaptable to persons of any fitness level, age, income, or physical ability.[45]

Qigong Research

Tai chi and qigong practices are so similar that they are often grouped together in research studies as tai chi and qigong (TCQ).[58] Correspondingly, systematic reviews on qigong establish comparable improvements in fall risk, depression, and QOL. A Cochrane review on TCQ for individuals with cancer showed an integrative approach resulted in broad benefits to both psychological and physical health. TCQ led to improvements in sleep disturbance, depression, fatigue, pain, and QOL. TCQ may even have a role in reducing the inflammatory response that causes progression of cancer.[58]

Qigong Therapy in Summary

A comprehensive review by the National Institutes of Health on TCQ shows consistent, significant results for several health benefits in RCTs and infers equivalence of the 2 mindful martial arts practices.[46]

FELDENKRAIS
The Feldenkrais Method

The Feldenkrais method (FM), founded by a physicist and engineer, is a system that uses movement exploration for somatic learning through 2 major techniques (**Table 6**).[59] Series of movements force the practitioner to use body sensation and perceptual feedback to choose between favorable (easy, comfortable) and unfavorable (painful, straining) positions. With practice, discernment between favorable and unfavorable movements improves, and movement modifications develop and become engrained. The FM fosters self-efficacy in a group setting and theoretically provides sustained health benefits.[60]

Feldenkrais Research

Although often compared with TCQ, the health benefits of Feldenkrais are less established in research studies. Despite this, the FM is used to modify motor behavior of

Table 6 Feldenkrais techniques	
Feldenkrais Technique	**Brief Description**
Awareness through movement	Group class with participants learning through verbally guided movements
Functional integration	Individual lessons with practitioners learning by gentle touch/manipulation from an instructor to manually guide movements

people ranging in age and ability. An RCT demonstrated that Feldenkrais resulted in more relaxed supine posture due to changes in muscle tone. This study implied that Feldenkrais may alleviate chronic tension based pain.[59] A second RCT showed the FM has comparable efficacy to back school for the treatment of chronic low back pain.[61] Another RCT found improvements in balance testing in middle-aged individuals with intellectual disability. Given the commonality of functional decline in this population, Feldenkrais may play a role in improving physical activity and maintaining a level of independence in patients with intellectual disability.[62]

Feldenkrais Therapy in Summary

The FM has broad applications for changing bodily perceptions; easing function; and promoting awareness, self-efficacy, and health. Yet, there is a paucity of scientific evidence validating the benefits of Feldenkrais. At this time, clinicians may only offer Feldenkrais as a supplementary therapy to patients interested in efficient physical performance and self-efficacy.[60]

DISCUSSION

Ancient philosopher Plato posed, "Lack of activity destroys the good condition of every human being, while movement and methodical physical exercise save it and preserve it."[63] Current research advances this aged notion, "exercise is medicine," and contends that mindful movement is effective whole-person medicine. Movement-based therapies (1) decrease fear avoidance and empower individuals to take a proactive role in their own health and wellness; (2) can benefit patients of any ability; practices are customizable to the individual's needs and health; (3) are safe, cost-effective, and potent adjunct treatments used to supplement (not replace) standard care; (4) deliver patient-centered, integrative care that accounts for the physical, psychological, social, and spiritual aspects of health and illness; (5) and have diverse, evidence-based benefits, including reduction in pain, stress, and debility and improvements in ROM, strength, balance, coordination, cardiovascular health, physical fitness, mood, and cognition.

Strong Evidence for Mind-Body Therapies

Mind-body therapies facilitate a unique interaction between psychological and physiologic processes, and psychoneuroimmunology has flourished with empirical findings during recent decades. For example, studies show that psychosocial stress promotes gene transcription expressed during inflammation and impairs leukocyte function.[64] Likewise, reviews conclude that meditation and deep-breathing practices, commonly used in movement therapies, alter gene expression to protect against cell injury from chronic stress.[65] This is consistent clinically, as yoga practitioners experience significantly less depression than the groups using only physical yoga poses without the usual meditation or relaxation breathing techniques.[66] Importantly, research has suggested that mind-body practices enhance the psychoneuroimmunity against novel coronavirus disease 2019.[67]

Movement Therapy Benefits

Movement-based therapies are well tolerated across diverse patient populations. International guidelines across specialties recommend these nonpharmacologic integrative approaches.[68–70] For instance, clinical practice guidelines from the American College of Physicians makes a strong recommendation for initial treatment of chronic low back pain with exercises, multidisciplinary rehabilitation, mindfulness-based stress reduction, tai chi, yoga, motor control relaxation, or progressive relaxation.[71] The United Kingdom National Guidelines also recommends Feldenkrais, yoga, tai chi, and Pilates as exercise therapies.[69] As movement therapies become mainstream, some health insurance plans recognize the cost-effectiveness of movement practices and have begun subsidizing their cost as part of preventive care. Moreover, movement-based therapies can sometimes offer an alternative therapeutic option for populations wishing to avoid pharmacologic treatments. For example, prenatal yoga for pregnant women may be effective in partly reducing depressive symptoms. A meta-analysis showed a yoga group had lower rates of depression than comparison groups that included prenatal care, exercise, social support, and massage.[66] A systematic review deemed yoga during pregnancy as safe and more effective than walking or standard prenatal exercises based on findings of lower incidences of prenatal disorders, lower levels of pain and stress, and higher relationship scores.[72]

Movement Therapy: Safety and Precautions

Strong evidence maintains that mind-body practices are safe or safer when compared with other exercise types.[4,45] Nevertheless, the recommended intensity and style of movement-based therapy should be customized to the individual's needs and health. Selecting a movement therapy is analogous to pharmacologic treatment, in which medication type, dose, uses, and contraindications should be carefully reviewed. For example, patients with glaucoma should avoid exercises that increase intraocular pressure (IOP), such as inverted yoga poses that position the head below the heart. Alternatively, another yoga technique, called Tratak kriya, offers ocular exercises that may lower IOP in patients with glaucoma.[73] Furthermore, medical knowledge of instructors is widely variable with some teacher trainings including cadaver laboratory dissection, whereas others only include an hour lecture on anatomy.

SUMMARY

Movement therapy delivers patient-centered integrative care that includes health and wellness practices that best serve each individual. Mind-body practices include a diverse group of techniques for a wide variety of conditions. A review solely on yoga included 46 different styles of yoga practice.[4] Although contemporary literature strongly supports mind-body practices, its adaptability does not lend itself well to the rigidity required by the scientific gold standard of randomized control trials. Consequently, movement-based therapies are recommended as potent treatments to supplement, not replace, standard care.

CLINICS CARE POINTS

- Movement-based therapies can be used to facilitate behavior change and reduce kinesiophobia.
- Movement therapies can be used to decrease pain, stress, and debility and improve ROM, strength, balance, coordination, cardiovascular health, physical fitness, mood, and cognition.
- Movement therapies can only be used as adjunct treatments to supplement the standard-of-care treatment.
- Movement therapies can be particularly valuable for conditions that affect both physical and mental health, such as cancer or chronic pain exacerbated by psychosocial factors.
- The addition of yoga to stand-of-care treatment is more effective in reducing depression symptoms than standard care alone.

- Pilates is a powerful supplement to traditional physical therapy programs for low back pain.
- Tai Chi and Qigong can be used for fall prevention in community dwelling elderly and patients with Parkinson disease.
- Movement therapies are adaptable to persons of any fitness level, age, income, or physical ability.

ACKNOWLEDGMENTS

Special thanks to Dr Dixie Aragaki for her support throughout this project.

DISCLOSURE

The authors have nothing to disclose.

REFERENCES

1. Hattori Y, Tomonaga M. Rhythmic swaying induced by sound in chimpanzees (Pan troglodytes). Proc Natl Acad Sci U S A 2020;117(2):936–42.
2. Constitution of the World Health Organization. Addendum to the Forty-Fifth Edition. Am J Public Health 2006;1–18.
3. Jeter PE, Slutsky J, Singh N, et al. Yoga as a Therapeutic Intervention: A Bibliometric Analysis of Published Research Studies from 1967 to 2013. J Altern Complement Med 2015;21(10):586–92.
4. Field T. Yoga research review. Complement Ther Clin Pract 2016;24:145–61.
5. Mooventhan A, Nivethitha L. Evidence based effects of yoga in neurological disorders. J Clin Neurosci 2017;43:61–7.
6. Kwong JS, Lau HL, Yeung F, et al. Yoga for secondary prevention of coronary heart disease. Cochrane Database Syst Rev 2015;(7):CD009506.
7. Wieland LS, Shrestha N, Lassi ZS, et al. Yoga for treating urinary incontinence in women. Cochrane Database Syst Rev 2019;(2):CD012668.
8. Broderick J, Crumlish N, Waugh A, et al. Yoga versus non-standard care for schizophrenia. Cochrane Database Syst Rev 2017;(9):CD012052.
9. Hartley L, Dyakova M, Holmes J, et al. Yoga for the primary prevention of cardiovascular disease. Cochrane Database Syst Rev 2014;(5):CD010072.
10. Cramer H, Lauche R, Klose P, et al. Yoga for improving health-related quality of life, mental health and cancer-related symptoms in women diagnosed with breast cancer. Cochrane Database Syst Rev 2017;(1):CD010802.
11. Yang ZY, Zhong HB, Mao C, et al. Yoga for asthma. Cochrane Database Syst Rev 2016;(4):CD010346.
12. Panebianco M, Sridharan K, Ramaratnam S. Yoga for epilepsy. Cochrane Database Syst Rev 2017;(10):CD001524.
13. Lawrence M, Celestino Junior FT, Matozinho HH, et al. Yoga for stroke rehabilitation. Cochrane Database Syst Rev 2017;(12):CD011483.
14. Felbel S, Meerpohl JJ, Monsef I, et al. Yoga in addition to standard care for patients with haematological malignancies. Cochrane Database Syst Rev 2014;(6):CD010146.
15. Wieland LS, Skoetz N, Pilkington K, et al. Yoga treatment for chronic non-specific low back pain. Cochrane Database Syst Rev 2017;(1):CD010671.
16. Pascoe MC, Bauer IE. A systematic review of randomised control trials on the effects of yoga on stress measures and mood. J Psychiatr Res 2015;68:270–82.

17. de Manincor M, Bensoussan A, Smith CA, et al. Individualized yoga for reducing depression and anxiety, and improving well-being: a randomized controlled trial. Depress Anxiety 2016;33(9):816–28.
18. Kinser PA, Elswick RK, Kornstein S. Potential long-term effects of a mind-body intervention for women with major depressive disorder: sustained mental health improvements with a pilot yoga intervention. Arch Psychiatr Nurs 2014;28(6):377–83.
19. Meister K, Becker S. [Yoga for mental disorders]. Nervenarzt 2018;89(9):994–8.
20. Sherman KJ, Wellman RD, Cook AJ, et al. Mediators of yoga and stretching for chronic low back pain. Evid Based Complement Alternat Med 2013;2013:130818.
21. Cramer H, Klose P, Brinkhaus B, et al. Effects of yoga on chronic neck pain: a systematic review and meta-analysis. Clin Rehabil 2017;31(11):1457–65.
22. Lauche R, Hunter DJ, Adams J, et al. Yoga for Osteoarthritis: a Systematic Review and Meta-analysis. Curr Rheumatol Rep 2019;21(9):47.
23. Anheyer D, Klose P, Lauche R, et al. Yoga for Treating Headaches: a Systematic Review and Meta-analysis. J Gen Intern Med 2020;35(3):846–54.
24. Akyuz G, Kenis-Coskun O. The Efficacy of Tai Chi and Yoga in Rheumatoid Arthritis and Spondyloarthropathies: A narrative biomedical review. Rheumatol Int 2018;38(3):321–30.
25. Villemure C, Ceko M, Cotton VA, et al. Insular cortex mediates increased pain tolerance in yoga practitioners. Cereb Cortex 2014;24(10):2732–40.
26. Lee M, Moon W, Kim J. Effect of yoga on pain, brain-derived neurotrophic factor, and serotonin in premenopausal women with chronic low back pain. Evid Based Complement Alternat Med 2014;2014:203173.
27. Cramer H, Lauche R, Hohmann C, et al. Randomized-controlled trial comparing yoga and home-based exercise for chronic neck pain. Clin J Pain 2013;29(3):216–23.
28. Lynton H, Kligler B, Shiflett S. Yoga in stroke rehabilitation: a systematic review and results of a pilot study. Top Stroke Rehabil 2007;14(4):1–8.
29. Moriello G, Proper D, Cool S, et al. Yoga therapy in an individual with spinal cord injury: A case report. J Bodyw Mov Ther 2015;19(4):581–91.
30. Panjwani U, Selvamurthy W, Singh SH, et al. Effect of Sahaja yoga practice on seizure control & EEG changes in patients of epilepsy. Indian J Med Res 1996;103:165–72.
31. Panjwani U, Gupta HL, Singh SH, et al. Effect of Sahaja yoga practice on stress management in patients of epilepsy. Indian J Physiol Pharmacol 1995;39(2):111–6.
32. Cramer H, Lauche R, Haller H, et al. Effects of yoga on cardiovascular disease risk factors: a systematic review and meta-analysis. Int J Cardiol 2014;173(2):170–83.
33. Cramer H. The Efficacy and Safety of Yoga in Managing Hypertension. Exp Clin Endocrinol Diabetes 2016;124(2):65–70.
34. Bhavanani AB, Ramanathan M, Balaji R, et al. Comparative immediate effect of different yoga asanas on heart rate and blood pressure in healthy young volunteers. Int J Yoga 2014;7(2):89–95.
35. Eliks M, Zgorzalewicz-Stachowiak M, Zenczak-Praga K. Application of Pilates-based exercises in the treatment of chronic non-specific low back pain: state of the art. Postgrad Med J 2019;95(1119):41–5.
36. Mazzarino M, Kerr D, Wajswelner H, et al. Pilates Method for Women's Health: Systematic Review of Randomized Controlled Trials. Arch Phys Med Rehabil 2015;96(12):2231–42.

37. Fleming KM, Herring MP. The effects of pilates on mental health outcomes: A meta-analysis of controlled trials. Complement Ther Med 2018;37:80–95.

38. Miranda S, Marques A. Pilates in noncommunicable diseases: A systematic review of its effects. Complement Ther Med 2018;39:114–30.

39. Yamato TP, Maher CG, Saragiotto BT, et al. Pilates for low back pain. Cochrane Database Syst Rev 2015;(7):CD010265.

40. Joyce AA, Kotler DH. Core training in low back disorders: role of the Pilates method. Curr Sports Med Rep 2017;16(3):156–61.

41. Herrington L, Davies R. The influence of Pilates training on the ability to contract the Transversus Abdominis muscle in asymptomatic individuals. J Bodyw Mov Ther 2005;(9):52–7.

42. Campos de Oliveira L, Goncalves de Oliveira R, Pires-Oliveira DA. Effects of Pilates on muscle strength, postural balance and quality of life of older adults: a randomized, controlled, clinical trial. J Phys Ther Sci 2015;27(3):871–6.

43. Yamato TP, Maher CG, Saragiotto BT, et al. Pilates for Low Back Pain: Complete Republication of a Cochrane Review. Spine (Phila Pa 1976) 2016;41(12):1013–21.

44. Huston P, McFarlane B. Health benefits of tai chi: What is the evidence? Can Fam Physician 2016;62(11):881–90.

45. Braddom RL, Chan L, Harrast MA. Physical medicine and rehabilitation. Philadelphia: Saunders/Elvier; 2011.

46. Jahnke R, Larkey L, Rogers C, et al. A comprehensive review of health benefits of qigong and tai chi. Am J Health Promot 2010;24(6):e1–25.

47. Church J, Goodall S, Norman R, et al. An economic evaluation of community and residential aged care falls prevention strategies in NSW. N S W Public Health Bull 2011;22(3–4):60–8.

48. Sherrington C, Fairhall NJ, Wallbank GK, et al. Exercise for preventing falls in older people living in the community. Cochrane Database Syst Rev 2019;(1):CD012424.

49. Cwiekala-Lewis KJ, Gallek M, Taylor-Piliae RE. The effects of Tai Chi on physical function and well-being among persons with Parkinson's Disease: A systematic review. J Bodyw Mov Ther 2017;21(2):414–21.

50. Li F, Harmer P. Economic Evaluation of a Tai Ji Quan Intervention to Reduce Falls in People With Parkinson Disease, Oregon, 2008-2011. Prev Chronic Dis 2015;12:E120.

51. Wu S, Chen J, Wang S, et al. Effect of Tai Chi Exercise on Balance Function of Stroke Patients: A Meta-Analysis. Med Sci Monit Basic Res 2018;24:210–5.

52. Li GY, Wang W, Liu GL, et al. Effects of Tai Chi on balance and gait in stroke survivors: A systematic meta-analysis of randomized controlled trials. J Rehabil Med 2018;50(7):582–8.

53. Howe TE, Rochester L, Neil F, et al. Exercise for improving balance in older people. Cochrane Database of Systematic Reviews 2011;11:CD004963.

54. Kendrick D, Kumar A, Carpenter H, et al. Exercise for reducing fear of falling in older people living in the community. Cochrane Database of Systematic Reviews 2014;11:CD009848.

55. Hall A, Copsey B, Richmond H, et al. Effectiveness of Tai Chi for Chronic Musculoskeletal Pain Conditions: Updated Systematic Review and Meta-Analysis. Phys Ther 2017;97(2):227–38.

56. Kolasinski SL, Neogi T, Hochberg MC, et al. 2019 American College of Rheumatology/Arthritis Foundation Guideline for the Management of Osteoarthritis of the Hand, Hip, and Knee. Arthritis Rheumatol 2020;72(2):220–33.

57. Wang C, Schmid CH, Fielding RA, et al. Effect of tai chi versus aerobic exercise for fibromyalgia: comparative effectiveness randomized controlled trial. BMJ 2018;360:k851.
58. Wayne PM, Lee MS, Novakowski J, et al. Tai Chi and Qigong for cancer-related symptoms and quality of life: a systematic review and meta-analysis. J Cancer Surviv 2018;12(2):256–67.
59. Brummer M, Walach H, Schmidt S. Feldenkrais 'Functional Integration' Increases Body Contact Surface in the Supine Position: A Randomized-Controlled Experimental Study. Front Psychol 2018;9:2023.
60. Hillier S, Worley A. The effectiveness of the feldenkrais method: a systematic review of the evidence. Evid Based Complement Alternat Med 2015;2015:752160.
61. Paolucci T, Zangrando F, Iosa M, et al. Improved interoceptive awareness in chronic low back pain: a comparison of Back school versus Feldenkrais method. Disabil Rehabil 2017;39(10):994–1001.
62. Torres-Unda J, Polo V, Dunabeitia I, et al. The Feldenkrais Method improves functioning and body balance in people with intellectual disability in supported employment: A randomized clinical trial. Res Dev Disabil 2017;70:104–12.
63. Burnyeat M, Leavett MJ, Plato. The Theaetetus of Plato. Indianapolis (IN): Hackett; 1990.
64. Littrell J. The mind-body connection: not just a theory anymore. Soc Work Health Care 2008;46(4):17–37.
65. Muehsam D, Lutgendorf S, Mills PJ, et al. The embodied mind: A review on functional genomic and neurological correlates of mind-body therapies. Neurosci Biobehav Rev 2017;73:165–81.
66. Gong H, Ni C, Shen X, et al. Yoga for prenatal depression: a systematic review and meta-analysis. BMC Psychiatry 2015;15:14.
67. Kim SW, Su KP. Using psychoneuroimmunity against COVID-19. Brain Behav Immun 2020;87:4–5.
68. Wong JJ, Cote P, Sutton DA, et al. Clinical practice guidelines for the noninvasive management of low back pain: A systematic review by the Ontario Protocol for Traffic Injury Management (OPTIMa) Collaboration. Eur J Pain 2017;21(2):201–16.
69. National Guideline Centre. National Institute for Health and Care excellence: clinical guidelines. In: Ashmore K, Bartlett M, King B, editors. Low back pain and Sciatica in over 16s: assessment and management. London: National Institute for Health and Care Excellence (UK) Copyright (c) NICE; 2016. p. 154–758.
70. Negrini S, Giovannoni S, Minozzi S, et al. Diagnostic therapeutic flow-charts for low back pain patients: the Italian clinical guidelines. Eur Med 2006;42(2):151–70.
71. Qaseem A, Wilt TJ, McLean RM, et al. Noninvasive treatments for acute, subacute, and chronic low back pain: a clinical practice guideline from the American College of Physicians. Ann Intern Med 2017;166(7):514–30.
72. Jiang Q, Wu Z, Zhou L, et al. Effects of yoga intervention during pregnancy: a review for current status. Am J Perinatol 2015;32(6):503–14.
73. Sankalp DT, Yadav RK, Faiq MA. Effect of yoga-based ocular exercises in lowering of intraocular pressure in glaucoma patients: an affirmative Proposition. Int J Yoga 2018;11(3):239–41.

Spinal Manipulation and Select Manual Therapies
Current Perspectives

Nathan Hinkeldey, DC, DACRB[a,b,]*, Casey Okamoto, DC[c,d],
Jamal Khan, DO[c,d]

KEYWORDS

- Spinal manipulation • Massage • Human touch • Manual therapy
- Osteopathic manipulation • Chiropractic manipulation

KEY POINTS

- Human touch has demonstrated contextual therapeutic effects.
- Massage therapy is one of the most common application of human touch.
- Spinal manipulative therapy is an evidence-based treatment of musculoskeletal spinal pain.
- Populations engaging in manual therapy tend to use fewer health care dollars.
- Manual therapy, including spinal manipulative therapy, is safe and associated with mild adverse events.

HUMAN TOUCH

The application of touch as medicine is depicted in hieroglyphics from the 2200s BCE on walls of the tomb of Ankhmahor in Egypt. Techniques recognizable as massage are described within *The Cong Fou of Tao-Tse*, Homer's *Odyssey*, and ancient ayurvedic texts.[1] Touch is a fundamental part of human experience, as demonstrated by catastrophic outcomes in children who are denied it. Children raised from infancy in Romanian orphanages have lower gray and white matter volume compared with noninstitutionalized children. The effect can be mitigated, although not reversed, by moving them to high-quality foster care before age 2.[2] Neglected children experience disruptions of the hypothalamic-pituitary-adrenal axis, specifically as it pertains to

[a] VA Central Iowa Health Care System, 3600 30th Street, Des Moines, IA 50310, USA; [b] Palmer College of Chiropractic, 1000 Brady Street, Davenport, IA 52803, USA; [c] Minneapolis VA Health Care System, 1 Veterans Drive, Minneapolis, MN 55417, USA; [d] Department of Rehabilitation Medicine, 500 Boynton Health Service Bridge, Minneapolis, MN 55455, USA
* Corresponding author. VA Central Iowa Health Care System, 3600 30th Street, Des Moines, IA 50310.
E-mail address: Nathan.hinkeldey@va.gov

Phys Med Rehabil Clin N Am 31 (2020) 593–608
https://doi.org/10.1016/j.pmr.2020.07.007
1047-9651/20/Published by Elsevier Inc.

pmr.theclinics.com

cortisol rhythm, which can result in stunted growth and social responsiveness.[3] Conversely, preterm infants with low birth weight who receive touch therapy gain significantly more weight than those with standard treatment. Particularly in the newborn period, the benefit of skin-to-skin contact has been shown to improve sleep, reduce anxiety, and facilitate brain development. Mothers benefit as well, experiencing less postpartum stress and depression.[4] For those living with dementia, manual massage has been shown to reduce agitation and depression, conditions that affect approximately half of that population.[5] Hippocrates, often regarded as the "father of medicine," advocated for the laying on of hands. He wrote, "It is believed by experienced doctors that the heat which oozed out of the hand, on being applied to the sick, is highly salutary."[6]

Despite popularity abroad, manual therapies did not become a feature of Western medicine until the mid-nineteenth century. Massage techniques from Sweden were imported to the United States by brothers and physicians, George Taylor and Charles Taylor. In the late nineteenth century, osteopathy and chiropractic were codified by Andrew Taylor Still and Daniel David Palmer, respectively, and both professions were founded on the use of the human hand for both diagnosis and treatment, with specific emphasis in spinal manipulative therapy (SMT).

Scientific Evidence

The mechanisms by which touch exerts its effects remain only partially understood; the most current explanations suggest that effects can be subcategorized into analgesic, affective, and somatoperceptual domains.[7]

Analgesic

Melzack and Wall[8] described the gate control theory as a mechanism by which touch may produce analgesia. The sensation of touch activates mechanoreceptors in the skin, resulting in depolarization of large-diameter non-nociceptive A-beta fibers that synapse in the dorsal horn of the spinal cord before proceeding to the brain. Activation of inhibitory interneurons by the depolarization of A-beta fibers results in diminution or gating of signals from smaller-diameter A-delta and C-fibers, both of which transmit nociception, and effectively blocks nociceptive transmission.

Affective

The tactile experience typically is explained in terms of discriminative touch, mediated by A-delta and A-beta fibers, and nociception transmitted along unmyelinated C-fibers. C-tactile (CT) fibers represent a subgroup of C-fibers that are low-threshold, activated by gentle touch and temperature approximating that of human skin. Although projections associated with discriminative touch synapse in the primary somatosensory cortex, CT afferents project to the insula, a brain region critical to imbuing sensory information with emotion.[9] Affective touch has been shown to be not only pleasant but also protective against pain. For example, contact to the arm, provided by a caring partner, results in increased activity in the ventral striatum, the reward region in the brain, and, for those with low self-esteem, a comforting touch on the shoulder has been associated with reduced anxiety. Touch can alter neuroendocrine signaling, influencing dopaminergic, oxytocin, and endogenous opioid systems. Salivary α-amylase and cortisol are biomarkers that have been associated with stress and have been demonstrated to decrease in study participants after massage therapy. This effect is, of course, contextual. If the touch is perceived to be unsympathetic or otherwise not friendly, the effect can be quite different.[10]

Somatoperceptual

Patients suffering from chronic pain can develop a condition known as cortical smudging or somatotopic reorganization, whereby the homuncular map of the body in the brain becomes less sharp, and localization of nociception to a specific area or anatomic structure becomes more difficult. Touch can be a key component in helping patients to conceptualize their body and its position in space. This practice is especially beneficial for parts of the body that are not easily visualized, such as the spine.[7]

MASSAGE/MYOFASCIAL TECHNIQUES

According to the American Massage Therapy Association, in the 12-month period beginning July 2017, approximately 50 million Americans had at least 1 massage. Massage has grown into an $18 billion industry, with 62% of clients seeking massage for "medical or health reasons." Massage is widely available and used both as recreational medicine and as an adjunct to rehabilitation programs. Dozens of massage techniques exist (Acupressure, Reflexology, Myofascial Release, Lymphatic Drainage, Trigger Point Therapy, Swedish Massage), each aiming to reduce pain and improve function, but the mechanisms by which they are purported to do so vary.

Acupressure

As a subcategory of traditional Chinese medicine, acupressure is predicated on the notion that qi, or life energy, flows along meridians/pathways within the body. The flow of qi can become stagnant or otherwise disrupted, resulting in disease processes and pain. It is proposed that by pressing on various acupressure points, the flow of qi can be regulated, resulting in equilibration of the qi and resolution of the disease process.

Reflexology

Reflexology is similar to acupressure in that practitioners manipulate the body's qi by gently stimulating points on the foot or hand. The plantar and palmar aspects of the foot and hand are partitioned to correlate to visceral and musculoskeletal parts of the body, respectively.

Myofascial Release

Stretching is applied to muscles to induce relaxation, improve blood and lymphatic circulation, and disrupt adhesions between muscle and fascia, a connective tissue sheath surrounding skeletal muscle. Rolfing is another manual therapy claiming to exert an effect on fascia, elongating it to counter the shortening effects of gravity.

Lymphatic Drainage

Rhythmic strokes are applied to a limb to promote drainage of lymphatic channels away from the periphery and toward the heart. Lymphatic drainage is used most commonly to mitigate lymphedema after mastectomy or other surgical intervention that may disrupt the lymphatic system.

Trigger Point Therapy

Manual pressure is applied to a myofascial trigger point (MTrP), defined as a hyperirritable spot in skeletal muscle that is associated with a hypersensitive palpable nodule in a taut band. The spot is tender when pressed and can give rise to characteristic referred pain, motor dysfunction, and autonomic phenomena.

Swedish Massage

Swedish massage is the most widely practiced massage technique, often available in spas, and is used for treatment of specific conditions, recreation, and relaxation. Swedish massage is structured around 5 fundamental strokes:

- Effleurage—a gentle pressure applied by gliding the palmar surface of the hand over soft tissue
- Petrissage—firm pressure is applied while kneading, rolling, wringing, and lifting with the palmar surface of the hand
- Tapotement—rhythmic forces applied with the fingers, edge of the hand, or a cupped hand
- Friction—applied in a circular or transverse fashion to isolated muscles, usually using the fingertips or thumbs
- Vibration—manual vibration of soft tissues accomplished with the palm or knuckles

Scientific Evidence

Evidence maps, published in 2016[11] and 2019,[12] investigating the efficacy of massage for treating various painful conditions using high-quality systematic reviews, indicated low strength of evidence suggesting massage may be beneficial for low back pain (LBP), neck pain, shoulder pain, fibromyalgia, temporomandibular joint disorder, and pain related to labor. The research revealed significant limitations in the differentiation of massage types and providers. Although the concept of qi and meridians remains controversial, acupuncture and acupressure have been used for millennia and have demonstrated efficacy for treating certain musculoskeletal conditions.[13–15] Contemporary explanations have been offered regarding the role of neuromodulation in producing analgesia once attributed to manipulation of qi,[16] with diffuse noxious inhibitory control, descending inhibition, and endogenous opioid and endocannabinoid systems playing potentially important roles. Mathematical models for deformation of fascia suggest that fascia is too robust to be deformed by forces applied during manual therapy,[17] although that is not to say that myofascial release and similar techniques cannot be effective. Most likely, relief is achieved by some combination of the analgesic, affective, and somatoperceptual effects of touch. Evidence has been mixed regarding the efficacy of lymphatic drainage for postmastectomy lymphedema. Two of the 10 randomized controlled trials (RCTs) assessing prevention of lymphedema found no significant difference between groups receiving standard treatment and those receiving manual lymphatic drainage (MLD). Seven of 10 RCTs assessed reduction in arm volume and also failed to demonstrate a significant difference between MLD and standard treatment.[18]

A review of the literature suggests that MTrPs are real and measurable and that their cause and maintenance likely are multifactorial.[19] Microdialysis studies found MTrPs amid an acidic milieu and higher concentrations of inflammatory mediators like calcitonin gene–related peptide and substance P, implicating peripheral sensitization. Ultrasound studies have revealed hypoechoic regions within MTrPs that may represent regions of local muscle contraction, injury, or ischemia. Elicitation of a local twitch response seems to reduce the concentration of nociceptive substances, at least in the short term.

Complications and Concerns

Adverse events typically are limited to post-treatment soreness that resolves over days; however, there are case reports detailing serious adverse events, including vertebral and carotid artery dissection, neurologic compromise, and soft tissue injury. The risk of massage applied to the low back seems to be exceedingly low whereas techniques applied to the neck are of relatively higher risk. The specific technique and provider type are not always identified in the literature, making it difficult to assess the safety of one massage technique relative to others.[20]

Summary

The efficacy of massage is difficult to assess; however, what high-quality studies exist suggest massage may provide relief for some musculoskeletal conditions, including LBP and neck pain, which are major contributors to the global burden of disease,[21] and the risk of serious adverse event is low. Although precautions should vary by the type of massage used, in general massage is contraindicated in acute thrombosis, acute infections, bleeding and open wounds; and certain conditions, such as fragility, atrophy, malignancy, inflammatory muscle disease, and pregnancy, warrant individual assessment. It has not been assessed how massage might augment the effect of other rehabilitative treatments. Because persistent pain frequently is found with and perhaps maintained by central sensitization, fear-avoidance, catastrophizing, and somatotopic reorganization, deliberate and sympathetic touch, including when applied via manual therapy, may be leveraged to reduce fear, improve somatoperception and mitigate the impact of central sensitization. Massage applied as a monotherapy can result in over-reliance on passive modalities; thus, it should be used as an adjunct to active treatments, such as exercise and mind-body strategies, that foster self-efficacy and result in more durable improvement.

SPINAL MANIPULATIVE THERAPY

Musculoskeletal disorders represent a significant public health concern, with neck pain and LBP ranking among the top 5 disorders in terms of burden of disability and expense worldwide. A 2016 trend analysis from the Global Burden of Disease Study revealed an increase of 30 million people affected with musculoskeletal pain between 1990 and 2016.[21] Over the past decade, numerous evidence-based guidelines have been published, using care pathways to assist clinicians and patients in navigating potential treatment options. Most recent guidelines support manual therapies, including SMT, as effective treatments of acute, subacute, and chronic spinal disorders.[22–27] The remainder of this article provides an update of the evidence published over the past decade pertaining to SMT and mechanisms of action, responder characteristics, dose-response, impact on the health care system, and functional performance.

Current Evidence

Mechanism of action
Many mechanisms have been proposed for the systemic impact of SMT. **Table 1** summarizes the literature published prior to 2010.[28] A contemporary systematic review describes the effects of SMT as hypoalgesia, sympathoexcitation, decreased spinal stiffness, and increased muscle strength and endurance.[29]

No effect was found with respect to temperature pain threshold. One study notes increased nociception spinal flexion reflex, salivary substance P concentration, and improved sway index.[30] Autonomic effects of SMT include changes in heart rate variability and skin conductance.[31] Heart rate variability changes depend on region, with upper thoracic and lower cervical SMT increasing variability and the inverse occurring with upper cervical SMT in asymptomatic volunteers. In individuals with acute neck pain, heart rate variability decreases post-SMT, regardless of cervical spine location.

Table 1 Summary of neurophysiologic effects of manual therapy	
Peripheral mechanisms	Significant reduction in blood and serum level cytokines in joint-biased manual therapy[32] Changes of blood levels of β-endorphin, anandamide, N-palmitoylethanolamide, serotonin[33] Endogenous cannabinoids[34]
Spinal mechanisms	Joint-biased manual therapy is speculated to bombard the central nervous system with sensory input from the muscle proprioceptors[35] Hypoalgesia[36,37] Afferent discharge[38,39] Motoneuron pool activity[40,41] Changes in muscle activity[42,43]
Supraspinal mechanisms	Joint-biased manual therapy to the lower extremity of rats after capsaicin injection. Functional MRI of the supraspinal region quantified the response of the hind paw to light touch after the injection. A trend was noted toward decreased activation of the supraspinal regions responsible for central pain processing.[44] Autonomic responses[37,45,46] Opioid responses[47,48] Expectation of effectiveness of manual therapy is associated with functional outcomes[49] Joint-biased manual therapy is associated with improved psychological outcomes[50] Dopamine production[51] Central nervous system[52]

Data from Refs. [28,32-52]

Skin conductance increases post-SMT. Importantly, specific therapeutic effects are not solely responsible for the patient outcome, and nonspecific effects play a significant role.

Predicting a patient's response

Advancing technology and a marketplace eager for efficiencies incentivizes patient outcomes; thus, patient-centered care models encourage clinicians to provide care that is respectful of and responsive to individual patient preferences, needs, and values, and ensures that patient values guide all clinical decisions, according to the Institute of Medicine.[53] A patient's clinical outcome depends on the following: patient expectations, conditioned response, and unconditioned response.

Patient expectations Optimistic patient expectation improves outcomes in the following domains: pain reduction,[54,55] self-reported functional scores,[56] return to work, and disability.[57,58] Eklund and colleagues[59] studied the impact patient expectations had on pain outcomes at visit 4 noted that patients were 9% more likely to improve per 1-point increase on the 10-point expectation scale. They also noted that three-quarters of patients with a high expectation (74.2%) of LBP improvement after SMT reported a definite improvement at the fourth visit compared with just under half of those with low expectations. Also, those with high expectation were 58% more likely to endorse "definite improvement" compared with those with low expectation.[59]

Nonconditioned response Although numerous clinical variables have been assessed for their ability to predict response to SMT, results should be interpreted carefully

Table 2
Factors negatively affecting fourth visit outcome

Social and general health	1. Total fee subsidization
	2. Total duration of pain in the past year more than 30 d
	3. General health less than OK
Mental health	4. Anxiety
	5. Depression

because application to the general population may be limited by the scientific rigor and necessarily narrow scope of RCTs as well as confounding factors, such as patient demographics and comorbid conditions.

Lack of short-term improvement (definite improvement by visit 4) can be predicted by a lack of definitive improvement by the second treatment, presence of leg pain, and a minimum total duration of pain of 30 days over the past year.[60] Further analyses identified social and health factors (**Table 2**) that have an additive impact on predictive variables (**Table 3**). The strongest predictor of recovery at 3 months and 12 months was being pain-free at visit 4.[61] The presence of some or all of these potentially confounding factors should prompt a clinician to consider an interdisciplinary approach over monotherapy.

Some investigators have assessed predictive models by combining patient information and examination findings. Flynn and colleagues[62] validated a clinical prediction rule (CPR) defining patients with LBP who demonstrate short-term relief with SMT using the following factors that were found to be additive (**Table 4**): less than 16 days of symptoms, greater than 35° of hip internal rotation in 1 hip, lumbar hypomobility, lack of symptoms distal to the knee, and Fear-Avoidance Beliefs Questionnaire work score less than 19. Dougherty and colleagues[63] omitted the duration variable in order to test validity in a chronic pain population but no significant differences were appreciated between the populations (positive or negative CPR), suggesting that this particular CPR may not be useful in chronic LBP populations.

Advanced imaging has been used in the development of CPRs for comparing patient response to SMT with severity of degenerative changes, apparent diffusion coefficients (ADCs), dynamic muscle thickness, and Modic changes. Responders to SMT present with the following: lower prevalence of severely degenerated facets,[64] higher baseline ADC,[64] increased dynamic muscle thickness,[64] decreased post-SMT spinal stiffness,[65] and increased post-SMT multifidus thickness ratio.[65] Annen and colleagues[66] investigated response to SMT in patients with magnetic resonance imaging (MRI)-confirmed lumbar disk herniation with and without Modic changes. Patients with Modic changes outperformed those without and had larger decreases in

Table 3
Additive impact of predictive variables in Table 2 have on patient outcome

Domain	Social and General Health			+ Mental Health			
# of variables	0	1	2 or 3	1	2	3	4 or 5
% of patients with good outcome at Visit 4	79	64	45	82	75	60	36

Table 4
Low back pain clinical prediction rule

# Variables	Probability of Success (%)
5	—
4+	95
3+	68
2+	49
1+	46

leg pain and disability at 2 weeks, 3 months, and 6 months. At 1-year follow-up, Modic II–positive patients were improved significantly over Modic I–positive patients, which provides a new direction for investigation of variables affecting outcomes of SMT.[66]

Therapeutic dose response In medicine, dosages often are initiated at low thresholds and titrated based on response (positive or negative). If an effective dose has been established, patients may be maintained/supported on that dose. Manual therapy serves primarily as a bridging modality; however, consideration of a supportive role is appropriate in cases of therapeutic withdrawal resulting in declining function. Although the relationship between SMT dose, frequency, and treatment outcomes remains undefined, evidence has emerged pertaining to treatment of cervicogenic headache, LBP, and neck pain.[67]

Cervicogenic headaches
There are 3 RCTs evaluating the dose-frequency response of cervicogenic headaches to SMT over 3-week, 6-week, and 8-week time periods. In the 3-week treatment study, a frequency of 3 visits/wk to 4 visits/wk was found superior to 1 visit/wk in decreasing headache disability and pain.[68] In the 6-week treatment study, 4 groups (0 SMT + 18 light massage [LM], 6 SMT + 12 LM, 12 SMT + 6 LM, and 18 SMT) were followed and all 3 SMT groups significantly outperformed LM; however, no significant differences were noted between manipulation groups.[69] In the 8-week treatment study, 8 visits and 16 visits of SMT alone significantly decreases headache days compared with LM of the same frequency; however, no frequency effect was observed between SMT groups.[70] In summary, current evidence suggests SMT significantly decreases headache days, disability, and pain compared with LM for cervicogenic headaches; however, no significant difference was noted when comparing treatment frequencies of 8 visits/8 wk and 16 visits/8 wk or 6 visits/6 wk, 12 visits/6 wk, and 18 visits/6 wk.

Chronic low back pain
There are 3 RCTs evaluating the dose-frequency response of chronic LBP to SMT. Haas and colleagues[71] demonstrated that SMT applied at 3 visits/wk and 4 visits/wk over 12 weeks produces significantly greater decreases in pain compared with 1 visit/wk and 2 visits/wk. The effect of SMT also was assessed over a 6-week time period at a frequency of 1 treatment visits/wk, 2 treatment visits/wk, and 3 treatment visits/wk compared with a control of LM, and all 3 SMT groups demonstrated significant improvements in number of back pain days and severity compared with LM; however, no between-group differences were appreciated.[72] Cambron and colleagues[73] assessed the efficacy of flexion-distraction manipulation for patients with lumbar spinal stenosis at frequencies of 8 treatments, 12 treatments, or 18 treatments over 6 weeks. Symptom severity and disability were followed for 6 months post-treatment, improved at course

completion, and were maintained at 3 months and 6 months in the high-frequency groups (12–18 visits). Discussion of SMT treatment plans often involves some mention of "maintenance or supportive care." The effect of maintenance care (MC) in reducing flares and recurrences of LBP has not been well-studied; however, 1 RCT comparing MC to condition-based care exists. Analysis revealed 12.8 fewer days of bothersome LBP, which was achieved at the cost of 1.7 additional visits to the chiropractor.[74] The limited available data support the theory that MC may be appropriate for certain populations of patients; however, further study is required.[75]

No significant difference was appreciated between 12 visits and 18 visits. In summary, the treatment of chronic LBP with SMT should begin with higher frequency, tapering off as symptoms improve.

Spinal manipulative therapy in nonpain populations and functional outcomes

Health care providers are becoming more aware of the impact of SMT on domains of disability, pain, and function, but impact on functional performance is less understood. SMT has been shown to improve sports performance testing by reducing time for special operations forces qualified personnel to complete complex whole-body motor response tasks, reducing spasticity of participants with cerebral palsy, enhancing forced vital capacity and forced expiratory volumes, improving lung function and exercise performance in patients with chronic obstructive pulmonary disease, possibly having an impact on neuropathic pain mechanisms, increasing muscle strength and corticospinal excitability to ankle plantar flexor muscles in elite tae kwon do athletes, and augmenting lumbar proprioception.[76-84] Despite improvements in sports performance testing, the preponderance of evidence fails to demonstrate an effect of SMT on in-game outcomes compared with sham, with the exception of increasing free-throw accuracy.

Health care system impact

Often the impact of a modality is viewed within a single frame of reference, the effect on the patient's pain and function; however, there often are downstream effects that are not appreciated. The following public health implications relating to the impact of SMT have been demonstrated: patients who saw a chiropractor had half the risk of filling an opioid prescription[85]; patients participating in chiropractic care were 64% less likely to receive an opioid prescription than nonusers[86]; the cost per episode of care for LBP was 20% less when care was initiated with a chiropractor rather than a physician[87]; when care was initiated with a chiropractor, patients saw fewer total health care providers throughout their episode of care[88]; in Medicare-aged patients, expenditure was greatest among those who used medical care alone whereas patients engaging in SMT had the lowest overall expenditure, shorter episode of care, and lower cost per episode-day[89]; patients who received chiropractic in addition to usual medical care reported a statistically significant moderate improvement in LBP intensity and disability at 6 weeks compared with those with usual medical care alone[90]; and approximately one-third of post-9/11 war veterans receiving Veterans Affairs chiropractic services also received an opioid prescription, but the frequency of opioid prescriptions was lower after the index chiropractic visit.[91]

Complications and Concerns

The risk of injury from SMT has been extensively studied. Whedon and colleagues[92] evaluated risk of injury to the Medicare population and found that the risk of injury within 7 days of patients receiving SMT from a chiropractor was lower (40/100,000) compared with the primary care cohort (153/100,000). In particular, the risk for a neuromusculoskeletal problem (eg, injury to the head, neck, or trunk) within 7 days was 76% lower among subjects who underwent chiropractic care.[92] The risk was elevated in patients with osteoporosis, inflammatory arthritis, chronic coagulation defect, aortic aneurysm and dissection, or long-term coagulation therapy. The risk of stroke was studied in the same population and, of 1.12 million patients, the specific incidence of vertebrobasilar stroke was too small to report, thus precluding further analysis per Medicare guidelines. The likelihood of stroke 30 days after chiropractic cervical manipulation was significantly lower than after evaluation by a primary care provider.[93] Thus, SMT generally is a safe modality to include in musculoskeletal spine treatment and was associated with rare minor, musculoskeletal harms, including transient soreness.[94]

Summary

When considering SMT as part of a treatment plan for acute and chronic spine pain, the best available evidence, treatment goals, and patient's value system should be taken into account. The research supports that SMT should be used in the treatment of acute, subacute, and chronic musculoskeletal spine pain.[27] SMT assists patients in obtaining their treatment goals, including pain modulation.[23] Importantly, 78% of patients reported preferring nonpharmacologic approaches for treating pain[95] and SMT is a good alternative. Passive treatments, such as SMT, traditionally have been used to provide windows of relief that facilitate return to work and meaningful engagement with active rehabilitation; however, emerging evidence exploring the role of SMT maintenance care has been shown to result in fewer days of bothersome LBP.[73] SMT has become an attractive modality due, in part, to its apparent role in mitigating cost,[89] decreasing opioid prescriptions,[85] and shortening episodes of care.[88] Clinicians seeking guidance regarding which patients will respond to SMT will find the literature sparse, and the greatest predictor of a good outcome is positive patient expectation. Risk associated with SMT seems to be low, with most common adverse events being minor, musculoskeletal trauma.

CLINICS CARE POINTS

- Human touch is an important part of the evaluation and development of the doctor-patient relationship. At minimum, touching a patient in the area of complaint can contextually build trust and affirm that the clinician has heard the patient.
- Massage and myofascial techniques are options for clinicians to incorporate into care plans for treatment of LBP and neck pain, shoulder pain, fibromyalgia, temporomandibular disorder, and labor pain.
- SMT should be a treatment option for patients with cervicogenic headaches, LBP, and neck pain.
- An initial trial of care for SMT of 12 visits over 6 weeks to 8 weeks is appropriate; however, re-evaluation should occur and include assessment of functional improvement.
- Manual therapies are generally of low risk.
- Care should be taken to ensure that these therapies are used to assist patients in engaging in active therapy in goal-directed care.

ACKNOWLEDGMENTS

The authors would like to acknowledge the following for their contributions in editing and guidance on this project: (1) Franz Macedo, DO, Comprehensive Pain Center & Headache Center of Excellence, and Program Director, University of Minnesota

Pain Medicine Fellowship; and (2) Michael Tunning, DC, MS, ATC, Associate Dean of Clinical Sciences, Palmer College of Chiropractic.

DISCLOSURE

N. Hinkeldey: (1) VA Central Iowa Health Care System. The views expressed in the following are the views of the authors only and do not represent the views of the Veteran Health Care Administration or the local affiliate. (2) Palmer College of Chiropractic Board of Trustees. The views expressed in the following do not represent the views of the Palmer College of Chiropractic Board of Trustees or Palmer College of Chiropractic. C. Okamoto, J. Khan: no disclosures.

REFERENCES

1. Cetkin M, Bahsi I, Orhan M. The massage approach of Avicenna in the canon of medicine. Acta Med Hist Adriat 2019;17(1):103–14.
2. Sheridan MA, Fox NA, Zeanah CH, et al. Variation in neural development as a result of exposure to institutionalization early in childhood. Proc Natl Acad Sci U S A 2012;109(32):12927–32.
3. Johnson AE, Bruce J, Tarullo AR, et al. Growth delay as an index of allostatic load in young children: predictions to disinhibited social approach and diurnal cortisol activity. Dev Psychopathol 2011;23(3):859–71.
4. Field T, Diego M, Hernandez-Reif M. Preterm infant massage therapy research: a review. Infant Behav Dev 2010;33(2):115–24.
5. Margenfeld F, Klocke C, Joos S. Manual massage for persons living with dementia: a systematic review and meta-analysis. Int J Nurs Stud 2019;96:132–42.
6. Tardy MEJ. "Until Mary Ellen held my hand..." The critical importance of touch in medicine. Braz J Otorhinolaryngol 2015;81(3):229–30.
7. Geri T, Viceconti A, Minacci M, et al. Manual therapy: exploiting the role of human touch. Musculoskelet Sci Pract 2019;44:102044.
8. Melzack R, Wall PD. Pain mechanisms: A new theory. Science 1965;150:971–9.
9. Cascio CJ, Moore D, McGlone F. Social touch and human development. Dev Cogn Neurosci 2019;35:5–11.
10. Ellingsen D-M, Leknes S, Loseth G, et al. The neurobiology shaping affective touch: expectation, motivation, and meaning in the multisensory context. Front Psychol 2015;6:1986.
11. Miake-Lye I, Lee J, Lugar T, et al. Massage for Pain: An Evidence Map. Washington, DC: Department of Veteran Affairs; 2016.
12. Miake-Lye IM, Mak S, Lee J, et al. Massage for pain: an evidence map. J Altern Complement Med 2019;25(5):475–502.
13. Li LW, Harris RE, Tsodikov A, et al. Self-acupressure for older adults with symptomatic knee osteoarthritis: a randomized controlled trial. Arthritis Care Res (Hoboken) 2018;70(2):221–9.
14. Hempel S, Taylor SL, Solloway MR, et al. Evidence Map of Acupuncture. Washington, DC: Department of Veteran Affairs; 2014.
15. Chaillet N, Belaid L, Crochetiere C, et al. Nonpharmacologic approaches for pain management during labor compared with usual care: a meta-analysis. Birth 2014; 41(2):122–37.
16. Hannah RE, Morrison JB, Chapman AE. Prostheses alignment: effect on gait of persons with below-knee amputations. Arch Phys Med Rehabil 1984;65(4): 159–62.

17. Chaudhry H, Schleip R, Ji Z, et al. Three-dimensional mathematical model for deformation of human fasciae in manual therapy. J Am Osteopath Assoc 2008; 108(8):379–90.

18. Huang TW, Tseng SH, Ch Li, et al. Effect of manual lymphatic drainage on breast cancer related lymphedema: a systematic review and meta-analysis of randomized controlled trials. World J Surg Oncol 2013;11:15.

19. Shah JP, Thaker N, Heimur J, et al. Myofascial trigger points then and now: a historical and scientific perspective. PM R 2015;7(7):746–61.

20. Paul Posadzki EE. The safety of massage therapy: an update of a systematic review. Focus Altern Complement Ther 2013;18(1):27–32.

21. GBD 2016 Disease and Injury Incidence and Prevalence Collaborators. Global, regional, and national incidence, prevalence, and years lived with disability for 328 diseases and injuries for 195 countries, 1990-2016: a systematic analysis for the Global Burden of Disease Study 2016. Lancet 2017;390(10100):1211–59.

22. Qaseem A, Wilt TJ, McLean RM, et al. Noninvasive treatments for acute, subacute, and chronic low back pain: a clinical practice guideline from the American College of Physicians. Ann Intern Med 2017;166(7):514–30.

23. Chou R, Huffman LH. Nonpharmacologic therapies for acute and chronic low back pain: a review of the evidence for an American Pain Society/American College of Physicians clinical practice guideline. Ann Intern Med 2007;147(7): 492–504.

24. Pangarkar SS, Kang DG, Sandbrink F, et al. VA/DoD clinical practice guideline: diagnosis and treatment of low back pain. J Gen Intern Med 2019;34(11):2620–9.

25. Bussieres AE, Stewart G, Al-Zoubi F, et al. Spinal manipulative therapy and other conservative treatments for low back pain: a guideline from the Canadian Chiropractic Guideline Initiative. J Manipulative Physiol Ther 2018;41(4):265–93.

26. Bronfort G, Haas M, Evans R, et al. Effectiveness of manual therapies: the UK evidence report. Chiropr Osteopat 2010;18:3.

27. Clar C, Tsertsvadze A, Court R, et al. Clinical effectiveness of manual therapy for the management of musculoskeletal and non-musculoskeletal conditions: systematic review and update of UK evidence report. Chiropr Man Therap 2014; 22(1):12.

28. Bialosky JE, Bishop MD, Price DD, et al. The mechanisms of manual therapy in the treatment of musculoskeletal pain: a comprehensive model. Man Ther 2009;14(5):531–8.

29. Wirth B, Gassner A, de Bruin ED, et al. Neurophysiological effects of high velocity and low amplitude spinal manipulation in symptomatic and asymptomatic humans: a systematic literature review. Spine (Phila Pa 1976) 2019;44(15):E914–26.

30. Lascurain-Aguirrebena I, Newham D, Critchley DJ. Mechanism of action of spinal mobilizations: a systematic review. Spine (Phila Pa 1976) 2016;41(2):159–72.

31. Gyer G, Michael J, Inklebarger J, et al. Spinal manipulation therapy: is it all about the brain? A current review of the neurophysiological effects of manipulation. J Integr Med 2019;17(5):328–37.

32. Teodorczyk-Injeyan JA, Injeyan HS, Ruegg R. Spinal manipulative therapy reduces inflammatory cytokines but not substance P production in normal subjects. J Manipulative Physiol Ther 2006;29(1):14–21.

33. Degenhardt BF, Darmani NA, Johnson JC, et al. Role of osteopathic manipulative treatment in altering pain biomarkers: a pilot study. J Am Osteopath Assoc 2007; 107(9):387–400.

34. McPartland JM, Giuffrida A, King J, et al. Cannabimimetic effects of osteopathic manipulative treatment. J Am Osteopath Assoc 2005;105(6):283–91.

35. Pickar JG, Wheeler JD. Response of muscle proprioceptors to spinal manipulative-like loads in the anesthetized cat. J Manipulative Physiol Ther 2001;24(1):2–11.

36. Mohammadian P, Gonsalves A, Tsai C, et al. Areas of capsaicin-induced secondary hyperalgesia and allodynia are reduced by a single chiropractic adjustment: a preliminary study. J Manipulative Physiol Ther 2004;27(6):381–7.

37. Vicenzino B, Paungmali A, Buratowski S, et al. Specific manipulative therapy treatment for chronic lateral epicondylalgia produces uniquely characteristic hypoalgesia. Man Ther 2001;6(4):205–12.

38. Colloca CJ, Keller TS, Gunzburg R, et al. Neurophysiologic response to intraoperative lumbosacral spinal manipulation. J Manipulative Physiol Ther 2000;23(7): 447–57.

39. Colloca CJ, Keller TS, Gunzburg R. Neuromechanical characterization of in vivo lumbar spinal manipulation. Part II. Neurophysiological response. J Manipulative Physiol Ther 2003;26(9):579–91.

40. Bulbulian R. Endogenous opioid effects on motoneuron pool excitability: potential analgesic effect of acute exercise. J Manipulative Physiol Ther 2002;25(4): 209–15.

41. Dishman JD, Burke J. Spinal reflex excitability changes after cervical and lumbar spinal manipulation: a comparative study. Spine J 2003;3(3):204–12.

42. Herzog W, Scheele D, Conway PJ. Electromyographic responses of back and limb muscles associated with spinal manipulative therapy. Spine (Phila Pa 1976) 1999;24(2):146–52 [discussion:153].

43. Symons BP, Herzog W, Leonard T, et al. Reflex responses associated with activator treatment. J Manipulative Physiol Ther 2000;23(3):155–9.

44. Malisza KL, Stroman PW, Turner A, et al. Functional MRI of the rat lumbar spinal cord involving painful stimulation and the effect of peripheral joint mobilization. J Magn Reson Imaging 2003;18(2):152–9.

45. Moulson A, Watson T. A preliminary investigation into the relationship between cervical snags and sympathetic nervous system activity in the upper limbs of an asymptomatic population. Man Ther 2006;11(3):214–24.

46. Sterling M, Jull G, Wright A. Cervical mobilisation: concurrent effects on pain, sympathetic nervous system activity and motor activity. Man Ther 2001;6(2): 72–81.

47. Kaada B, Torsteinbo O. Increase of plasma beta-endorphins in connective tissue massage. Gen Pharmacol 1989;20(4):487–9.

48. Vernon HT, Dhami MS, Howley TP, et al. Spinal manipulation and beta-endorphin: a controlled study of the effect of a spinal manipulation on plasma beta-endorphin levels in normal males. J Manipulative Physiol Ther 1986;9(2):115–23.

49. Kalauokalani D, Cherkin DC, Sherman KJ, et al. Lessons from a trial of acupuncture and massage for low back pain: patient expectations and treatment effects. Spine (Phila Pa 1976) 2001;26(13):1418–24.

50. Williams NH, Hendry M, Lewis R, et al. Psychological response in spinal manipulation (PRISM): a systematic review of psychological outcomes in randomised controlled trials. Complement Ther Med 2007;15(4):271–83.

51. de la Fuente-Fernandez R, Lidstone S, Stoessl AJ. Placebo effect and dopamine release. J Neural Transm Suppl 2006;(70):415–8.

52. Matre D, Casey KL, Knardahl S. Placebo-induced changes in spinal cord pain processing. J Neurosci 2006;26(2):559–63.

53. IOM. Crossing the quality chasm: A new health system for the 21st century. Washington, DC: National Academy Press; 2001.

54. Gross DP, Battie MC. Work-related recovery expectations and the prognosis of chronic low back pain within a workers' compensation setting. J Occup Environ Med 2005;47(4):428–33.

55. Boersma K, Linton SJ. Expectancy, fear and pain in the prediction of chronic pain and disability: a prospective analysis. Eur J Pain 2006;10(6):551–7.

56. Myers SS, Phillips RS, Davis RB, et al. Patient expectations as predictors of outcome in patients with acute low back pain. J Gen Intern Med 2008;23(2): 148–53.

57. Opsommer E, Rivier G, Crombez G, et al. The predictive value of subsets of the Orebro Musculoskeletal Pain Screening Questionnaire for return to work in chronic low back pain. Eur J Phys Rehabil Med 2017;53(3):359–65.

58. Ebrahim S, Malachowski C, Kamal El Din M, et al. Measures of patients' expectations about recovery: a systematic review. J Occup Rehabil 2015;25(1):240–55.

59. Eklund A, De Carvalho D, Page I, et al. Expectations influence treatment outcomes in patients with low back pain. A secondary analysis of data from a randomized clinical trial. Eur J Pain 2019;23(7):1378–89.

60. Axen I, Jones JJ, Rosenbaum A, et al. The Nordic Back Pain Subpopulation Program: validation and improvement of a predictive model for treatment outcome in patients with low back pain receiving chiropractic treatment. J Manipulative Physiol Ther 2005;28(6):381–5.

61. Leboeuf-Yde C, Gronstvedt A, Borge JA, et al. The nordic back pain subpopulation program: demographic and clinical predictors for outcome in patients receiving chiropractic treatment for persistent low back pain. J Manipulative Physiol Ther 2004;27(8):493–502.

62. Flynn T, Fritz J, Whitman J, et al. A clinical prediction rule for classifying patients with low back pain who demonstrate short-term improvement with spinal manipulation. Spine (Phila Pa 1976) 2002;27(24):2835–43.

63. Dougherty PE, Karuza J, Savino D, et al. Evaluation of a modified clinical prediction rule for use with spinal manipulative therapy in patients with chronic low back pain: a randomized clinical trial. Chiropr Man Therap 2014;22(1):41.

64. Wong AYL, Parent EC, Dhillon SS, et al. Differential patient responses to spinal manipulative therapy and their relation to spinal degeneration and post-treatment changes in disc diffusion. Eur Spine J 2019;28(2):259–69.

65. Wong AYL, Parent EC, Dhillon SS, et al. Do participants with low back pain who respond to spinal manipulative therapy differ biomechanically from nonresponders, untreated controls or asymptomatic controls? Spine (Phila Pa 1976) 2015;40(17):1329–37.

66. Annen M, Peterson C, Leemann S, et al. Comparison of outcomes in MRI confirmed lumbar disc herniation patients with and without modic changes treated with high velocity, low amplitude spinal manipulation. J Manipulative Physiol Ther 2016;39(3):200–9.

67. Pasquier M, Daneau C, Marchand A-A, et al. Spinal manipulation frequency and dosage effects on clinical and physiological outcomes: a scoping review. Chiropr Man Therap 2019;27:23.

68. Haas M, Groupp E, Aickin M, et al. Dose response for chiropractic care of chronic cervicogenic headache and associated neck pain: a randomized pilot study. J Manipulative Physiol Ther 2004;27(9):547–53.

69. Haas M, Bronfort G, Evans R, et al. Dose-response and efficacy of spinal manipulation for care of cervicogenic headache: a dual-center randomized controlled trial. Spine J 2018;18(10):1741–54.

70. Haas M, Spegman A, Peterson D, et al. Dose response and efficacy of spinal manipulation for chronic cervicogenic headache: a pilot randomized controlled trial. Spine J 2010;10(2):117–28.
71. Haas M, Groupp E, Kraemer DF. Dose-response for chiropractic care of chronic low back pain. Spine J 2004;4(5):574–83.
72. Haas M, Vavrek D, Peterson D, et al. Dose-response and efficacy of spinal manipulation for care of chronic low back pain: a randomized controlled trial. Spine J 2014;14(7):1106–16.
73. Cambron JA, Schneider M, Dexheimer JM, et al. A pilot randomized controlled trial of flexion-distraction dosage for chiropractic treatment of lumbar spinal stenosis. J Manipulative Physiol Ther 2014;37(6):396–406.
74. Eklund A, Jensen I, Lohela-Karlsson M, et al. The Nordic Maintenance Care program: effectiveness of chiropractic maintenance care versus symptom-guided treatment for recurrent and persistent low back pain-A pragmatic randomized controlled trial. PLoS One 2018;13(9):e0203029.
75. Eklund A, Jensen I, Leboeuf-Yde C, et al. The Nordic Maintenance Care Program: does psychological profile modify the treatment effect of a preventive manual therapy intervention? A secondary analysis of a pragmatic randomized controlled trial. PLoS One 2019;14(10):e0223349.
76. Botelho MB, Alvarenga BAP, Molina N, et al. Spinal manipulative therapy and sports performance enhancement: a systematic Review. J Manipulative Physiol Ther 2017;40(7):535–43.
77. DeVocht JW, Vining R, Smith DL, et al. Effect of chiropractic manipulative therapy on reaction time in special operations forces military personnel: a randomized controlled trial. Trials 2019;20(1):5.
78. Kachmar O, Kushnir A, Matiushenko O, et al. Influence of spinal manipulation on muscle spasticity and manual dexterity in participants with cerebral palsy: randomized controlled trial. J Chiropr Med 2018;17(3):141–50.
79. Joo S, Lee Y, Song C-H. Immediate effects of thoracic spinal manipulation on pulmonary function in stroke patients: a preliminary study. J Manipulative Physiol Ther 2018;41(7):602–8.
80. Wearing J, Beaumont S, Forbes D, et al. The use of spinal manipulative therapy in the management of chronic obstructive pulmonary disease: a systematic review. J Altern Complement Med 2016;22(2):108–14.
81. Galletti J, Mcheileh G, Hahne A, et al. The clinical effects of manipulative therapy in people with chronic obstructive pulmonary disease. J Altern Complement Med 2018;24(7):677–83.
82. Onifer SM, Sozio RS, DiCarlo DM, et al. Spinal manipulative therapy reduces peripheral neuropathic pain in the rat. Neuroreport 2018;29(3):191–6.
83. Christiansen TL, Niazi IK, Holt K, et al. The effects of a single session of spinal manipulation on strength and cortical drive in athletes. Eur J Appl Physiol 2018;118(4):737–49.
84. Cerqueira MS. Response to "spinal manipulative therapy and sports performance enhancement: a systematic review". J Manipulative Physiol Ther 2019;42(5):382.
85. Whedon JM, Toler AWJ, Kazal LA, et al. Impact of chiropractic care on use of prescription opioids in patients with spinal pain. Pain Med 2020. https://doi.org/10.1093/pm/pnaa014.
86. Corcoran KL, Bastian LA, Gunderson CG, et al. Association between chiropractic use and opioid receipt among patients with spinal pain: a systematic review and meta-analysis. Pain Med 2020;21(2):e139–45.

87. Liliedahl RL, Finch MD, Axene DV, et al. Cost of care for common back pain conditions initiated with chiropractic doctor vs medical doctor/doctor of osteopathy as first physician: experience of one Tennessee-based general health insurer. J Manipulative Physiol Ther 2010;33(9):640–3.

88. Kosloff TM, Elton D, Shulman SA, et al. Conservative spine care: opportunities to improve the quality and value of care. Popul Health Manag 2013;16(6):390–6.

89. Weeks WB, Leininger B, Whedon JM, et al. The association between use of chiropractic care and costs of care among older medicare patients with chronic low back pain and multiple comorbidities. J Manipulative Physiol Ther 2016;39(2):63–75.e2.

90. Goertz CM, Long CR, Vining RD, et al. Effect of usual medical care plus chiropractic care vs usual medical care alone on pain and disability among US service members with low back pain: a comparative effectiveness clinical trial. JAMA Netw Open 2018;1(1):e180105.

91. Lisi AJ, Corcoran KL, DeRycke EC, et al. Opioid use among veterans of recent wars receiving veterans affairs chiropractic care. Pain Med 2018;19(suppl_1):S54–60.

92. Whedon JM, Mackenzie TA, Phillips RB, et al. Risk of traumatic injury associated with chiropractic spinal manipulation in Medicare Part B beneficiaries aged 66 to 99 years. Spine (Phila Pa 1976) 2015;40(4):264–70.

93. Whedon JM, Song Y, Mackenzie TA, et al. Risk of stroke after chiropractic spinal manipulation in medicare B beneficiaries aged 66 to 99 years with neck pain. J Manipulative Physiol Ther 2015;38(2):93–101.

94. Paige NM, Miake-Lye IM, Booth MS, et al. Association of spinal manipulative therapy with clinical benefit and harm for acute low back pain: systematic review and meta-analysis. JAMA 2017;317(14):1451–60.

95. Gallup Inc. Gallup-Palmer College of Chiropractic Annual Report: Americans' Views of Prescription Pain Medication and Chiropractic Care. 2017.

Performing Arts Medicine

Jovauna Currey, MD[a], Dana Sheng, MD[b], Alyssa Neph Speciale, MD[b],
Camilla Cinquini, DPT[c], Jorge Cuza, MD[b], Brandee L. Waite, MD[d],*

KEYWORDS

- Performing arts • Music therapy • Dance • Musician • Injury • Sports
- Rehabilitation • Prevention

KEY POINTS

- Although music may be used by artists during performances to connect with the audience, it may also be used by physicians and therapists to rehabilitate cognitive, sensory, and motor dysfunction in patients.
- The evaluation of each injury should be comprehensive, including evaluation of problematic movements, technique, muscle strength imbalances, and environmental factors.
- When providing medical care for performers, it is ideal, whenever possible, to recommend strategies that allow them to keep performing.

INTRODUCTION

Traditional athletes move for a purpose. For performers, the movement is the purpose.

Performing artists exist at the intersection between art and athletics. They must bring to life the vision of the choreographer or director and are expected to repeat this high level of perfection numerous times a week. They are a unique patient population because they are both artists and athletes. However, it can be difficult for performers to define what optimal performance is for them, because there is no winning in the performing arts. Many performing artists do their best to perform through the pain of an injury[1] because competition for roles and pressure from directors can be fierce. Circumstances vary from studio rehearsals and home performances to traveling with a tour, when access to normal medical care, nutrition, and support may be challenging.

Musculoskeletal and medical issues of performers should be addressed with special attention to their unique physical demands. Some performing artists are

a Department of Sports and Physical Medicine, Kaiser Permanente, The Permanente Medical Group, 3975 Old Redwood Highway, MOB 5, Suite 152, Santa Rosa, CA 95403, USA; b Department of Physical Medicine and Rehabilitation, UC Davis, UC Davis Health, 4860 Y Street, Suite 3850, Sacramento, CA 95817, USA; c Kaiser Permanente Rehabilitation, The Permanente Medical Group, 3975 Old Redwood Highway, MOB 5, Suite 154, Santa Rosa, CA 95403, USA; d Department of Physical Medicine and Rehabilitation, UC Davis School of Medicine, UC Davis Sports Medicine, 3301 C Street, Suite 1600, Sacramento, CA 95816, USA
* Corresponding author.
E-mail address: blwaite@ucdavis.edu
Twitter: @jcurreymd (J.C.); @brandeewaite (B.L.W.)

Phys Med Rehabil Clin N Am 31 (2020) 609–632
https://doi.org/10.1016/j.pmr.2020.08.001
1047-9651/20/© 2020 Elsevier Inc. All rights reserved.

diagnosed with neurologic medical issues that can affect cognitive, sensory, and motor functions. However, music has been shown to be a successful rehabilitation treatment of these issues.

MUSIC AS THERAPY

Music has long been used to foster emotional expression and support, help build personal relationships, facilitate positive group behaviors, and support other forms of learning.[2] Around the early 1990s, music therapy evolved from a social science model to a neuroscience model of clinical practice and research.[3] Music has been found not only to activate brain areas that are unique to music (eg, Broca area)[4] but to lead to changes in the brain.[5] These findings led to a new approach to music therapy known as neurologic music therapy (NMT). NMT is a neuroscience-based clinical application of music to address cognitive, sensory, and motor dysfunctions.

Initially, research was focused on efforts to find shared mechanisms between musical and nonmusical functions in motor control. One of the most important shared mechanisms is rhythm and timing.[2] A technique known as rhythmic auditory stimulation (RAS) was studied in patients with stroke and Parkinson disease.[6] Rhythmic auditory cues were used to give an external sensory timer to synchronize walking. In 1 study, patients showed improvement in stride time and stride length symmetry, weight-bearing time on paretic limb, and more balanced muscular activation patterns on electromyograms between the paretic and nonparetic limbs.[7] RAS also proved to be superior to other standard physical therapy interventions.[8] RAS for upper extremity rehabilitation after stroke showed a decrease in compensatory reaching movements.[9] Within the Parkinson disease population, RAS proves to be beneficial by quickening movement and preventing freezing,[10] improving mean gait velocity, cadence, and stride length,[11] and reducing the number of falls.[12]

Other applications of NMT in neurorehabilitation are in speech and cognitive recovery. Singing was first studied for speech apraxia in 1975.[13] Singing relies mainly on the right-hemisphere and can bypass injured left-hemisphere speech centers.[14] Melodic intonation therapy (MIT) is a technique used in NMT that engages the right frontotemporal network through melodic intonation (singing of words and phrases) and left-hand tapping.[15] Studies found functional and structural changes in right frontotemporal networks with MIT.[16,17] Music can also serve as an effective mnemonic device to facilitate verbal learning and recall. Learning word lists in a song activates temporal and frontal brain areas on both sides of the brain, whereas spoken-word learning activates only areas in the left hemisphere.[18] Musical memories provide a tool to enhance access to nonmusical recall and knowledge.[19] Studies have also shown that music has a neurohormonal effect by increasing serotonin release when listening to pleasant music.[20]

The mechanisms and the role of music as therapy in neurorehabilitation are becoming clearer with continued advances in science and technology. NMT is a promising complex multisensory modality for neurorehabilitation. Thanks to new insights from research into music and brain function, music therapy is beginning to prove itself a viable, evidence-based modality, specifically for neurorehabilitation.

MUSCULOSKELETAL ISSUES IN PERFORMING ARTISTS
Musicians

To attain professional proficiency, musicians spend 10,000 hours in 10 years of deliberate practice[21] involving nonphysiologic body positions and countless repetitions, creating an environment for muscle injury.[22] Musculoskeletal injuries may be caused by a specific injury or related to overuse in the setting of sudden increased practice or performance intensity or from poor technique and ergonomics. Prevalence of instrument-related musculoskeletal issues is as high as 87%.[23,24] Patterns of involvement vary with instrument dimensions, posture required, and technical demands of the repertoire. Musicians most often localized pain to the neck/spine, shoulders, and hands/wrists,[24–27] with postural disorders being 54%.[25] String, keyboard, and female musicians are most often affected.[24,26,28–31] Motor dysfunction, primarily fine motor, develops and ranges along a continuum, from fatigue-related transient/subtle deficits to more permanent deficits.[26,32] Importantly, studies have shown that better-trained musicians produce less excessive muscle recruitment during skilled repetitive movements, and this isolation ability improves with training.[24] For example, advanced trumpeters have more muscle activity in the muscles surrounding the lips instead of recruiting muscles in and around the lips equally.[24]

Evaluation and treatment

Motor fatigue Motor fatigue is short-lived loss of motor control while playing caused by overuse or lack of practice. Mental or bodily fatigue is associated, but pain is not. Symptoms include loss of regularity in scales, trills, and other fast repetitive movements, and deterioration of sound quality.[32] Muscle fatigue can lead to dysfunctional movement (eg, dysfunctional finger movements caused by compensatory intrinsic hand muscle use).[32] Usually, the fatigue is short lasting, often resolves overnight, and does not compromise overall performance.

Overuse injury Overuse refers to excessive limb use beyond anatomic and physiologic tolerance, causing local tissue inflammation, pain mediator release, and abnormal muscle tone, and leading to deterioration of motor control.[24,32] Recent unaccustomed or prolonged practice is often associated.[32] Pain is the predominant symptom. Overuse injury usually resolves with rest in 2 days to 4 weeks.[32] Relative rest, specifically from playing the instrument, is the only treatment that has proved to be effective. Other treatments without significant supportive data include splinting, antiinflammatories, analgesics, muscle relaxants, and stretching.[24,32]

Focal dystonias Although dystonia affects only 1% of professional musicians, they are the most disabling dysfunctions, often ending musicians' careers.[32] Focal dystonia (so-called musician's cramp) is persistent muscular incoordination during specific highly trained/overlearned movements of instrument playing. Major forms include focal dystonia of the hand and embouchure dystonia, related to the way in which a player applies the mouth to the mouthpiece of a brass or wind instrument.[32,33] Symptoms include subtle loss of control during fast passages, irregularity of trills, finger curling (**Fig. 1**), fingers sticking to keys, and loss of embouchure control.[32] Cocontraction of agonist and antagonist muscles often occurs. Pain is usually not a major feature unless the musician attempts to compensate for dystonia by overactivating antagonist muscles, causing muscular strain.[32] However, most musicians believe their reduced precision is caused by lack of technique and subsequently intensify their practice, exacerbating the problem. Sensory and proprioceptive input, including skin stroking, slight position changes, and weighted gloves, may provide temporary relief.[24] Medications include selective serotonin reuptake inhibitors, anticholinergics (particularly trihexyphenidyl), local botulinum toxin injections, and antiepileptics.[32] Neuromuscular reeducation and intensive task-specific training for 6 months or more have shown long-lasting effects.[34–36]

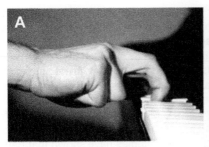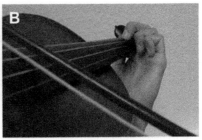

Fig. 1. Focal dystonias in musicians: finger curling as seen in (*A*) a pianist, (*B*) a violinist. (*From* Altenmüller E, Ioannou CI, Lee A. Apollo's curse: neurological causes of motor impairments in musicians. In: Altenmüller E, Finger S, Boller F, eds. Music, Neurology, And Neuroscience: Evolution, The Musical Brain, Medical Conditions, And Therapies, Volume 217. 1st ed. Waltham, MA: Elsevier; 2015:89-106; with permission.)

Entrapment neuropathies Entrapment neuropathies are common in musicians, predominantly median followed by ulnar disorder. Predisposing factors include pressure from hypertrophied finger, wrist flexor, or pronator muscles; nerve traction from extreme playing position; and repetitive motion friction trauma.[24] Treatment includes splinting, physical therapy, steroid injections, and surgical release.

Joint hypermobility Joint hypermobility can present technical issues in performance. It is most commonly seen in the first metacarpophalangeal (MCP)/proximal interphalangeal (PIP) joints.[24,30] Laxity not only causes inherent joint instability, leading to recurrent subluxation, but may also cause the musician to use other muscles for dynamic joint stabilization (eg, recruiting intrinsic thenar muscles to compensate for first MCP/carpometacarpal laxity), leading to fatigue and pain.[24] Management includes muscle strengthening for joint stability. Ring splints can prevent hyperextension and provide proprioceptive feedback to retrain finger positioning (**Fig. 2**), but it should not be a substitute for strengthening.[24] Extreme cases with painful instability may

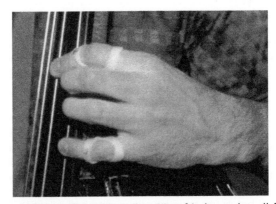

Fig. 2. Bass player with ring splints supporting PIPs of index and small fingers to address joint hypermobility. (*From* Brandfonbrener AG. Musculoskeletal problems of instrumental musicians. Hand Clin. 2003;19(2):231-239; with permission.)

require surgery (eg, reconstruction of the ulnar collateral ligament of the first MCP using the palmaris longus).

Instrument-specific musculoskeletal issues

String players Posture-associated pain occurs in string instrumentalists and is worse with larger instruments. Poor shoulder positioning leads to a phenomenon known as upper crossed syndrome (**Fig. 3**).[25] Injuries affect the fingering arm (usually left) wrist flexors, finger extensors, and abductors more than the bowing arm/hand (usually right) finger flexors and wrist extensors.[24,33] Musicians who hold their instruments between the chin and shoulder may have temporomandibular joint (TMJ) dysfunction.[22,24] Treatment includes shoulder or chin rest modifications, occlusal splinting, and physical therapy. Hypermobile musicians may also have TMJ subluxation.[24] String instrumentalists also develop some less common nerve injuries, including radial neuropathy, digital nerve compression, and so-called gamba leg compression of the saphenous nerve from lower leg position supporting the large string instrument.[24,37,38]

Brass players and wind instrumentalists Brass instrumentalists have many issues related to embouchure.[24,39] In wind instrumentalists, the supporting hand is often affected. Other injuries include TMJ dysfunction/malocclusion, de Quervain tenosynovitis in English horn players,[22,38] and thoracic outlet syndrome in flutists[24] (**Table 1**).

Pianists The bilateral wrist and finger extensors, lumbricals (especially fourth and fifth), and right hand interossei are frequently affected in pianists.[24] Tendinitis/tenosynovitis frequently affects the nondominant hand.[22] Degenerative changes occur at the second to fifth MCP joints, particularly on the right.[24] Individual anatomy may also predispose to injury, with small hand span requiring larger digit abduction angles and wrist range of motion in order to play chords and octaves.[24,40]

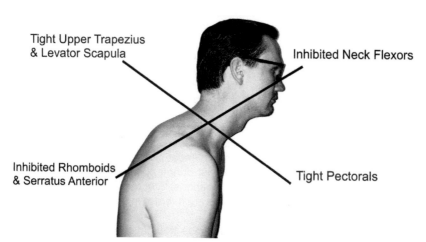

Tight Upper Trapezius & Levator Scapula

Inhibited Neck Flexors

Inhibited Rhomboids & Serratus Anterior

Tight Pectorals

Fig. 3. Upper crossed syndrome: overactivation of the trapezius and levator scapulae leads to shortening of the pectoralis, causing subsequent weakening of the surrounding counter muscles (neck flexors, scapular stabilizers). The intersection, or crossing, of these opposing muscle forces leads to forward shifting of the head and protraction of the shoulders.

Table 1 Musculoskeletal issues in wind and brass players related to supporting arm and embouchure	
Players	**Unique Musculoskeletal Issues**
Brass players	Embouchure-related issues: • TMJ disorders caused by the mandibular displacement required to form the embouchure • Satchmo syndrome (orbicularis oris rupture, a unique injury seen in trumpet players)
Wind instrumentalists	Supporting hand injury related to weight of the instrument and awkward positioning: • Clarinet, oboe, English horn players: overuse of right first web space muscles • Flutists: left upper extremity issues related to left wrist hyperextension • Bassoonists: left thumb sprain and basal joint arthritis

Guitarists Guitarists often have injuries related to extreme positioning, including hyperflexion of the wrist potentially causing hand/forearm strain of the fingering arm.[33] Focal dystonia often involves flexion of the third digit.[24]

Percussionists Drummers get stress fractures.[33] Cymbal players can get bicipital tenosynovitis (known as cymbal player's shoulder).[38]

Singers Although musculoskeletal issues in vocalists have not been well addressed, a unique injury is vocal cord dystonia.[33] Singers also experience hip, knee, and foot issues, perhaps related to prolonged standing.[38]

Marching band musicians Additional injury occurs because of the increased strength, coordination, and endurance required for transporting and supporting instruments, especially the larger instruments.[33] Heat-related illness and lower extremity stress fractures also occur.

Dancers

Dancers are at high risk for musculoskeletal injuries given the countless hours of rigorous training and performances. Although ballet is the most studied, most injuries are seen across dance styles. Acute injuries occur from macrotrauma where normal or insufficient tissue is subject to sudden stress beyond the tissue's capacity at a single point in time (eg, during lifting maneuvers, jumps, or landings).[41] Chronic/overuse injuries arise from repetitive microtrauma, wherein recurrent injury recurs without enough time for healing between, or without elimination of, the causative factor.[41] There are many contributors to chronic injury, grouped into intrinsic (related to the dancer) or extrinsic (environmental) causes (**Table 2**). Dance injury prevalence is as high as 95% in professional companies,[33,41] most commonly in the ankle/foot and then the knee.[33,41–43] Injury rates are highest during opening months of the season as well as during rehearsal/performance periods.[41] Acute injuries include sprains, strains, and tendinitis.[41] Most dance injuries are overuse injuries, including tendinosis and stress fractures.[33,41] Reinjury is common.[44]

Younger dancers more frequently experience traumatic injuries and hip/back injuries, whereas older dancers are prone to more leg, ankle, and foot injuries.[41] Certain maneuvers require extreme body alignments, such as fifth position or en pointe in ballet, wrist spins in breakdancing, or splits positioning in many styles of dance. Incorrect technique leads to compensatory misalignments that increase risk for injury.

Table 2 Intrinsic and extrinsic causes for chronic injury in dancers		

Intrinsic Factors	Physiologic	• Anatomic deformity such as genu recurvatum:
		  ○ May lead to posterior capsular strain and discomfort
		• Anatomic variation such as length of toes:
		  ○ A ballerina with 1 toe longer than the rest has less stability on pointe and more force transmitted through that base compared with a dancer with similar lengths of the first to third toes

	Technical	• Extreme moves like grand plie, which involves extreme deep flexion required of the knees and hips: ○ Repetition of this contributes to extensor mechanism overuse injuries • Improper dance technique; eg, forcing turnout
Extrinsic Factors	—	• Footwear (including amount of support provided, age, and wear of the shoe) • Dance floor surface (sprung vs not, amount of friction provided): ○ Changing dance floor surfaces (from flat to raked stages) changes how dancers must adjust their balance, which can predispose to injury

Unique injuries in growing dancers include growth plate fractures and osteochondroses.[45] These injuries often occur at nonarticular locations caused by repetitive stress at tendon/ligament attachments. Acute injury or overuse can also lead to apophyseal injuries in young dancers. Treatment of Osgood-Schlatter disease at the tibial tuberosity, Sinding-Larsen-Johansson syndrome at the inferior pole of the patella, and Sever disease at the calcaneus may include relative rest, focal bracing/heel lift, and strengthening/stretching for the associated muscles. Immobilization is occasionally needed if the condition is severe.

Common musculoskeletal issues in dancers

Some dance style–specific injuries along with explanation for injury profile variation are explored in **Table 3**.

Hip Extreme hip ranges of motion are seen in many dance maneuvers[55] (**Fig. 4**) and can be associated with femoral acetabular impingement, subluxation, and strain on the acetabular labrum.[55,56] Labral tears may cause anterior hip/groin pain with mechanical catching. Symptoms occur with pivoting on the hip joint, standing from seated position, or performing side leg extensions.[41] Other hip injuries include snapping hip, osteoarthritis, sacroiliac joint (SIJ) dysfunction, and stress fractures. Snapping hip can be caused by various snapping tendons (lateral or medial) but can also occur from intra-articular cartilage/labrum injury. Snapping tendons are usually painless but can become painful over time. Osteoarthritis causes anterior groin pain and limited internal rotation/flexion. SIJ dysfunction may cause local/referred posterior hip pain with jumps and limited hip extension.[57] Stress fractures can occur at the femoral neck in this population as well. Inferior (compression side) femoral neck stress fractures may be treated conservatively, whereas superior (tension side) injuries pose a significant risk of progression to fracture and require non–weight-bearing status and surgical consultation.[41]

Knee/lower leg Patellofemoral pain is common, may be worse in dancers with increased Q angle, and can be exacerbated by turnout technique.[41] Excess tibial torsion from forcing turnout stresses the medial knee and can lead to meniscal/ligament

Table 3
Notable style-specific musculoskeletal issues in dancers

Style of Dance	Unique Musculoskeletal Issues
Hip hop	• Knee (most common; 36%) > lumbar spine (19%) > foot and ankle[42,46,47] • Meniscal injury: more common in men • Patellofemoral pain: more common in women • Lumbar disc injuries: occur at the L5/S1 level

Modern	• Back injuries: related to significant flexion and extension of the spine at all levels[48]
	• Knee injuries: related to floor work, including kneeling positions[48]
	• Specific modern styles are associated with more or less frequent knee injury[49]:
	  ○ More frequent in styles that compress and hyperextend the knee (eg, Graham style)
	  ○ Less frequent in styles that flex the knee and strengthen the quadriceps (eg, Horton style)
	• Cervical and thoracic strain: seen twice as frequently in modern dance students compared with in ballet students[50]

International modern and Latin dancesport	• Highest prevalence: neck, back, shoulder, knee, lower leg, ankle, and foot: ○ Neck injury likely because of female dancers' positioning, which requires extension of the upper body and neck with further neck rotation to the left[51]

Flamenco	Injury profile varies depending on level of training:
	• Students: foot is the most common site of injury
	  ○ Stress fractures, sesamoiditis
	• Professional dancers: back (especially lumbar) and knee injuries are more common than foot injuries:
	  ○ Possibly related to younger dancers focusing on dynamic and fast footwork with several repetitions of escobias, whereas older dancers with more experience focus on subtle details of artistry, including angles and level changes[52]
	  ○ The more experienced may also wear nonflamenco shoes with more support and shock absorption

Belly dancing	• Lower limb and trunk injuries most common[53]
	• Some variation by experience level:
	  ○ Lower limbs more involved (especially the knee) in more experienced belly dancers
	  ○ Lower back more involved in less experienced dancers
	• Knee injuries: thought to be related to the repeated loading of the knees while flexed causing more knee instability as well as more cumulative fatigue
	• Frequent back injuries (including stress fractures): thought to be related to the repetitive movements initiated at or involving the spine as well as the positions of extreme spinal extension, as in backbends[53]

Russian Cossack dancing	• Meniscal tears: thought to be related to the rapid flexion and extension required at the knee joints while in the squatting position[48]
Broadway dance	Injuries reflect the types of dance represented within the Broadway dance. Broadway dance is a combination of the other main classifications of theatrical dance: classical ballet, classical modern dance, and cultural dance forms[48] • Lower extremities > back and neck ○ Lower extremity injuries: knee > ankle > foot > hip > calf[54]

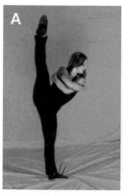
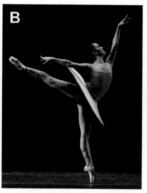
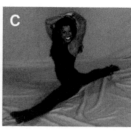

Fig. 4. Dancers showing various positions involving extreme hip end ranges of motion: (*A*) développé à la seconde, (*B*) arabesque, (*C*) grand écart lateral (splits). ([A] *Courtesy of* A. Hinman, Berkeley, CA.; [B] B. Truitt Covert, Portland, OR. and M. Dore, New York, NY. [C] S. Andrews, Berkeley, CA.)

injury.[49,58] Genu recurvatum stretches the posterior capsule, puts tension on the anterior cruciate ligament, and is commonly associated with quadriceps weakness.[58] Tendon overuse injuries include patellar tendinitis (jumper's knee) resulting from chronic eccentric quadriceps use during jumps (more common in male ballet dancers, some modern/jazz dancers).[49,59] Iliotibial band (ITB) friction syndrome features pain where the ITB moves over the lateral femoral epicondyle and can be worse in dancers with insufficient hip turnout.[49] Tibial/fibular stress fractures are often caused by improper technique or repetitive stress. Tibial stress fractures are the second most common stress fractures in ballet dancers, after the second metatarsal.[60] Fibular stress fractures are related to inadequate strength of intrinsic foot muscles and sickling of the foot.[60] Stress fracture risk may be increased after lateral ankle sprain if ankle-stabilizing muscles were not properly strengthened. Fatigue of the foot muscles also causes increased force transmission through the tibia.[61]

Ankle Lateral/inversion ankle sprains are the most common acute injury[41] and most commonly occur during plantarflexion-inversion in demi-pointe or during landing of a jump. Anterior ankle impingement of bony/soft tissue between the anterior distal tibia and the talus can cause chronic ankle pain. Repetitive ankle dorsiflexion is associated with multiple disorders, including hypertrophic scar tissue involving the anterior talofibular ligament, traction spurs, stretched joint capsule, avulsion fractures, loose bodies, and calcium deposition.[41] Posterior ankle impingement of bony/soft tissue between the posterior tibial plafond and the calcaneus can cause acute or chronic injury from repetitive plantarflexion.[41] Although many causes exist,[62] the most common are os trigonum, flexor hallucis longus (FHL) tendinitis (dancer's tendinitis), and Achilles tendinitis (**Fig. 5**).[41]

Foot Acute injuries include fractures and subluxations. Dancer's fracture (acute spiral fracture of the fifth metatarsal neck) is caused by twisting inversion of the foot in demi-pointe.[41] Cuboid subluxation, often concurrent with lateral ankle sprain, occurs during inversion-plantarflexion, such as during landing from a jump in pronation or during repetitive alternation between plantarflexion and dorsiflexion.[41] Subtalar dislocation occurs during ankle hyperplantarflexion, external rotation, and slight inversion, such as during a grand plié en pointe or landing in demi-pointe from a jump.[41] The most common overuse injuries of the foot are stress fractures. Stress fracture of the second

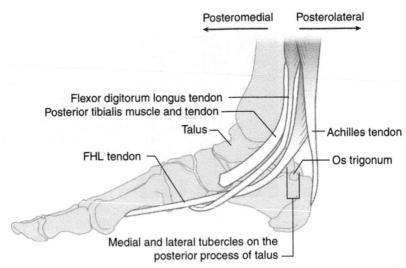

Posteromedial → ← Posterolateral →

Flexor digitorum longus tendon
Posterior tibialis muscle and tendon
Talus
FHL tendon

Achilles tendon
Os trigonum

Medial and lateral tubercles on the
posterior process of talus

Fig. 5. Posteromedial view of the ankle, with locations of the most common causes of posterior ankle impingement labeled, including os trigonum, FHL tendon, and Achilles tendon. (*From* Motta-Valencia K. Dance-related injury. Phys Med Rehabil Clin North Am. 2006;17(3):697-723; with permission.)

metatarsal is the most common stress fracture in ballet dancers.[41] Navicular stress fractures are also seen. Plantar fasciitis is usually caused by repetitive grand plié or relevé, abnormal pronation, and tight gastrocnemius-soleus/Achilles complex.[63,64] It can also occur with cavus foot caused by altered shock absorption.

Great toe Common injuries include hallux rigidus, hallux valgus, and bunions, especially from dancing en pointe.[63,65] Hallux saltans may develop in FHL tendinitis.[63] Subungual hematoma is common in pointe dancers.[63,65] Sesamoid injuries include stress fractures and sesamoiditis, with the medial sesamoid most commonly injured.[63]

Treatment and rehabilitation
Protocols for evaluation and treatment of each injury are beyond the scope of this article. However, evaluation should be comprehensive, including evaluation of problematic movements, technique, muscle strength imbalances, and environmental factors. Complete rest from dance may not be realistic or necessary, because injuries often improve with alterations in technique, degree, speed, or style of movements.[64] Rehabilitation protocols mimicking/enhancing dance exercises in a pool or with resistance bands, for example, are likely to be well received.[64] When considering return to dance, specific technique requirements must be considered in addition to the injury itself. Although much of the research available pertains to ballet and contemporary dancers, this information can reasonably be extrapolated to other techniques. Most dance forms require a certain amount of flexibility, all require precise motor control, and, for mastery, all require extensive training. Because flexibility is required for success with many dance styles, it is common to find that dancers have some hypermobility. Understanding of hypermobility helps clinicians be better able to guide the patients through recovery. Educating patients about hypermobility in general is important, as is discussing that related decreased proprioception[66] may slow recovery. This information may help to alleviate some of the negative stress associated with absence from dance.[66]

Box 1
Rehabilitation progression following generalized dance injury

Phase 1: early phase, acute injury, or early postoperative

Goals: reduce pain
  Reduce swelling
  Activity modification

Use of modalities as needed for pain

Use of bracing, taping, protective padding as needed to restrict range of motion, minimize swelling, provide support

Range of motion to other joints as appropriate

Cross-training when appropriate to maintain endurance

Therapeutic exercise for joints distant to the injury as appropriate

In phase 1, floor barre or pool activity may be appropriate

Phase 2: moderate restriction, protected movement

Goals: continue to manage pain and swelling
  Start to return to modified class

Continue with floor barre if instituted

Begin return to barre in class, limiting specific positions or activities as needed depending on the nature of the injury; that is, for foot/ankle injuries, start without releve; for hip injuries, only allow tendu initially; for back injuries, limit the overall motion in cambre

For most lower extremity injuries, it may be best to limit the dancer to first and second positions only initially

For most lower extremity injuries, initially allow only demi plie

Continue to work on cross-training as able for cardiovascular endurance

Work on balance and proprioception bilaterally then unilaterally (balance board, foam) on flat foot

Phase 3: minimal restriction, progression of movement

Goals: progress to center work
  Increase endurance

Progress positions allowed at barre (third, fourth, fifth)

Progress to grande plie if not already performing

Increase height of leg to degage, grand battements as appropriate

Progress to center: initially with adagio and petit allegro (the topple test and airplane test can help determine readiness)

Consider increasing cross-training for improved cardiovascular endurance

Phase 4: progression to full center, pointe, partnering

Goals: return to pain-free dance

Progress work in center to include higher jumps (grand allegro) (the saute test can help determine readiness)

Progress to partnering work when appropriate

Return to preinjury cross-training if an alternative was instituted because of injury

For each step in the return-to-dance progression, the dancer should show pain-free, dance-specific skills with proper biomechanics before receiving clearance to perform those skills in the classroom.

For injuries with established rehabilitation protocols, those should be followed with modifications made to include dance-specific activities when appropriate. When managing other common injuries, conservative approaches typically start with restricting movement and activity and slowly adding these back as the athlete heals. Especially with hypermobility, initially it is important to help the dancer strengthen within a protected range of motion and ultimately to develop strength for the end ranges of motion that they will need. Because there are few written objective criteria for return to dance,[67] it is invaluable to have clinicians with working knowledge of the demands of different dance styles. Improper or poor technique can often be the ultimate cause of injury[67]; therefore, assessment of technique by a trained clinician or therapist before return to class and performance is important. **Box 1** provides a general rehabilitation management template that can be applied to many types of dance injuries. At present, return to sport following knee surgery shows a trend where progression to the next phase of rehabilitation is patient specific and based on achievement of certain functional tests rather than being solely time based.[68] This approach can be applied to the dancer; following completion of any weight-bearing restrictions, the patient is expected to progress based on functional achievement. One case report following rehabilitation after os trigonum excision detailed return-to-dance tests being used to establish appropriate return-to-class progression (**Box 2**[66] and **Fig. 6**).

Injury prevention

Dance and music are art forms that require the ability to perform complex sequences of movement, sometimes in extreme ranges of motion. It is vital to have solid technique for both injury prevention and pleasing performance.[69] Performing arts injuries are frequently chronic, associated with years of training many hours per week, resulting in overuse and microtrauma.[70–73] Cross-training is an important aspect of injury prevention to allow the body to balance some of the effects of these microtraumas. Performing artists may cross-train to improve specific aspects of their technique, such as plyometric training, aerobic exercise, and fine motor control. Musicians, particularly those working in an asymmetrical posture, should cross-train to balance their overall posture and support systems. Both musicians and dancers must show significant control, so working on core stability and local stabilization is

---

Box 2
Return-to-dance tests

Pencil test: while in long sitting, the dancer performs maximal plantarflexion. A straight edge is placed along the top of the dorsal talar neck; if it clears the most distal part of the tibia, it is considered a pass, meaning the dancer has enough plantarflexion for pointe work.

Airplane test: the dancer stands on 1 leg with the trunk and nonsupporting leg extended parallel to the ground. The dancer then performs 5 controlled single-leg squats with the arms reaching for the ground. A pass is indicated by completion of 4 successful repetitions.

Topple test: the dancer performs a pirouette. A pass is indicated when it is performed successfully with the standing leg in full knee extension; the gesture leg is in full, correct passe position; the trunk remains vertical; and the dancer is able to control the deceleration and descent from the pirouette.

Single-leg saute test: the dancer performs 16 consecutive single-leg jumps. A pass is when at least 8 are completed with a neutral pelvis, upright and stable trunk, proper alignment of the lower extremity, and proper heel-toe landing.

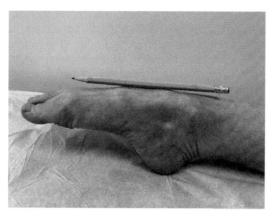

Fig. 6. Pencil test.

important. It is also recommended that performing artists cross-train with aerobic exercise.

Dancers often stretch as part of their preclass warmup to help them achieve flexibility and prevent compensations that may lead to injury. However, studies of the effects of static stretching on power have shown a decrease in strength performance following static stretching.[74] Extrapolating this information to performing artists in general, the artists might put themselves at a relative risk for injury caused by muscle inhibition if they are going into class, rehearsal, or performance having just spent a significant time stretching. At the Australian Ballet, dancers are no longer encouraged to maintain static stretch positions but are encouraged to work on eccentric strengthening, allowing them to achieve improved control at end ranges.[75] Performing artists may use myofascial tools to address tissue flexibility. Static stretches may be useful when executed separately from performance.

Pilates has been used by dancers as a method for cross-training for many years. The Pilates method is a technique focused on initiating movement from a central core of stability.[69,76–79] The exercises have goals of control, flexibility, mind-body awareness, and strength.[78] There are many variations of Pilates, some of which incorporate tenets from physical therapy and biomechanics to modify exercises for use with injury.[78] One study of Pilates mat work and apparatus training in young female dancers showed improvements in posture, flexibility in the ITB and hamstrings, and improved abdominal muscle strength.[69] Thus, Pilates may be a good technique to include for cross-training to help with general injury prevention in performing artists.

MEDICAL CONCERNS AND TREATMENT
Vocalists and Musicians

Singing requires synergy of many body systems for proper functioning.[80] Many factors, such as overuse, singing out of the comfortable range (tessitura), improper vocal technique, venue acoustics and allergens, performance anxiety, travel, respiratory illness, medication use, and substance abuse, may affect the voice. The otolaryngologist and speech pathologist are important members of the team for proper diagnosis and treatment for rapid return to performance. Professional musicians are at high risk of developing noise-induced hearing loss caused by chronic exposure to loud sounds. Musicians and vocalists also experience similar stressors to athletes, leading to risk of depression, anxiety, and substance abuse.

Voice

Essential tremor is the most common vocal action tremor and is present in both phonation and nonphonation, whereas dystonic tremor does not occur in nonphonation.[81] Treatment of dystonic tremor involves botulinum toxin injections into the thyroarytenoid and interarytenoid muscles.[81] Essential tremor does not respond well to botulinum toxin injections, but there may be mild benefit with oral propranolol, although the responses are not as robust as those seen in treatment of essential tremor of the extremities.

Laryngopharyngeal reflux (LPR), or silent reflux, occurs because of reflux of gastric contents (pepsin, bile salts, trypsin, proteins) onto the laryngeal mucosa. The refluxed chemicals reduce mucosal thickness, and also cause inflammation, vocal fold dehydration, and increased risk of epithelial injury, leading to benign vocal fold lesions.[82] Singers are at high risk for LPR because of higher intra-abdominal pressure, stress, and frequently poor nutrition. LPR presents with dysphonia, cough, vocal fatigue, and throat clearing and can progress to greater vocal limitations. Efficacy of treatment with proton pump inhibitors varies widely, from 18% to 87%.[83] Other treatment options include H2 blockers, alginate, prokinetics,[83] and the less well-studied combination of oral hyaluronic acid and chondroitin sulfate.[84]

Traumatic vocal fold lesions caused by vocal overuse are composed of mucus stranding, nodules, polyps, hematomas, cysts, and contact hyperplasia. These lesions result in mucosal thickening, hyperkeratosis, and fusiform swelling.[85] Vocal nodules develop after prolonged misuse of the voice and present with bilateral asymmetric intraepithelial thickening, whereas polyps are inflammatory unilateral growths characterized by hemorrhages and may limit glottal closure, prolong the open phase of vibratory cycles, and cause asynchronous and asymmetric vibratory movements. Acute vocal overuse can also cause vocal cord hematoma. Treatment of vocal lesions involves voice therapy/reeducation to eliminate the source of the lesion, steroids in acute cases, and phonomicrosurgery with lesion excision.[85,86] Complete voice rest is required after surgery for 2 to 3 weeks with progression through voice therapy and return to singing by week 4 to 5.[87] Most singers are able to return to prior or an enhanced level of performance after surgical treatment.[88]

The most common cause of dysphonia in singers is laryngitis, often associated with voice fatigue or viral and bacterial organisms associated with a respiratory illness. Chronic laryngitis is associated with smoking, chronic tonsillitis, asthma, and gastroesophageal reflux disease.[89] Treatment of laryngitis requires treatment of the underlying source with antacids, antibiotics, smoking cessation, and so forth.

Hearing

Noise-induced hearing loss (NIHL) is a sensorineural disorder affecting the cochlear hair cells in the inner ear.[90] The higher frequencies (3000–6000 Hz) are preferentially affected, with greater prevalence among pop/rock musicians than classical musicians. The most common auditory symptom is tinnitus, described as ringing in the ears without external auditory stimulus, and has prevalence as high as 35% to 77% in those with NIHL.[90] Tinnitus has been associated with higher rates of depression among rock musicians.[90,91] Hyperacusis (decreased tolerance to noises of average intensity and painful sensitivity to usual environmental sounds) is more common among pop/rock musicians, whereas diplacusis (a hearing abnormality in which the same tone is perceived as a different pitch in each ear) is more prevalent in classical musicians.[90] Risks for NIHL include higher-intensity and higher-frequency sounds without proper ear protection. Musicians that regularly use hearing protection have a statistically significant lower mean hearing threshold than those that did not wear protection.[92] With daily exposure to sound levels greater than 85 dB over 8 hours, hearing loss progresses rapidly during the first few years of exposure.[33] Pop/rock musicians are exposed to an average of 103 dB versus 94 dB for classical musicians, correlating with the higher prevalence of NIHL in pop/rock music. The level of exposure is highly variable among musicians but there is a dose-response effect with weekly hours having a greater effect compared with years playing.[93,94] In addition to protective equipment, strict regulations on time and quantity of noise exposure are imperative because these symptoms can be career ending.[90]

Psychology

Unhealthy eating in musicians is precipitated by depression and anxiety, stress, unpredictable schedules, low income, and frequent travel. The self-reported lifetime prevalence of disordered eating/eating disorder (ED) in musicians is as high as 32.3%.[95] Auxiliary members, including color guard, majorettes, and dancers, are also at high risk of ED, amenorrhea, and body dysmorphia because of demanding performance schedules, high fitness requirements, revealing uniforms, and societal pressures, with a prevalence of 29.7% in division I auxiliary members.[96]

Music performance anxiety (MPA) is a social anxiety experienced by musicians manifesting as tachycardia, hypertension, vocal tremor, abdominal pain, dry mouth, chest pain, shortness of breath, and sweating, among many other symptoms.[97] The cause is multifactorial because of hyperactivity of the sympathetic nervous system with release of adrenaline as well as cognitive influences of inherent perfectionism, fear of failure, catastrophizing, poor coping skills, and self-doubt.[98] The condition may be debilitating and lead to performance avoidance and early retirement. Prevalence is estimated at 15% to 25%,[97] and it is more common in women and younger musicians, although some studies have quoted much higher estimates.[99–101] Many treatments have been recommended for MPA, including β-blockers, mindfulness and meditation, cognitive behavior therapy, hypnosis, music therapy, psychotherapy, yoga, relaxation, deep breathing, and biofeedback/neurofeedback therapy, all with variable efficacy.[98,101]

High stress and excessive travel by musicians can lead to an unhealthy lifestyle and substance abuse, resulting in a shortened life expectancy.[102] Compared with the general US population, musicians were found to have 2 times higher mortality, greatest in the mid–20-year age group, with reduced rates thereafter. Suicide and liver-related disease secondary to substance abuse were more common in country, metal, and rock musicians, whereas homicides were more common in hip hop and rap musicians.[103] Therefore, it is important to thoroughly address all aspects of the performer's mental health, especially after an injury or setback.

Dancers

Involvement in sports with an emphasis on aesthetics, such as dance, gymnastics, figure skating, and running, creates an increased risk for ED. Often, EDs are associated with preexisting depression and anxiety as well as an immense pressure to stay lean. Substance abuse and misuse is also high to help cope with stress and weight loss.[104] These unhealthy behaviors place dancers at greater risk for injury because of impaired energy stores, menstrual dysfunction, and low bone density, resulting in female athlete triad (FAT) or relative energy deficiency in sport (RED-S).[105]

Psychology

Substance use is prevalent among professional ballet dancers. A study of female Croatian ballet dancers found that 25% smoke cigarettes on a daily basis, 90% use analgesics, 35% use illicit drugs, and 26% binge drink at least once per month.[104] Alcohol consumption was higher among dancers who used analgesics as well as those who had a history of disordered eating.

In dancers, the estimated point prevalence of ED is 15%, with a lifetime prevalence of 50% to 80%.[106–108] FAT and RED-S involve low energy availability often resulting from disordered eating, menstrual dysfunction, and low bone mineral density. More than 95% of total bone mineral density in women is acquired by the age of 18 years, with more than 50% gained during adolescence (age 11–14 years).[109] Secondary amenorrhea occurs because of inhibition of the hypothalamic axis in a low energy state, leading to low estrogen levels. RED-S increases the risk of stress fractures and soft tissue/tendon injuries because of impaired healing capabilities. The Low Energy Availability in Females–Questionnaire (LEAF-Q) was developed to identify female athletes at risk for FAT and has a sensitivity of 78% and specificity of 90% in female dancers and endurance athletes. It is a brief and easy-to-administer 25-item self-reported symptom questionnaire that may be considered for use to detect early FAT.[110]

One-third of elite ballet dancers were found to have low bone mineral density (Z score < −1.0) with values lowest in the arm and highest in the leg because of the osteogenic effect of bone loading sites.[111] Of these dancers, 39% had oligomenorrhea.[112] Given the high risk of FAT on athlete health, it is extremely important to screen for this disorder in any athlete with concern for fatigue, chronic or frequent injuries, weight loss, or menstrual dysfunction. After completion of laboratory work and dual energy x-ray absorptiometry scan, as indicated, the athlete may be referred to a nutritionist for guidance on improving energy availability. Reversal of menstrual irregularities and increase in bone mineral density lag behind improvements in energy availability and hormonal axis.[105,112] Referral to endocrinology may also be considered in complex cases.

RECOMMENDATIONS FOR CARE PROVIDERS

When providing medical care for performers, it is ideal to recommend strategies that allow them, whenever possible, to keep performing. Ideally, care providers should have an understanding of the artist's specific genre/style of performance. If unfamiliar, watching brief online videos of the performer, or the genre in general, can be enlightening. National organizations for performing arts medicine can be a good resource for physician education/assistance (**Box 3**). Providers should consider speaking with the performer's teacher/choreographer/director to discuss accommodations, just as team doctors speak with athletic trainers or coaches in traditional sports. If there is no feasible way of accommodating continued performance, it is important to have the artist watch rehearsal for mental health reasons, to prevent feelings of isolation or depression related to removal from the social aspects of the art. Also, research has shown that watching class is beneficial in assisting the brain in recall by stimulating neurons as they transition back into active participation.[113–115]

Continuing medical education (CME) specific to performing arts enhances providers' ability to care for this unique population. Unlike many organized sports, performers generally do not get screened before performing. The DIVA (dancer, instrumentalist, vocalist, and actor) screen is a preparticipation screening examination that was developed by the Performing Arts Medical Association (PAMA). It is designed to include various sections that are relevant to specific performing artists. Certification in this screening technique is offered at PAMA and American College of Sports Medicine (ACSM) conferences.

Box 3
Performing arts organizations

- Artists' Health Alliance
- The Actors Fund
- Association for Applied Sport Psychology
- Athletes and the Arts
- Dancers Alliance
- Dance/USA Task Force on Dancer Health
- Doctors for Dancers
- Drum Corps International
- Harkness Center for Dance Injuries
- Health Promotion in Schools of Music
- Healthcare for Artists
- International Association for Dance Medicine and Science
- MusiCares
- Music Teachers National Association
- National Association of Schools of Music
- National Association of Teachers of Singing
- National Hearing Conservation Association
- National Dance Education Organization
- New Orleans Musician's Clinic
- Performing Arts Medicine Association
- The Screen Actors Guild
- SHAPE America
- Trinity Laban Health
- The Voice Foundation

To promote themselves among performing artists, providers should consider providing community educational presentations at local studios about injury prevention, treatment, or other related topics. Another strategy is to cultivate and share a list of local resources, including medical doctors, physical therapists, physicians' assistants, chiropractors, nurse practitioners, psychologists, and nutritionists with an interest/knowledge in treating performers. Because many performers have limited access to care for financial reasons, clinicians may consider partnering with a local free or low-cost clinic on an intermittent basis and advising communities when/where performing arts medicine services will be available.

Clinics Care Points

- Music therapy has proved itself a viable, evidence-based modality for neurorehabilitation.
- Musicians localize pain to neck/spine, shoulders, and hands/wrists, mostly because of postural/ergonomic disorders and overuse.

- Dance injuries are highest during the opening months of a season, are most common in the foot/ankle, and are experienced by up to 95% of the population within professional companies.
- Psychological stress of performing and touring can create specific physical and mental health risks for performers.
- The LEAF-Q is a highly sensitive and specific screening questionnaire for use in performing artists with concern for fatigue, chronic/frequent injuries, weight loss, or menstrual dysfunction.
- Whenever possible, use of preperformance screenings, injury prevention techniques, and access to performing arts–trained clinicians optimizes health and wellness in this community.

DISCLOSURE

J. Currey, D. Sheng, A. Neph, C. Cinquini, J. Cuza: none. B.L. Waite, consultant with Level42AI.

REFERENCES

1. Shah S, Weiss DS, Burchette RJ. Injuries in professional modern dancers: incidence, risk factors, and management. J Dance Med Sci 2012;16(1):17–25.
2. Thaut M, McIntosh G. How music helps to heal the injured brain: therapeutic use crescendos thanks to advances in brain science. New York: Dana Foundation; 2010. Available at: https://dana.org/article/how-music-helps-to-heal-the-injured-brain/. Accessed April 27, 2020.
3. de l'Etoile SK. Processes of Music Therapy: Clinical and Scientific Rationales and Models. In: Hallam S, Cross I, Thaut M, editors. The Oxford Handbook of Music Psychology. 2nd edition. Oxford: Oxford University Press; 2016. p. 805–18.
4. Maess B, Koelsch S, Gunter TC, et al. Musical syntax is processed in Broca's area: an MEG study. Nat Neurosci 2001;4(5):540–5.
5. Pascual-Leone A. The brain that plays music and is changed by it. Ann N Y Acad Sci 2001;930:315–29.
6. Thaut MH, McIntosh GC, Hoemberg V. Neurobiological foundations of neurologic music therapy: rhythmic entrainment and the motor system. Front Psychol 2014;5:1185.
7. Thaut MH, McIntosh GC, Prassas SG, et al. Effect of rhythmic auditory cuing on temporal stride parameters and EMG. patterns in hemiparetic gait of stroke patients. Neurorehabil Neural Repair 1993;7(1):9–16.
8. Thaut MH, Leins AK, Rice RR, et al. Rhythmic auditory stimulation improves gait more than NDT/Bobath training in near-ambulatory patients early poststroke: a single-blind, randomized trial. Neurorehabil Neural Repair 2007;21(5):455–9.
9. Malcolm MP, Massie C, Thaut M. Rhythmic auditory-motor entrainment improves hemiparetic arm kinematics during reaching movements: a pilot study. Top Stroke Rehabil 2009;16(1):69–79.
10. Thaut MH, McIntosh GC, Rice RR, et al. Rhythmic auditory stimulation in gait training for Parkinson's disease patients. Mov Disord 1996;11(2):193–200.
11. McIntosh GC, Brown SH, Rice RR, et al. Rhythmic auditory-motor facilitation of gait patterns in patients with Parkinson's disease. J Neurol Neurosurg Psychiatry 1997;62(1):22–6.

12. Thaut MH, Rice RR, Braun Janzen T, et al. Rhythmic auditory stimulation for reduction of falls in Parkinson's disease: a randomized controlled study. Clin Rehabil 2019;33(1):34–43.

13. Keith RL, Aronson AE. Singing as therapy for apraxia of speech and aphasia: report of a case. Brain Lang 1975;2(4):483–8.

14. Belin P, Van Eeckhout P, Zilbovicius M, et al. Recovery from nonfluent aphasia after melodic intonation therapy: a PET study. Neurology 1996;47(6):1504–11.

15. Schlaug G, Norton A, Marchina S, et al. From singing to speaking: facilitating recovery from nonfluent aphasia. Future Neurol 2010;5(5):657–65.

16. Schlaug G, Marchina S, Norton A. Evidence for plasticity in white-matter tracts of patients with chronic Broca's aphasia undergoing intense intonation-based speech therapy. Ann N Y Acad Sci 2009;1169:385–94.

17. Glasser MF, Rilling JK. DTI tractography of the human brain's language pathways. Cereb Cortex 2008;18(11):2471–82.

18. Thaut MH, Peterson DA, McIntosh GC. Temporal entrainment of cognitive functions: musical mnemonics induce brain plasticity and oscillatory synchrony in neural networks underlying memory. Ann N Y Acad Sci 2005;1060:243–54.

19. Rainey DW, Larsen JD. The effect of familiar melodies on initial learning and long-term memory for unconnected text. Music Percept 2002;20(2):173–86.

20. Evers S, Suhr B. Changes of the neurotransmitter serotonin but not of hormones during short time music perception. Eur Arch Psychiatry Clin Neurosci 2000; 250(3):144–7.

21. Ericsson KA, Krampe RT, Tesch-Romer C. The role of deliberate practice in the acquisition of expert performance. Psychol Rev 1993;100(3):363–406.

22. Elbaum L. Musculoskeletal problems of instrumental musicians*. J Orthop Sports Phys Ther 1986;8(6):285–97.

23. Zaza C. Playing-related musculoskeletal disorders in musicians: a systematic review of incidence and prevalence. Can Med Assoc J 1998;158(8):1019–25.

24. Bejjani FJ, Kaye GM, Benham M. Musculoskeletal and neuromuscular conditions of instrumental musicians. Arch Phys Med Rehabil 1996;77(4):406–13.

25. Barczyk-Pawelec K, Sipko T, Demczuk-Włodarczyk E, et al. Anterioposterior spinal curvatures and magnitude of asymmetry in the trunk in musicians playing the violin compared with nonmusicians. J Manipulative Physiol Ther 2012;35(4): 319–26.

26. Kok LM, Nelissen RGHH, Huisstede BMA. Prevalence and consequences of arm, neck, and/or shoulder complaints among music academy students: a comparative study. Med Probl Perform Art 2015;30(3):163–8.

27. Sousa CM, Machado JP, Greten HJ, et al. Occupational diseases of professional orchestra musicians from Northern Portugal: a descriptive study. Med Probl Perform Art 2016;31(1):8–12.

28. Kok LM, Vlieland TPMV, Fiocco M, et al. A comparative study on the prevalence of musculoskeletal complaints among musicians and non-musicians. BMC Musculoskelet Disord 2013;14:9.

29. Kok LM, Groenewegen KA, Huisstede BMA, et al. The high prevalence of playing-related musculoskeletal disorders (PRMDs) and its associated factors in amateur musicians playing in student orchestras: a cross-sectional study. PLoS One 2018;13(2):e0191772.

30. Brandfonbrener AG. Musculoskeletal problems of instrumental musicians. Hand Clin 2003;19(2):231–9, v.

31. Hoppmann RA, Patrone NA. A review of musculoskeletal problems in instrumental musicians. Semin Arthritis Rheum 1989;19(2):117–26.

32. Altenmüller E, Ioannou CI, Lee A. Apollo's curse: neurological causes of motor impairments in musicians. Prog Brain Res 2015;217:89–106.

33. Dick RW, Berning JR, Dawson W, et al. Athletes and the arts–the role of sports medicine in the performing arts. Curr Sports Med Rep 2013;12(6):397–403.

34. Berque P, Gray H, McFadyen A. A combination of constraint-induced therapy and motor control retraining in the treatment of focal hand dystonia in musicians: a long-term follow-up study. Med Probl Perform Art 2013;28(1):33–46.

35. Enke AM, Poskey GA. Neuromuscular re-education programs for musicians with focal hand dystonia: a systematic review. Med Probl Perform Art 2018;33(2):137–45.

36. Tubiana R. Prolonged neuromuscular rehabilitation for musician's focal dystonia. Med Probl Perform Art 2003;18(4):166–9.

37. Jepsen JR. Posterior interosseous neuropathy in the distal radial tunnel in a contrabassoon musician. Med Probl Perform Art 2014;29(1):23–6.

38. Panush RS. Occupational and recreational musculoskeletal disorders. In: Firestein GS, Budd RC, Gabriel SE, et al, editors. Kelley and Firestein's Textbook of Rheumatology. Vol 1. 10th ed. Philadelphia: Elsevier; 2017. p. 520–32.

39. Storms PR, Elkins CP, Strohecker EM. Embouchure dysfunction in air force band brass musicians. Med Probl Perform Art 2016;31(2):110–6.

40. Lai K-Y, Wu S-K, Jou I-M, et al. Effects of hand span size and right-left hand side on the piano playing performances: exploration of the potential risk factors with regard to piano-related musculoskeletal disorders. Int J Ind Ergon 2015;50:97–104.

41. Motta-Valencia K. Dance-related injury. Phys Med Rehabil Clin N Am 2006;17(3):697–723.

42. Liederbach M. General considerations for guiding dance injury rehabilitation. J Dance Med Sci 2000;4(2):54–65.

43. Byhring S, Bø K. Musculoskeletal injuries in the Norwegian National Ballet: a prospective cohort study. Scand J Med Sci Sports 2002;12(6):365–70.

44. Fuller M, Moyle GM, Hunt AP, et al. Ballet and contemporary dance injuries when transitioning to full-time training or professional level dance: a systematic review. J Dance Med Sci 2019;23(3):112–25.

45. Luke A, Micheli LJ. Management of injuries in the young dancer. J Dance Med Sci 2000;4(1):6–15.

46. Jubb C, Bell L, Cimelli S, et al. Injury patterns in hip hop dancers. J Dance Med Sci 2019;23(4):145–9.

47. Ursej E, Sekulic D, Prus D, et al. Investigating the prevalence and predictors of injury occurrence in competitive hip hop dancers: prospective analysis. Int J Environ Res Public Health 2019;16(17). https://doi.org/10.3390/ijerph16173214.

48. Washington EL. Musculoskeletal injuries in theatrical dancers: site frequency, and severity. Am J Sports Med 1978;6(2):75–98.

49. Jenkinson DM, Bolin DJ. Knee overuse injuries in dance. J Dance Med Sci 2001;2(1):2–10.

50. Revere GD, Webb LX, Gristina AG, et al. Musculoskeletal injuries in theatrical dance students. Am J Sports Med 1983;11(4):195–8.

51. McCabe TR, Wyon M, Ambegaonkar JP, et al. A bibliographic review of medicine and science research in dancesport. Med Probl Perform Art 2013;28(2):70–9.

52. Pederson ME, Wilmerding V. Injury profiles of student and professional flamenco dancers. J Dance Med Sci 1998;2(3):108–14.

53. Milner SC, Gray A, Bussey M. A retrospective study investigating injury incidence and factors associated with injury among belly dancers. J Dance Med Sci 2019;23(1):26–33.

54. Evans RW, Evans RI, Carvajal S, et al. A survey of injuries among Broadway performers. Am J Public Health 1996;86(1):77–80.

55. Kern-Scott R, Peterson JR, Morgan P. Review of acetabular labral tears in dancers. J Dance Med Sci 2011;15(4):149–56.

56. Merckaert S, Zambelli P-Y. Acetabular labral tear secondary to repeated lateral "grand écart" split exercises in an adolescent ballet dancer: case report and review of the literature. J Dance Med Sci 2019;23(3):126–32.

57. DeMann LE. Sacroiliac dysfunction in dancers with low back pain. Man Ther 1997;2(1):2–10.

58. Scioscia TN, Giffin JR. Knee ligament and meniscal injuries in dancers. J Dance Med Sci 2001;5(1):11–5.

59. Teitz CC. Hip and knee injuries in dancers. J Dance Med Sci 2000;4(1):23–9.

60. Bolin DJ. Evaluation and management of stress fractures in dancers. J Dance Med Sci 2001;5(2):37–42.

61. Howse J. Dance Technique and Injury Prevention. In: Howse J, McCormack M, editors. 3rd edition. New York: Routledge; 2000. https://doi.org/10.4324/9780203826119.

62. Yasui Y, Hannon CP, Hurley E, et al. Posterior ankle impingement syndrome: a systematic four-stage approach. World J Orthop 2016;7(10):657–63.

63. Conti SF, Wong YS. Foot and ankle injuries in the dancer. J Dance Med Sci 2001; 5(2):43–50.

64. Grossman G, Wilmerding V. Dance physical therapy for the leg and foot: plantar fasciitis and achilles tendinopathy. J Dance Med Sci 2000;4(2):66–72.

65. Tuckman AS, Werner FW, Bayley JC. Analysis of the forefoot on pointe in the ballet dancer. Foot Ankle 1991;12(3):144–8.

66. Filipa A, Barton K. Physical therapy rehabilitation of an adolescent preprofessional dancer following os trigonum excision: a case report. J Orthop Sports Phys Ther 2018;48(3):194–203.

67. Vosseller JT, Dennis ER, Bronner S. Ankle injuries in dancers. J Am Acad Orthop Surg 2019;27(16):582–9.

68. Sherman SL, DiPaolo ZJ, Ray TE, et al. Meniscus injuries: a review of rehabilitation and return to play. Clin Sports Med 2020;39(1):165–83.

69. Ahearn EL, Greene A, Lasner A. Some effects of supplemental pilates training on the posture, strength, and flexibility of dancers 17 to 22 years of age. J Dance Med Sci 2018;22(4):192–202.

70. Gamboa JM, Roberts LA, Maring J, et al. Injury patterns in elite preprofessional ballet dancers and the utility of screening programs to identify risk characteristics. J Orthop Sports Phys Ther 2008;38(3):126–36.

71. Smith TO, Davies L, de Medici A, et al. Prevalence and profile of musculoskeletal injuries in ballet dancers: a systematic review and meta-analysis. Phys Ther Sport 2016;19:50–6.

72. Costa MSS, Ferreira AS, Orsini M, et al. Characteristics and prevalence of musculoskeletal injury in professional and non-professional ballet dancers. Braz J Phys Ther 2016;20(2):166–75.

73. Rickman AM, Ambegaonkar JP, Cortes N. Core stability: implications for dance injuries. Med Probl Perform Art 2012;27(3):159–64.

74. Lima CD, Brown LE, Ruas CV, et al. Effects of static versus ballistic stretching on hamstring:quadriceps strength ratio and jump performance in ballet dancers and resistance trained women. J Dance Med Sci 2018;22(3):160–7.

75. Pilcher LB. Why The Australian Ballet dancers quit stretching. Dance Informa. Available at: https://dancemagazine.com.au/2019/09/why-the-australian-ballet-dancers-quit-stretching/. Accessed February 27, 2020.

76. Armstrong C, Bergeron CS, Boucher T. Effectiveness of Pilates training vs dance-based plyometric training on dancers' vertical and horizontal jump. Natl Dance Soc J 2018;3(1):37–44.

77. Bernardo LM, Nagle EF. Does Pilates training benefit dancers? An appraisal of Pilates research literature. J Dance Med Sci 2006;10(1&2):46–50.

78. Bergeron CS, Greenwood M, Smith T, et al. Pilates training for dancers: a systemic review. Natl Dance Soc J 2017;2(1):66–77.

79. Stolze LR, Allison SC, Childs JD. Derivation of a preliminary clinical prediction rule for identifying a subgroup of patients with low back pain likely to benefit from Pilates-based exercise. J Orthop Sports Phys Ther 2012;42(5):425–36.

80. Bird HA. Performing arts medicine in clinical practice. Cham (Switzerland): Springer International Publishing; 2016. https://doi.org/10.1007/978-3-319-12427-8.

81. Guglielmino G, Moraes BT de, Villanova LC, et al. Comparison of botulinum toxin and propranolol for essential and dystonic vocal tremors. Clinics (Sao Paulo) 2018;73:e87.

82. Lechien JR, Schindler A, Robotti C, et al. Laryngopharyngeal reflux disease in singers: pathophysiology, clinical findings and perspectives of a new patient-reported outcome instrument. Eur Ann Otorhinolaryngol Head Neck Dis 2019; 136(3S):S39–43.

83. Martinucci I, de Bortoli N, Savarino E, et al. Optimal treatment of laryngopharyngeal reflux disease. Ther Adv Chronic Dis 2013;4(6):287–301.

84. Chmielecka-Rutkowska J, Tomasik B, Pietruszewska W. The role of oral formulation of hyaluronic acid and chondroitin sulphate for the treatment of the patients with laryngopharyngeal reflux. Otolaryngol Pol 2019;73(6):38–49.

85. Milutinović Z, Bojić P. Functional trauma of the vocal folds: classification and management strategies. Folia Phoniatr Logop 1996;48(2):78–85.

86. Ropero Rendón MDM, Ermakova T, Freymann M-L, et al. Efficacy of phonosurgery, logopedic voice treatment and vocal pedagogy in common voice problems of singers. Adv Ther 2018;35(7):1069–86.

87. Zeitels SM. The art and craft of Phonomicrosurgery in Grammy award-winning elite performers. Ann Otol Rhinol Laryngol 2019;128(3_suppl):7S–24S.

88. Bastian RW. Vocal fold microsurgery in singers. J Voice 1996;10(4):389–404.

89. Stepanova YE, Konoplev OI, Gotovyakhina TV, et al. Acute and chronic laryngitis in the subjects engaged in the voice and speech professions. Vestn Otorinolaringol 2019;84(1):68–71 [in Russian].

90. Di Stadio A, Dipietro L, Ricci G, et al. Hearing loss, tinnitus, hyperacusis, and diplacusis in professional musicians: a systematic review. Int J Environ Res Public Health 2018;15(10). https://doi.org/10.3390/ijerph15102120.

91. Stormer CCL, Sorlie T, Stenklev NC. Tinnitus, anxiety, depression and substance abuse in rock musicians a norwegian survey. Int Tinnitus J 2017;21(1):50–7.

92. Schmuziger N, Patscheke J, Probst R. Hearing in nonprofessional pop/rock musicians. Ear Hear 2006;27(4):321–30.

93. Pouryaghoub G, Mehrdad R, Pourhosein S. Noise-Induced hearing loss among professional musicians. J Occup Health 2017;59(1):33–7.

94. Halevi-Katz DN, Yaakobi E, Putter-Katz H. Exposure to music and noise-induced hearing loss (NIHL) among professional pop/rock/jazz musicians. Noise Health 2015;17(76):158–64.

95. Kapsetaki ME, Easmon C. Eating disorders in musicians: a survey investigating self-reported eating disorders of musicians. Eat Weight Disord 2019;24(3): 541–9.

96. Torres-McGehee TM, Green JM, Leeper JD, et al. Body image, anthropometric measures, and eating-disorder prevalence in auxiliary unit members. J Athl Train 2009;44(4):418–26.

97. Spahn C. Diagnosis and therapy of performance anxiety. MMW Fortschr Med 2011;153(43):46–8 [in German].

98. Spahn C. Treatment and prevention of music performance anxiety. Prog Brain Res 2015;217:129–40.

99. van Kemenade JF, van Son MJ, van Heesch NC. Performance anxiety among professional musicians in symphonic orchestras: a self-report study. Psychol Rep 1995;77(2):555–62.

100. Medeiros Barbar AE. Kenny music performance anxiety inventory (KMPAI): transcultural adaptation for brazil and study of internal consistency. J Depress Anxiety 2014;03(04). https://doi.org/10.4172/2167-1044.1000167.

101. Nedelcut S, Leucuta D-C, Dumitrascu DL. Lifestyle and psychosocial factors in musicians. Clujul Med 2018;91(3):312–6.

102. Patalano F. Psychosocial stressors and the short life spans of legendary jazz musicians. Percept Mot Skills 2000;90(2):435–6.

103. Kenny DT, Asher A. Life expectancy and cause of death in popular musicians: is the popular musician lifestyle the road to ruin? Med Probl Perform Art 2016;31(1):37–44.

104. Wyon MA, Hutchings KM, Wells A, et al. Body mass index, nutritional knowledge, and eating behaviors in elite student and professional ballet dancers. Clin J Sport Med 2014;24(5):390–6.

105. Williams NI, Koltun KJ, Strock NCA, et al. Perspectives for progress - female athlete triad and relative energy deficiency in sport: a focus on scientific rigor. Exerc Sport Sci Rev 2019. https://doi.org/10.1249/JES.0000000000000200.

106. Liu C-Y, Tseng M-CM, Chang C-H, et al. Comorbid psychiatric diagnosis and psychological correlates of eating disorders in dance students. J Formos Med Assoc 2016;115(2):113–20.

107. Hincapié CA, Cassidy JD. Disordered eating, menstrual disturbances, and low bone mineral density in dancers: a systematic review. Arch Phys Med Rehabil 2010;91(11):1777–89.e1.

108. Arcelus J, Witcomb GL, Mitchell A. Prevalence of eating disorders amongst dancers: a systemic review and meta-analysis. Eur Eat Disord Rev 2014; 22(2):92–101.

109. Tosi M, Maslyanskaya S, Dodson NA, et al. The female athlete triad: a comparison of knowledge and risk in adolescent and young adult figure skaters, dancers, and runners. J Pediatr Adolesc Gynecol 2019;32(2):165–9.

110. Melin A, Tornberg AB, Skouby S, et al. The LEAF questionnaire: a screening tool for the identification of female athletes at risk for the female athlete triad. Br J Sports Med 2014;48(7):540–5.

111. Wewege MA, Ward RE. Bone mineral density in pre-professional female ballet dancers: a systematic review and meta-analysis. J Sci Med Sport 2018;21(8):783–8.

112. Wielandt T, van den Wyngaert T, Uijttewaal JR, et al. Bone mineral density in adolescent elite ballet dancers. J Sports Med Phys Fitness 2019;59(9):1564–70.

113. Ludden JA. A Dance Legend Who Still Finds New Directions. All Things Considered. 2004. Available at: https://www.npr.org/templates/story/story.php?storyId=4233100. Accessed March 27, 2020.
114. Mathon B. Mirror neurons: from anatomy to pathophysiological and therapeutic implications. Rev Neurol (Paris) 2013;169(4):285–90 [in French].
115. Sale P, Franceschini M. Action observation and mirror neuron network: a tool for motor stroke rehabilitation. Eur J Phys Rehabil Med 2012;48(2):313–8.

Autonomic Rehabilitation
Adapting to Change

Raouf S. Gharbo, DO

KEYWORDS

- Adaptation • Autonomic health and rehabilitation • Dysautonomia
- Heart rate variability and biofeedback • Parasympathetic health • Placebo analgesia
- Rehabilitation

KEY POINTS

- Adapting to environmental change or personal health change is not through maintaining autonomic balance for resilience, but rather understanding homeostasis is comprised of 2 autonomic levers in dynamic equilibrium prepared to adapt.
- Injury, poor health, and fear ruminations leading to persistent sympathetic activation fosters and cognitive inflexibility, increasing stickiness and reducing adaptability and health further.
- Focused breathing with heart rate variability biofeedback is the most pragmatic foundation for beginning a process cognitive and autonomic flexibility to improve for better adaptation.
- The emergence of medical use of wearable technology will foster paradigm shifts in the understanding of emotion such as energy is finite, and emotions are energy tools.
- The emergence of heart rate variability wearable technology will serve as a practical whole health biomarker of autonomic health for population health.

ODE FOR AUTONOMIA

Stuck, on the hopeless fear superhighway
Fear is the fuel,
our friend for survival
Cloaked as craving
Consuming and pursuing - illusionary control
Anger, the petulant fear
Harness her, knowing autonomic is not automatic
Hope is a process
Be open, nurture kindness
Not fear, nor anger

Department of Physical Medicine and Rehabilitation, Virginia Commonwealth University, 109 Elizabeth Meriwether, Williamsburg, VA 23185, USA
E-mail address: rsgharbo@gmail.com

Phys Med Rehabil Clin N Am 31 (2020) 633–648
https://doi.org/10.1016/j.pmr.2020.07.003
1047-9651/20/© 2020 Elsevier Inc. All rights reserved.

Embrace,
  Embrace your amygdala exactly as it is
  Let gratitude in
  Permit gratitude to be the parent
Feeling it, measuring it
Let go,
Trust is parasympathetic
Forgiveness is wellness
Over time, adapt by growing insular off ramps
Always, remain empathetic
Yet judicious with your heart's compassionate energy
Know a life of purpose entails conflict and
Kindness will always remain
  -the healer that conquers all

Courtesy of Raouf S. Gharbo.

INTRODUCTION

Lifespan and cardiovascular, metabolic, and psychological health in the United States have been declining for years. The 2008 federal parity law created to improve access for behavioral health has not been enforced, and most health care resources continue to be spent on treatment of physical comorbidities rather than behavioral disorders.[1] Even for those with access to behavioral health care, it is not clear that an effective model for changing health trajectory is being used. Additionally, addressing marginalized populations is crucial for improving health care delivery, and new more objective models of engagement are required to ensure equitable trajectory change.[2]

A fundamental health problem in the digital age is persistent sympathetic activation (PSA), which may also be the core feature of the concept of the chronic pain cycle.'[3] Persistent amygdala triggering[4] of the sympathoadrenal pathway frequently creates unnecessary cardiovascular arousal that is powerful, yet inefficient, and leads to further autonomic nervous system (ANS) inflexibility.[5] Persistent hypothalamus-pituitary-adrenal (HPA) axis triggering causes hormonal consequences leading to metabolic and immune changes. PSA also leads to reduced parasympathetic capacity, fatigue, burnout, and, eventually, helplessness and hopelessness. This combination of PSA, inflammation, and fatigue is a translational challenge for whole health. Additionally, population health programs frequently focus on specific behavioral change, such as smoking cessation, and frequently show only short-term success. Thus, society continues to fail in overall health, winning the battles but losing the war. Currently, standard medical chronic illness methodology is focused on an organ-based specialist pathogenesis model that is procedurally incentivized. The pharmacologic answers for poor psychological health and chronic pain have failed. Furthermore, although electrodes and other interventional procedures are alluring, they cannot teach how to adapt to PSA.

In the behavioral health arena, the *Diagnostic and Statistical Manual of Mental Disorders* (DSM-5) criteria and its vocabulary create confusion, preventing a cohesive team-oriented approach. Using industrial psychology approaches, the technology industry has helped create intricate habit formation algorithms that foster societal cravings. Although digital technology can improve access to behavioral health, a Cochrane review on cognitive behavioral therapy (CBT) defined its limitations and the need for a better mechanism for change theory.[6] Portions of CBT are known to be exhausting,[7] so decision fatigue remains problematic despite increasing access. All these factors contribute to a progression of passiveness, helplessness, and ultimately hopeless-ness. On the other hand, it is now also possible to utilize mobile sensing technologies to allow one to look beyond these positive and negative emotions that may have judg-mental barriers to treatment access, and to analyze ANS physiologic change during emotional episodes.[8] Although mindfulness-based wellness programs do have kind, value-based methods that can result in wellness trajectory, these approaches often lack rigorous scientific structure and reproducibility and commonly have low rates of worker engagement.[9]

This article offers a semantically accessible approach that incorporates enhanced team cohesion through a unified education model and introduces novel concepts for whole-health trajectory change. Practitioners of PM&R are innately positioned to lead a model of value-based health trajectory change with a wide span of impairments in type and severity, using a team-oriented approach. Additionally, experience with spinal cord and brain injury rehabilitation have familiarized physiatrists with autonomic dysregulation. This novel approach outlines how rehabilitation professionals can lead in the assessment of and adaptation to the digital age autonomic dysregulation with a true, value-based, biopsychosocial model of autonomic rehabilitation[10] for whole health, using wearable technology, remote monitoring, and telehealth. This methodol-ogy blends well with existing heart rate variability (HRV) parameters[11] that can serve as whole-health biomarkers, encompassing physiologic and psychological stress with subsequent forms of fatigue.[12–21] HRV, while extensively studied, is poorly understood clinically. HRV parameters are highly sensitive to physical and/or emotional distress but nonspecific. Properly structured, HRV parameters can move from nonspecific to unifying, value-based, whole-health lodestars. Those with autonomic inflexibility from PSA or in the chronic pain cycle may be referred to as stuck. Being stuck[22] can amplify each person's unique individual genetic and environmental physical health and behavioral vulnerabilities. The inefficient hyperarousal energy spent on survival decision making and then the subsequent decision fatigue leads to helplessness and disability. Autonomic rehabilitation emphasizes free will, energy allocation, deci-sion making over intricate habit formation techniques by targeting, 2 specific types of vulnerable decision making. This articles offer an integrative, energy allocation method based on HRV science with digital age applications targeting whole-health, population-based, trajectory change.

BASIC HEALTH CHOICES

HRV science can play an important role in 3 traditional basic healthy choices and high-lights the importance of focused breathing as a starting point.

Purposeful Movement

Exercise is the largest, long-term modifier of HRV, whole-health parameters and is essential to physical rehabilitation.[23–25] A life of purpose increases whole health[26] and leads to increased physical activity.[27] Fear avoidance, catastrophizing, and kine-sophobia frequently limit physical rehabilitation and are major factors in disability in those with otherwise minor physical impairments.[28–31] In this context, rehabilitation is the process of moving past one's fear of movement, with an awareness of one's realistic and dynamic limitations. This is analogous to yoga teaching one to move to one's barrier and holding that position with awareness and relaxation, and then gently re-engaging that boundary repeatedly. Tai Chi and the Feldenkrais and Alexander Techniques also include this moment-to-moment awareness combined with purpose-ful, muscular movement. With practice, incapacitating fears may be reduced, while moment-to-moment boundary awareness is increased. In another context, a parent stuck in PSA but devotes their purpose to break a childhood abuse cycle for their own child can benefit from partnership with a cohesive team.[32] Starting with diaphragm muscles exercises and physical activity guided by innovative wearable devices, one can shift with purpose from PSA towards whole-health progression.[33]

Thoughtful Intake

Being thoughtful, or mindful, about intake, including food, fluids, supplements, medications, and illicit substances, is vital. As cravings are the fundamental emotion of all addictions,[34] insulin rebound craving can be a primary target. For those stuck and vulnerable from PSA or impaired by any cravings, prioritizing diet plans that reduce insulin rebound cravings over total calorie consumption may be a meaningful initial approach. Despite being only 2% of body mass, the brain can burn greater than 20% of available carbohydrates under emotional stress.[35] With a few weeks of a low, simple sugar and/or periodic diet plan, insulin rebound cravings can be reduced, lessening feelings of helplessness and leading to other beneficial circadian and translational health outcomes.[36–38] Diet, medications, supplements, and chemotherapies can all affect HRV and be efficiently monitored with wearable ambient HRV focusing on the effects on circadian rhythm, leading to less decision fatigue and clearer thinking.[39,40]

Intentional Recovery

Postexercise heart rate (HR) recovery is an established measure of whole health, with HR passively lowering from load to a recovery state.[41,42] Similarly, early in sleep, impaired cardiac dipping of HR is a sign of circadian disruption and a translational sign of dysautonomia and whole health.[18,40,43–45] The diaphragm's secondary pump action strongly modulates HRV alterations during daytime and sleep recovery periods. HRV parameters are affected by the diaphragm, providing more information about the respiratory system and recovery states than HR alone.[39,40] The study of heart-diaphragm dynamic coupling during sleep has overemphasized the sympathetic system,[46] whereas inspiration is the most important driving force for cerebral spinal fluid flow.[47] HRV biofeedback (HRV-B) breathing methods are an active way of dipping into recovery daytime[48] and when used prior to sleep can improve nighttime parameters of health.[49] Intentional recovery is defined as valuing, understanding, and measuring recovery in a purposeful manner. Being intentional about recovery has the potential for mitigating disability-associated helplessness and decision fatigue.

Focused Breathing

Most mindful and holistic activities include focused breathing with a practice of reflective sensory awareness. Numerous studies have shown that focused breathing can improve decisions under duress.[50] Using HRV parameters to induce respiratory sinus arrhythmia and thus cardiorespiratory synchronization (CRS)[48] is the most studied and objective method of real-time, active neuromodulation that induces a physiologically efficient homeostatic state. Inducing vagal tone afferently with handheld devices via HRV-B is the most pragmatic and durable way to foster objective focused breathing habits and skills.[51] Although focused breathing cannot reverse spinal stenosis, HRV-B can durably reduce pain magnification at its most basic level and can be the starting point for a trajectory change in chronic illness, burnout, and whole health.[51] Combining HRV-B with creative ambient HRV, wearable monitoring tools can be an ideal starting point to coach moment-to-moment uncoupling of survival decision making while also reducing the risk of decision fatigue. The backbone of the model supports an objective HRV-B habit to achieve a generalized skill acquisition on demand. This can lead to more adaptive free will, healthy decision making of the basic wellness choices.

AUTONOMIC REHABILITATION

Much like bowel retraining of the ANS during spinal cord injury rehabilitation, attempts to restore circadian dysregulation with HRV-B could potentially rehabilitate the ANS after central autonomic network (CAN) dysregulation of the heart after concussion.[21,49] Two robust chronic pain and whole-health models are the Fear Avoidance Model and the Catastrophic Construct, the latter comprised of 3 components of magnification, rumination, and helplessness. Intrusive thoughts and catastrophizing have a bidirectional relationship maintaining chronic pain and anxiety.[52] Commonly, childhood or adult trauma can develop an exaggerated amygdala connectivity in the decision-making regions of the brain that correlate with depression and chronic pain, catastrophizing subscales of rumination and helplessness.[4,30,53] This hyperconnectivity, which can create fear superhighways, fosters PSA, hyperarousal survival decision making, and triggering of the CAN and HPA axis that can then lead to decision fatigue, dysautonomia, and ill health.[54]

Fear may simply be considered as the sole emotion of PSA. Often individuals are coached to accept fear is the fuel for survival decision making, leading to decision fatigue. Specifically, fear rumination[51] is targeted with HRV-B focused breathing to shift into an energy-efficient state that can increase more pliable thinking with afferent vagal influence and reduce pain-catastrophizing magnification. Amygdala connections are modulated by the salience network (SN) for detection of interoceptive and external changes in the environment and to maintain homeostasis by regulating the ANS activity and social-emotional function.[53,55] The insula is a core node of the SN and is linked to apathy/helplessness, arousal, rumination, anxiety, empathy, suicide, cravings, depression, and brain health. Individuals are coached to practice HRV-B to foster off-ramp rewiring of the fear superhighway over time,[53] improving energy utilization with voluntary CAN uncoupling of descending pathways. Incorporating acceptance-based models, individuals are coached that PSA triggering is inevitable after trauma; however, one can learn to defuel fears and possibly build off-ramps in the brain's salience network for free will, descending energy modulation.

INITIAL CLINICAL CONSULTATION

Initial clinical consultation begins much like any chronic pain or rehabilitation consultation, with the assumption that all chronic pain and chronic disorders have both physical and psychological components. Although initially prioritizing the physical evaluation can gain a therapeutic partnership, it is also important to specifically listen for fear words (eg, afraid, worried, scared, or terrified) throughout the evaluation. Fear is the emotional root driver of being stuck; therefore, avoidance behaviors and anger are rooted in fear. Listen patiently for fear words, not frustration, the nidus of ruminations. Asking "Why you are angry?" or "Why do you drink alcohol?" can waste time and energy. Rather, ask open-ended questions or specific questions,[56] such as "What do you fear?," "What do you crave?," or "Is your home or bedroom a sleep-recovery sanctuary?" Several validated psychological subjective scales are available, with the Pain Catastrophizing Scale being particularly ideal for chronic pain management.[57] When developing a treatment plan, passive treatments should take a secondary, supportive role to self-efficacy techniques that foster active engagement in a process for improved healthy decision making. Passive treatments are not divided into medical, psychological, or holistic silos, but rather divided into 2 integrative categories: supportive platforms to address the underlying physical component or autonomic resets to assist with short-term disruption of PSA.

Supportive Platforms

Bariatric surgery, insulin pumps, elective total joint replacements, and nicotine or buprenorphine transdermal patches are all ineffective long term without prioritizing PSA management. Not addressing catastrophizing is predictively associated with chronic pain and opioid utilization postoperatively in elective procedures.[30,58] All passive supportive platforms should be evaluated using a common set of metrics and priorities and updated regularly based on current literature and related criteria. Thematically, these always take on a secondary supportive role to minimize PSA. As objective signs of HRV-B engagement and therapeutic partnership are demonstrated, access to greater resources and risk exposure can be broadened. For instance, not all opioids are a high risk. Focused breathing addressing PSA coupled with a weekly buprenorphine patch could be an effective supportive platform over surgical intervention for chronic pain for severe spinal stenosis or with a traumatized joint.[58]

Autonomic Resets

Several weeks or months of HRV-B may be necessary to affect and rewire underlying chronic disease states, including chronic pain sensitization. Developing short-term goals for HRV-B is necessary when stuck. Successful short-term goals include defueling fear ruminations, cravings, panic attacks, phobias and what may be referred to as racing brain insomnia. Focused breathing can be backed up and individualized with exercise or passive modalities, such as massage, aromas, acupuncture, float tanks, stellate ganglion blocks, virtual reality, ketamine infusions, to spark ownership for defueling fear ruminations and healthy decision making. Passively stimulating the vagus nerve with an electrode, brain stimulation, intravenous infusions, and stellate ganglion blocks can temporarily reset the ANS or CAN. Clinical trials using medical grade, ambient HRV monitoring could tease out efficacy among various autonomic resets. Clinicians should develop evidence-based, annually updated, integrative matrixes of autonomic resets for their own practices and for the field. Given the high cost, limited durability, and passive nature of passive autonomic resets, the regular use of the active HRV-B remains the primary PSA self-efficacy method. Modulating these whole-health biomarkers in real time can lead to remarkable health outcomes.[59]

CLINIC VISIT 2: AUTONOMIC INTRODUCTION AND HEART RATE VARIABILITY ASSESSMENT

Homeostasis is typically described as autonomic balance, the parasympathetic system as the relaxation response, and HRV parameters as a dashboard of the 2 main ANS branches.[60] Although this may imply that these 2 branches have a linear relationship, homeostasis is an energy-efficient state of coengagement of 2 independent levers in dynamic equilibrium. HRV parameters are the best and relatively simple measures of the parasympathetic lever[61] and recovery, although other better measures of the sympathetic system and load are available. PSA impairs parasympathetic capacity, so whole-health trajectory change is guided toward parasympathetic health with HRV whole-health biomarkers. Staff can easily be trained to incorporate several basic validated HRV assessments introduced at the beginning of the second visit.

Heart Rate Variability Short Recordings

Five-minute resting, short recordings of HRV are nonspecific, easily manipulated and highly contextual to external environment changes[62] and must be interpreted with caution. Their value is for education of a 2 independent lever model in dynamic equilibrium. Short recordings can visually display different emotional physiologic categories:

- The stress response (high sympathetic throttle and low parasympathetic braking)
- Recovery (high braking and low throttle),
- Flow zone (high coengagement)
- An efficient set point (low coengagement homeostasis)
- Depleted autonomic states that portend translational whole health consequences

These short recordings can educate and increase insight in situations if

- One's current stress response is mismatched out of proportion to the current nonthreatening external environment
- An individual is outwardly calm but has limited interoceptive awareness to one's "still waters that run deep"

Ambient Heart Rate Variability Monitoring

HRV is predictive of post-traumatic stress disorder prior to deployment, preclinical viral illness, and early risk for sepsis mortality.[63–66] Adaptions to the post-COVID19 (coronavirus disease 2019) world may herald in the medical wearable age. Creative, color-coded, ambient monitoring can have a marked effect on moment-to-moment healthy decision making, by gaining insight into the decision of energy efficiency over needless energy expenditure during texting arguments, quarantine, or social distancing. Taken further, clinical trials could study the risk for decision fatigue of before, during, and after intensive counseling, prioritizing dissecting and restructuring past events. Obsessed perfectionists seeking zone performance, individuals stuck in craving, or those who are simply exhausted can all be redirected toward being intentional about recovery for sustainable high performance. Longitudinal nocturnal HRV monitoring may emerge in prominence with wearables, and over weeks and months can teach increasing battery capacity with exercise, detect incomplete battery recharging overnight, and guide how to induce deeper, steeper sleep recovery when combined with HRV-B.[49,60] For example, when stuck trying harder to be a good person and in conflict with one's morals, reducing alcohol consumption that impairs overnight HRV,[39] and instead focusing on improving HRV parameters for health and performance can be liberating. Organizational culture shift with tools and coaching is possible by fostering intentional recovery that playfully incentivizes skills of deeper, steeper, longer quality, recovery day or night.[67]

Heart Rate Variability Response to Deep Breathing

HRV-deep breathing (DB) is the most energy-efficient awake state and is the most basic and accepted evaluation, assessing parasympathetic capacity among autonomic laboratories.[36] HRV-DB entails diaphragmatic breathing at a rate of 5 seconds of inhalation, followed by 5 seconds of exhalation to induce CRS. At this frequency of approximately 0.1 Hz, there is an alignment of the cardiorespiratory and neurologic systems.[68] The literature is so robust for HRV-DB that the American Diabetic Association and American Academy of Neurology[69,70] recommend testing in all new diabetics, repeated again in 5 years, as the most sensitive predictor of long-term diabetic complications prior to the diagnosis of diabetes mellitus. To date, this recommendation has not been implemented in clinical practice because of cumbersome equipment and a lack of value-based incentives. Reduced HRV-DB findings can be explained as depleted brake pad thickness from persistent left foot braking the ANS from PSA.[10] This reduced brake pad thickness reduces one's ability to adapt to unpredictable twists and turns of life. Daily practice of the HRV-DB is the basis of HRV-B; thus, inducing CRS is not only an important assessment but is also the foundation to thicken brake pads.

Heart Rate Variability Biofeedback Introduction

The heart is the largest surface-measured electrical signal in the body by a factor of 10. Compared with other forms of biofeedback, HRV-B has the greatest immediate impact on whole-body physiology, and this acquired skill is durable. The diaphragm is modulated by both the autonomic and voluntary networks, so this muscle is the largest autonomic wedge; thus, autonomic is not automatic. HRV training can be done by any certified HRV-B trainer.[51] Purposeful movement of the diaphragm muscle with HRV-B focused breathing can be a natural fit for physical therapy that regularly engages kinesophobia and psychologically informed physical therapy.[71] Using HRV-B methodology and autonomic rehabilitation concepts for rural care with remote monitoring and telehealth could improve access and disparity of care in a cohesive manner with whole-health outcome measures to meet mental health parity law standards. There remains quality, equipment, and HRV parameter controversies that require resolving prior to fully launching the medical wearable age.[60,62,72,73]

CLINIC VISIT 3: INTRODUCE STOP, SHIFT, AND DECIDE METHODOLOGY

The third visit and a handful of future visits are loosely broken down to 50 minutes of HRV training followed by a 10-minute visit with the lead physician to answer questions, develop short-term goals, assess treatment appropriateness, and expand the therapeutic team, supportive platforms, and autonomic resets as appropriate. Moving forward the visits are tethered by novel stop, shift, and decide methodology based on cardiovascular anatomy. The sinoatrial (SA) node, the pacemaker, is innervated by both autonomic branches; however, the myocardium is only innervated by the sympathetic system. One can actively use the diaphragm to help the foster parasympathetic component to outcompete the slower sympathetic component[42] at the SA node for efficient CRS rhythms.[48] However, even in CRS, if PSA and fear rumination persist, powerful and potentially fatiguing contractions continue. After focused breathing, a process to let go of PSA triggering, from fear ruminations of the CAN is necessary to achieve stillness and recovery.

Stop the Racing Brain with a Necessary Diaphragm Habit

Everyone has their own resonant frequency, varying slightly around 0.1 Hz, that can be determined with highly skilled staff and sophisticated biofeedback equipment. Maintaining a diaphragmatic practice habit, inducing CRS twice per day with a simple HRV-B pulse wave handheld device, can more pragmatically obviate the use of those sophisticated measures. Over time, individuals can learn to sense the shift into CRS and develop heart awareness, regardless of aptitude with prior meditation experiences. HRV-B allows for prescribing focused breathing homework and monitoring, to assess both engagement and ability even remotely:

Prescription: Focused breathing 10 minutes twice daily and as needed
Dispense: #1 HRV-B device with remote HRV ambient monitoring

Diagnosis: PTSD with chronic low back pain
Precautions: none

Those open to a practice, demonstrating objective signs of engagement are identified as stuck and ready. An objective, focused breathing prescription can also allow for stratification of opioid risk prescribing and allocation of limited resources for supportive platforms and autonomic resets more equitably for vulnerable, marginalized populations.[2] Clinicians holding individuals to an objective focused breathing practice with mindful accountability, using patience and educational analogies seems to be a key component to success.[51,59]

During quiet meditation and meditative prayer, people with a history of prior trauma frequently have fearful intrusive thoughts and memories. For some who have been stuck on fear superhighways for many years, this physiologic shift into CRS for the first time can be unsettling. Feeling safe in the clinic is paramount to courageously breathe and sit in stillness to defuel fear ruminations. Similarly, those with obsessive disorders, high performers, and perfectionists have future-based, fearful intrusive thoughts. The core emotion that fuels all substance use disorders is craving.[34] Individuals suffering from cravings are coached that cravings are cloaked fear, because reward cycles ultimately trigger the same CAN. Mindful accountability is necessary to prevent panic, reassuring that this is a healthy, efficient state. Allowing one to avoid this feeling and moving onto another integrative modality will disrupt trajectory change. Individuals are coached to become comfortable with this new feeling, to help build off-ramps. Dissecting past events is not a primary goal, is fatiguing, and is done at an individual's own pace. During focused breathing, individuals are coached to identify and categorize all fear ruminations into past, future, or present fears. A home practice of defueling is prioritized, saving time and energy and building confidence. With time, individuals will recognize and prioritize defueling over control of past or future events to choose energy efficiency.

Addressing current fears, suffering, and pain requires a more involved approach. During focused breathing, one can practice scanning and sensing individually each of the 5 external and interoceptions above and below the diaphragm. The purpose is to improve SN awareness, to improve data acquisition and appraisal of the external world, to prevent injury, to mitigate wasted energy, and to recognize dynamic changes in internal capacity. Modern society values doing over listening. To teach active neuromodulation of both dynamic autonomic levers, society will need to value listening skills. Achieving a silent stillness, or simply stillness, under duress is an early essential skill to save energy and adapt to uncertainty and new threats that may require stressful social distancing. Stillness can be developed in a graded manner that can be assisted with wearable devices: first with physical movement (accelerometers), then physiologically (HRV wearables), and then perhaps even cognitively (EEG biofeedback). For team communication, this practice of fostering the 5 external and interoceptive skills can be encapsulated as afferent training for insular rewiring. Silent retreats are an ideal opportunity to improve afferent listening skills and stillness.

Shift Emotion on Demand by Acquiring a Heart Skill

The emotion of feeling appreciation can induce CRS.[74] This notion opens the door to a biopsychosocial model that categorizes emotions based on differing energy utilization profiles.[8] Distinguishing the difference between cognitively remembering to be grateful from physiologically feeling gratitude, by shifting into efficient CRS shift, is essential. Initially, this shifting skill is taught in a safe HRV-B clinic environment;

then, a practice habit, an acquired skill of shifting, can be generalized to the community without HRV-B devices under severe duress. This is subtly, but importantly, different from being positive or getting into one's happy place in truly horrible circumstances. Happiness is not a primary goal but a byproduct of an aligned energy efficient life of purpose. Integrative use of rituals can assist shifting skills. For instance, olfactory access to the brain is powerful. Rather than a confusing an array of aromas for each individual emotion, the author recommends limiting the number of aromas and being disciplined with their therapeutic use. One may purposefully choose 1 aroma for peaceful, humble, recovery (high PNS/low SNS) states, and another for courageous, flow zone (higher energy, high coengagement of PNS and SNS) states to modulate the CAN. Rituals can be individualized with any of the 5 external senses to trigger stillness, the important intermediate step, prior to making confusing, energy allocation decisions in the moment. Music and art can be helpful even in the darkest times to feel appreciation for health.[67,75,76] HRV science may have unlocked Cicero's words, "...gratitude is the parent of all virtues." In this vein, the author coaches that feeling gratitude is the parent of all PSA.

Decide with Free Will

As in physics and biochemistry, accept that emotional energy resources are finite in this biopsychosocial model.[8] If the notion of fear being the fundamental human emotion of the SNS is reasonable, then proposing that trust is parasympathetic[77] can be a key insight to scientifically unlock timeless body-mind-spirit concepts. The emotion of trust is basis of all partnerships, the herding response, the relaxation response,[78] hope, and faith. Free-will allocation of energy emotions to adapt to external threats from moment to moment can improve whole-health sustainably. Seeing emotions of fear, trust, craving, and gratitude as energy allocations choices, HRV as the energy meter, and HRV-B as the key to energy allocation is essential for whole-health. More simply stated, emotions are energy tools.

During quiet counseling sessions, individuals broadly define a personal and professional purpose and right and left value boundaries. One's purpose is used to tether HRV whole-health parameters for resolving or adapting to energy-draining conflicts. Having early, difficult value conversations in stillness about energy conflicts with people using focused breathing and stillness skills can prevent more draining conversations later about infringement of standards, policies, and laws. Values, such as do no harm, humility, forgiveness, and kindness, guide energy allocation decisions. Mindful accountability is difficult to teach. Individuals are coached to initially create a sanctuary of recovery in the bedroom, free of conflict and technological stimulus. To attain stillness, a critical milestone, an integrative ritual with focused breathing combined with single unique aroma of choice for cueing the emotion of courage can be utilized to hold new boundaries with other household members. Holding new boundaries with mindful accountability for health and energy restoration can be less personal and reduce unnecessary exhausting conflict.

Using an energy utilization premise, individuals are taught to distinguish between the risks and benefits of practicing empathy or compassion. Conceivably, empathy is a cognitive understanding and articulation of other people's suffering while valuing personal health, whereby compassion is associated with CAN physiologic triggering. If a lack of self-care awareness goes unchecked or if there is an absence of SN off ramps, PSA can lead to compassion fatigue, burnout, or depersonalization.[79] The author encourages always maintaining cognitive empathy with stillness and focused breathing to modulate CAN triggering with free will. More concisely, empathy always but be judicious with compassion.

Milestones

A hopeful moment, an ah ha moment, and a welcome back moment are documented throughout the process. Early on, how hope is guided by the team can ethically leverage the placebo response. Those suffering, vulnerable, and helpless often have hope directed toward yet to be established lucrative, passive treatments. Although, open-label placebo analgesia is possible with passive modalities, long-term benefits have not been established. Positive emotions are not necessary for the placebo response.[80–82] To ethically maximize the placebo response long term, a process of active neuromodulation is likely necessary followed by healthy energy allocation and restoration decisions. The goals and expectations need to be properly framed in partnership; educational analogies must be realistic and based on sound science. Hope should be guided toward a reproducible process for free-will decision making.

As the ah ha moment implies, there is a moment, with enough practice and understanding, of successful application in the real world. Typically, those moments easily identify themselves on review of remote HRV monitoring[51] with a story and a proud smile. Wearable accelerometers, ambient HRV monitoring, and HRV biofeedback software could all be incorporated in patient-centered medical homes (PCMHs) to scale these moments and help people adapt to an uncertain world. Personal ah ha moments are typically associated with an irreversible change to one's self-efficacy and self-confidence in the future.

A 2-lever, dynamic adaptation model of the ANS, based on energy restoration and allocation, allows one to argue ethically, spiritually, and scientifically that values like gentle forgiveness for others and for self are healthy. The model allows one to distinguish cognitive empathy from riskier compassion, free of DSM confusion. The model permits discussion about the physiologic difference between remembering gratitude and feeling gratitude, possibly even categorizing emotions based on energy utilization and neural networks, such as peace (high PNS/low SNS) and love (high coengagement with CRS). As more people live longer with the stress and uncertainty[35] of cancer, this model could provide a framework for spirituality studies,[8,83] linking cancer fatigue,[84] feeling gratitude for each moment,[85] and cancer outcomes.[14]

SUMMARY

The goal of autonomic rehabilitation is not attaining homeostatic balance, but rather recognizing and modulating energy, internal and external, moment-to-moment, sustainably, in line with one's purpose in an uncertain world. With regularity, over different time periods, there are welcome back moments. Not when all conflicts and ailments are resolved but rather when the person can be seen for who that person really is, no longer stuck in PSA, exhausted, and hopeless. This autonomic rehabilitation process, if scaled to every PCMH, can change health care trajectory for the masses of individuals with a series of welcome back moments, 1 person at a time, 1 moment at a time.

CLINICS CARE POINTS

- Fear ruminations lead to persistent sympathetic activation, fostering cognitive inflexibility and reducing health and adaptability. Adaptation to changes in external environment or internal health is not through maintaining autonomic balance for resilience, but rather actively modulating 2 independent autonomic levers in dynamic equilibrium in energy-efficient homeostasis.

- Focused breathing with HRV biofeedback is an objective, safe, and effective start point for lifestyle changes, improving cognitive and autonomic flexibility for healthy adaptation. The emergence of medical wearable technology into health care, accelerated by COVID-19, will create insights into emotion and physiology, fostering paradigm shifts, including the idea that energy utilization for emotion is finite and emotions are energy tools.

DISCLOSURE

Adviser and investor Peerbridge Health.

REFERENCES

1. Thorpe K, Jain S, Joski S. Prevalence and spending associated with patients who have a behavioral health disorder and other condition. Health Aff 2017;36(1): 124–132..
2. Moody L, Bridge E, Thakkar V, et al. Engaging under- and/or never-engaged populations in health services: a systematic review. Patient Exp J 2019;16–32.
3. Olsen K. History of pain: the nature of pain. Pract Pain Manag 2015;13(6). Available at: https://www.practicalpainmanagement.com/treatments/history-pain-brief-overview-19th-20th-centuries. Accessed August 20, 2020.
4. Jiang Y, Oathes D, Hush J, et al. Perturbed connectivity of the amygdala and its subregions with the central executive and default mode networks in chronic pain. Pain 2016;157(9):1970–8.
5. Feliu-Soler A, Montesinos F, Gutiérrez-Martínez O, et al. Current status of acceptance and commitment therapy for chronic pain: a narrative review. J Pain Res 2018;11:2145–59.
6. Williams ACDC, Eccleston C, Morley S. Psychological therapies for the management of chronic pain (excluding headache) in adults. Cochrane Database Syst Rev 2012;(11):CD007407.
7. McCracken LM, Eccleston C. A comparison of the relative utility of coping and acceptance-based measures in a sample of chronic pain sufferers. Eur J Pain 2006;1(10):23–9.
8. Siegel EH, Sands MK, Van den Noortgate W, et al. Emotion fingerprints or emotion populations? A meta-analytic investigation of autonomic features of emotion categories. Psychol Bull 2018;144(4):343–93.
9. Kachan D, Olano H, Tannenbaum SL, et al. Prevalence of mindfulness practices in the US workforce: National Health Interview Survey. Prev Chronic Dis 2017; 14:E01.
10. Gharbo R, Ginsberg JP. Heart rate variability, chronic pain and rehabilitating the autonomic nervous system. Pain Pract 2016;17–8.
11. Billman GE. Heart rate variability - a historical perspective. Front Physiol 2011; 2:86..
12. Tsuji H, Veditti FJ, Manders ES, et al. Reduced heart rate variability and mortality risk in an elderly cohort. The Framingham Heart Study. Circulation 1994;(2): 873–83.
13. Bissinger A. Cardiac autonomic neuropathy: why should cardiologists care about that? J Diabetes Res 2017;2017:5374176.
14. Kloter E, Barrueto K, Klein S, et al. Heart rate variability as a prognostic factor for cancer survival – a systematic review. Front Physiol 2018;9:623.
15. Binici Z, Mouridsen MR, Kober L, et al. Decreased nighttime heart rate variability is associated with increased stroke risk. Stroke 2011;42:3196–201.

16. Aeschbacher S, Schoen T, Dörig L, et al. Heart rate, heart rate variability and inflammatory biomarkers among young and healthy adults. Ann Med 2017;49(1): 32–41.

17. Tracy LM, Ioannou L, Baker KS, et al. A meta-analytic evidence for decreased heart rate variability in chronic pain implicating parasympathetic nervous system dysregulation. Pain 2016;157(1):7–29.

18. Chervin RD, Teodorescu M, Kushwaha R, et al. Objective measures of disordered sleep in fibromyalgia. J Rheumatol 2009;36(9):2009–16.

19. Chalmers JA, Quintana DS, Abbott MJ, et al. Anxiety disorders are associated with reduced heart rate variability: a meta-analysis. Front Psychiatry 2014;5:80.

20. Nagpal ML, Gliechauf K, Ginsberg JP. Meta-analysis of heart rate variability as a psychophysiological indicator of posttraumatic stress. disord. J Trauma Treat 2013;3:1.

21. Conder R, Conder A. Heart rate variability interventions for concussion and rehabilitation. Front Psychol 2014;5:890.

22. Borsook D, Youssef AM, Simons L, et al. When pain gets stuck: the evolution of pain chronification and treatment resistance. Pain 2018;159(12):2421–36.

23. Routledge FS, Campbell TS, McFetridge-Durdle JA, et al. Improvements in heart rate variability with exercise therapy. Can J Cardiol 2010;26(6):303–12.

24. Villafaina S, Collado-Mateo D, Fuentes JP, et al. Physical exercise improves heart rate variability in patients with type 2 diabetes: a systematic review. Curr Diab Rep 2017;17(11):110.

25. May R, McBerty V, Zaky A, et al. Vigorous physical activity predicts higher heart rate variability among younger adults. J Physiol Anthropol 2017;36:24..

26. Hooker SA, Masters KS, Park CL. A meaningful life is a healthy life: a conceptual model linking meaning and meaning salience to health. Rev Gen Psychol 2018; 22(1):11–24.

27. Hooker SA, Masters KS. Purpose in life is associated with physical activity measured by accelerometer. J Health Psychol 2016;21(6):962–71.

28. Sullivan MJL, Bishop SR, Pivik J. The pain catastrophizing scale: development and validation. Psychol Assess 1995;7(4):524–32.

29. Silva Guerrero AV, Maujean A, Campbell L, et al. A systematic review and meta-analysis of the effectiveness of psychological interventions delivered by physiotherapists on pain, disability and psychological outcomes in musculoskeletal pain conditions. Clin J Pain 2018;34(9):838–57.

30. Theunissen M, Peters ML, Bruce J, et al. Preoperative anxiety and catastrophizing: a systematic review and meta-analysis of the association with chronic postsurgical pain. Clin J Pain 2012;28(9):819–41.

31. Svensson GL, Lundberg M, Ostgaard HC, et al. High degree of kinesiophobia after lumbar disc herniation surgery: a cross-sectional study of 84 patients. Acta Orthop 2011;82(6):732–6.

32. Guerrero S, Vivian A, Annick M. Identification of functioning domains in the presurgical period and their relationships with opioid use and pain catastrophizing. Clin J Pain 2018;34(9):838–57.

33. Gevirtz R. The nerve of that disease: the vagus nerve and cardiac rehabilitation. Biofeedback 2013;41(1):32–8.

34. McHugh RK, Fitzmaurice GM, Carroll KM, et al. Assessing craving and its relationship to subsequent prescription opioid use among treatment-seeking prescription opioid dependent patients. Drug Alcohol Depend 2014;145::121–6.

35. Petes A, McEwen BS, Friston K. Uncertainty and stress: why it causes diseases and how it is mastered by the brain. Prog Neurobiol 2017;156::164–88.

36. Longo VD, Panda S. Fasting, circadian rhythms, and time-restricted feeding in healthy lifespan. Cell Metab 2016;23(6):1048–59.

37. Castro A, Gomez-Arbelaez D, Crujeiras A, et al. Effect of a very low-calorie ketogenic diet on food and alcohol cravings, physical and sexual activity, sleep disturbances, and quality of life in obese patients. Nutrients 2018;10(10):1348.

38. Buono R, Longo W. Starvation, stress resistance, and cancer. Trends Endocrinol Metab 2018;4(29):271–80.

39. Pietilä J, Helander E, Korhonen I, et al. Acute effect of alcohol intake on cardiovascular autonomic regulation during the first hours of sleep in a large real-world sample of Finnish employees: observational study. JMIR Ment Health 2018;5(1):e23.

40. Kadoya M, Koyama H, Kanzaki A, et al. Plasma brain-derived neurotrophic factor and reverse dipping pattern of nocturnal blood pressure in patients with cardiovascular risk factors. PLoS One 2014;9(8):e105977.

41. Ackland GL, Minto G, Clark M, et al. Autonomic regulation of systemic inflammation in humans: A multi-center, blinded observational cohort study. Brain Behav Immun 2018;67:47-53.

42. Peçanha T, Silva-Júnior ND, Forjaz CLdM. Heart rate recovery: autonomic determinants, methods of assessment and association with mortality and cardiovascular diseases. Clin Physiol Funct Imaging 2014;34:327–39.

43. Haley RW, Charuvastra E, Shell WE, et al. Cholinergic autonomic dysfunction in veterans with gulf war illness: Confirmation in a population-based sample. JAMA Neurol 2013;70(2):191–200.

44. Goldstein B, Toweill D, Lai S, et al. Uncoupling of the autonomic and cardiovascular systems in acute brain injury. Am J Physiol 1998;275(4):R1287–92.

45. Williamson JB, Heilman KM, Porges EC, et al. A possible mechanism for PTSD symptoms in patients with traumatic brain injury: central autonomic network disruption. Front Neuroeng 2013;6:13.

46. Zambotti M, Trinder J, Silvani A, et al. Dynamic coupling between the central and autonomic nervous systems during sleep: a review. Neurosci Biobehav Rev 2018; 90. https://doi.org/10.1016/j.neubiorev.2018.03.027.

47. Dreha-Kulaczewski S, Joseph AA, Merboldt KD, et al. Inspiration is the major regulator of human CSF flow. J Neurosci 2015;35(6):2485–91.

48. Lehrer P, Gevirtz R. Heart rate variability biofeedback: how and why does it work? Front Psychol 2014;5:756.

49. Sakakibara M, Hayano J, Oikawa LO, et al. Heart rate variability biofeedback improves cardiorespiratory synchronization resting function during sleep. Appl Psychophysiol Biofeedback 2013;38(4):265–71.

50. De Couck M, Caers R, Musch L, et al. How breathing can help you make better decision: two studies on the effects of breathing patterns on heart rate variability and decision-making in business cases. Int J Psychophysiol 2019;(139):1–9.

51. Gharbo R, Bagherpour R, Lazarus N. Untangling chronic pain and hyperarousal with heart rate variability: a case report. Pract Pain Manag 2019;9(7):33–6.

52. Ravn SL, Hartvigsen J, Hansen M, et al. Do post-traumatic pain and post-traumatic stress symptomatology mutually maintain each other? A systematic review of cross-lagged studies. Pain 2018;159(11):2159–69.

53. Uddin LQ. Functions of the salience network. In: Uddin LQ, editor. Salience network of the human brain. Cambridge: Academic Press; 2017. p. 11–6.

54. Benarroch E. The central autonomic network: functional organization, dysfunction, and perspective. Mayo Clin Proc 1993;68(10):988–1001.

55. Strum VE, Brown JA, Hua AY, et al. Network Architecture Underlying Basal Autonomic Outflow: Evidence from Frontotemporal Dementia. Journal of Neuroscience 2018;38(42):8943–55.

56. Resnicow K, McMaster F. Motivational interviewing: moving from why to how with autonomy support. Int J Behav Nutr Phys Act 2012;9:19.

57. Leung L. Pain catastrophizing: an updated review. Indian J Psychol Med 2012; 34(3):204–17.

58. Travaglini L, Highland KB, Rojas W, et al. Identification of functioning domains in the presurgical period and their relationships with opioid use and pain catastrophizing. Pain Med 2019;20(9):1717–27.

59. Gilman J, Gharbo R. Improved pain coping and arrhythmia mitigation with heart rate variability biofeedback training: a case report. Poster Abstract 508. Annual Conference of American Academy of Pain Medicine AAPM March 2020. Available at: http://annualmeeting.painmed.org/uploads/2020/aapm2020_posters_web.pdf. Accessed February 28, 2020.

60. Billman G. The LF/HF ratio does not accurately measure cardiac sympatho-vagal balance. Front Physiol 2013;4:26.

61. Low PA, Benarroch EE. Clinical autonomic disorders. 3rd edition. Baltimore: Lippincott Williams & Wilkins; 2008. p. 139–41.

62. Shaffer F, Ginsberg JP. An overview of heart rate variability metrics and norms. Front Public Health 2017;5:258.

63. Pyne J, Constans J,, Wiederhold M, et al. Heart rate variability: pre-deployment predictor of post-deployment PTSD symptoms. Biol Psychol 2016;121. https://doi.org/10.1016/j.biopsycho.2016.10.008.

64. Ahmad S, Tejuja A, Newman KD, et al. Clinical review: a review and analysis of heart rate variability and the diagnosis and prognosis of infection. Crit Care 2009;13(6):232.

65. Samsudin MI, Liu N, Prabhakar SM, et al. A novel heart rate variability based risk prediction model for septic patients presenting to the emergency department. Medicine (Baltimore) 2018;97(23):e10866.

66. Arbo JE, Lessing JK, Ford WJH, et al. Heart rate variability measures for prediction of severity of illness and poor outcome in ED patients with sepsis. Am J Emerg Med 2020. [Epub ahead of print].

67. Reimer MU, Catanzaro D, Gharbo R. An intervention to promote mind-body awareness in a university wind ensemble. Visions of research in music education 2017. 30. Available at:http: http://www.usr.rider.edu/~vrme/v30n1/visions/Reimer_Mind_Body_Awareness.pdf. Accessed August 22, 2020.

68. Shaffer F, McCraty R, Zerr CL. A healthy heart is not a metronome: an integrative review of the heart's anatomy and heart rate variability. Front Psychol 2014;5:1040.

69. Benichou T, Pereira B, Mermillod M, et al. Heart rate variability in type 2 diabetes mellitus: A systematic review and meta-analysis. PLoS One 2018;13:e0195166.

70. Gibbons C. Approved by AAN Board of Directors in October 2014. 2014. Available at: https://www.aan.com/siteassets/home-page/tools-and-resources/practicing-neurologist–administrators/billing-and-coding/model-coverage-policies/14autonomicmodel_tr.pdf. Accessed August 22, 2020.

71. Archer K, Coronado R, Wegener S. The role of psychologically informed physical therapy for musculoskeletal pain. Curr Phys Med Rehabil Rep 2018. https://doi.org/10.1007/s40141-018-0169-x.

72. Peake JM, Kerr G, Sullivan JP. A critical review of consumer wearables, mobile applications, and equipment for providing biofeedback, monitoring stress, and sleep in physically active populations. Front Physiol 2018;9:743.
73. 2019 8th International Conference on Affective Computing and Intelligent Interaction (ACII). Available at: https://arxiv.org/abs/1907.07327. Accessed August 21, 2020.
74. McCraty R, Atkinson M, Tiller W, et al. The effects of emotions on short-term power spectrum analysis of heart rate variability. Am J Cardiol 1995;76:1089–93. https://doi.org/10.1016/S0002-9149(99)80309-9.
75. Vickhoff B, Malmgren H, Aström R, et al. Music structure determines heart rate variability of singers [published correction appears in Front Psychol. 2013 Sep 05;4:599]. Front Psychol 2013;4:334.
76. Haiblum-Itskovitch S, Czamanski-Cohen J, Giora G. Emotional response and changes in heart rate variability following art-making with three different art materials. Front Psychol 2018;968.
77. Gharbo R. The chronic pain performance curve: a new model for our times. J Phys Med Rehab Sci 2013;26:2.
78. Stahl JE, Dossett ML, LaJoie AS, et al. Relaxation response and resiliency training and its effect on healthcare resource utilization [published correction appears in PLoS One. 2017 Feb 21;12 (2):e0172874]. PLoS One 2015;10(10):e0140212.
79. West CP, Dyrbye LN, Erwin PJ, et al. Interventions to prevent and reduce physician burnout: a systematic review and meta-analysis. Lancet 2016;388(10057): 2272–81.
80. Carvalho C, Caetano JM, Cunha L, et al. Open-label placebo treatment in chronic low back pain: a randomized controlled trial. Pain 2016;157(12):2766–72.
81. Evers AWM, Colloca L, Blease C, et al. Implications of placebo and nocebo effects for clinical practice: expert consensus. Psychother Psychosom 2018; 87(4):204–10.
82. Locher C, Nascimento AF, Kossowsky J, et al. Open-label placebo response – does optimism matter? A secondary-analysis of a randomized controlled trial. J Psychosom Res 2019;116:25–30.
83. Hulett JM, Armer JM. A systematic review of spiritually based interventions and psychoneuroimmunological outcomes in breast cancer survivorship. Integr Cancer Ther 2016;15(4):405–23.
84. Weis J. Cancer-related fatigue: prevalence, assessment and treatment strategies. Expert Rev Pharmacoecon Outcomes Res 2011;11(4):441–6.
85. Burch JB, Ginsberg JP, McLain AC, et al. Symptom management among cancer survivors: randomized pilot intervention trial of heart rate variability biofeedback. Appl Psychophysiol Biofeedback 2020;45(2):99–108.

Physical Activity, Exercise, Whole Health, and Integrative Health Coaching

Heather L. Malecki, PT, DPT[a],*, Jared M. Gollie, PhD[b,c,d], Joel Scholten, MD[e]

KEYWORDS

- Physical activity • Exercise • Integrative health coaching • Whole health
- Integrative medicine

KEY POINTS

- Physical activity plays a significant role in the management and prevention of more than 35 medical conditions.
- Both physical activity and exercise are considered primary preventative measures against chronic disease.
- The Whole Health model of care incorporates all aspects of care, including prevention, treatment, conventional, and complementary approaches resulting in care for the whole person.
- Integrative health coaching is an invaluable tool for clinicians seeking to achieve behavior changes for improved health, particularly in the areas of physical activity and exercise.

Physical inactivity is considered a primary cause for dozens of chronic health conditions,[1] and, therefore, engaging in physical activity and exercise is essential for maintaining health and function. Although current physical activity and exercise guidelines recommend engaging in $\geq$150 minutes per week of moderate-intensity or $\geq$75 minutes per week of vigorous-intensity aerobic activity, or some combination of both moderate- and vigorous-intensity aerobic activity, and muscle strengthening activities that are of moderate or high intensity involving all major muscle groups should be performed at least 2 days per week,[2–4] almost one-quarter of the global

[a] Washington DC VA Medical Center, Integrative Health & Wellness (117), 50 Irving Street NW, Washington, DC 20422, USA; [b] Washington DC Veterans Affairs Medical Center, Research Service (151), Building 14, Room 1044, 50 Irving Street NW, Washington, DC 20422, USA; [c] Department of Health, Human Function, and Rehabilitation Sciences, School of Medicine and Health Sciences, The George Washington University, Washington, DC, USA; [d] Department of Rehabilitation Science, School of Health and Human Services, George Mason University, Fairfax, VA, USA; [e] Department of Veterans Affairs, 810 Vermont Ave NW, Office 975 BB, Washington DC 20420, USA
* Corresponding author.
E-mail address: Heather.Malecki@va.gov

Phys Med Rehabil Clin N Am 31 (2020) 649–663
https://doi.org/10.1016/j.pmr.2020.06.001
1047-9651/20Published by Elsevier Inc.

adult population does not meet these recommended physical activity guidelines for health, and rates of physical inactivity are even higher in people with disabilities.[4] Initiatives to promote physical activity in health care settings have been established to address the health and economic concerns associated with physical inactivity,[3–5] which has led to suggesting physical activity be viewed as a vital sign and monitored by health care providers.[6] In addition, integrative health models, such as the Whole Health System (WHS), introduced by the Veterans Health Administration (VHA), use a combination of complementary and integrative medicine for health promotion. These models emphasize shifting the plan of care from a disease management focus to a more personalized, proactive, and patient-driven approach to prioritize healthy lifestyle change.[7] Integrative Health Coaching (IHC) is an effective tool to affect behavior changes that promote physical activity and exercise and is an important component of Whole Health (WH). IHC is a modality that can assist patients to effect behavior change and achieve goals encompassing physical activity, exercise, and other areas of self-care and overall health. Health Coaching is defined as a process that empowers individuals to make lasting health behavior changes that are the cornerstones of lifelong well-being. It bridges the gap between medical recommendations and patients' abilities to successfully implement those recommendations into their life.[8] The belief behind IHC is that behavior changes are sustainable when linked to one's personal values and sense of purpose.[9]

IMPORTANCE OF PHYSICAL ACTIVITY AND EXERCISE IN SPECIFIC POPULATIONS

Insufficient levels of physical activity are a major public health concern.[5] Estimates of adult physical inactivity in the United States range from 17.3% to 47.7% with all states and territories having more than 15% of adults identified as physically inactive (**Fig. 1**).[10] In adults with disabilities, the level of physical inactivity is likely to be even greater than that of the general population. For example, 47.1% of adults with disabilities were reported to be physically inactive compared with 26.1% of adults without disabilities.[11] According to data from the 2017 Behavioral Risk Factor Surveillance System, only 45.2% of adults with mobility limitations reported engaging in aerobic activity, and 39.5% reported meeting one or both components of the physical activity guidelines.[12] From a rehabilitation perspective, low levels of physical activity are reported to negatively impact treatment adherence and thus potential treatment outcomes.[13]

Physical inactivity ranks fourth among leading risk factors for mortality, behind only high blood pressure, tobacco use, and high blood glucose.[14] Strong evidence supports excessive amounts of sedentary behavior as an increased risk for all-cause and cardiovascular disease mortality.[15] The economic burden of inadequate physical activity levels is substantial. It is estimated that physical inactivity accounts for greater than 11% of health care expenditures in the United States.[16] In 2013, conservative estimates found that international health care costs owing to physical inactivity amounted to $53.8 billion.[17] Given the health and economic impact of physical inactivity, several global initiatives have been organized to prioritize increases in physical activity levels through strategies including education, policy, technology, community design, health care, public health, and mass media efforts.[3–5,18]

Physical activity is defined as any bodily movement produced by skeletal muscle that requires energy expenditure.[2] Exercise refers to a type of physical activity consisting of planned, structured, and repetitive bodily movement done to improve and/or maintain one or more components of physical fitness.[2] Both physical activity and exercise are considered primary preventative measures against many chronic diseases.[1,19] A

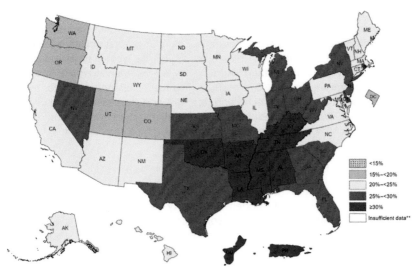

Fig. 1. Prevalence of self-reported physical inactivity among US adults by state and territory. Respondents were classified as physically inactive if they responded "no" to the following question: "During the past month, other than your regular job, did you participate in any physical activities or exercises such as running, calisthenics, golf, gardening, or walking for exercise?" ** Sample size <50 or the relative standard error (dividing the standard error by the prevalence) ≥30%. (*Courtesy of* Centers for Disease Control and Prevention, Atlanta, GA. Available at https://www.cdc.gov/physicalactivity/data/inactivity-prevalence-maps/index. html#overall. Accessed July 24, 2020.)

systematic review of 24 systematic reviews and metaanalyses found that physically active, older adults experienced reduced risk of all-cause and cardiovascular mortality, breast and prostate cancer, fractures, recurrent falls, activities of daily living disability and functional limitation, and cognitive decline, dementia, Alzheimer disease, and depression.[20] It was also reported that active older adults experience healthier aging trajectories, better quality of life, and improved cognitive functioning.[20]

THE ROLE OF HEALTH CARE PRACTITIONERS

Health care professionals represent a first line of defense to address the physical inactivity crisis. Despite the known benefits of physical activity, physical activity counseling by health care professionals is inconsistently implemented. For example, over the course of 12 months, 56% of adults aged 18 to 64 years with a disability who visited a health professional reported not receiving a recommendation for physical activity.[11] In addition, incorporating physical activity as part of routine health management has proven to be challenging because of a variety of factors. Time constraints during visits limit health care professionals' ability to incorporate physical activity counseling and assessment while attending to other health concerns.[18] Lack of incentive within the health care system for providers to counsel and educate patients on the importance of physical activity presents another barrier to implementation.[18] In addition, health care professionals may not feel confident in their ability to appropriately prescribe and counsel patients in physical activity because most medical schools do not offer physical activity–related courses.[18]

The Exercise Medicine initiative focuses on encouraging clinicians to evaluate patient physical activity levels during each clinic encounter, comparing each patient's current physical activity level with national physical activity guidelines, and providing counseling and/or referrals to each patient who does not meet the national guidelines.[18] Health care providers are encouraged to view physical activity as a vital sign (PVAS), similar to traditionally used vital signs, such as blood pressure and heart rate.[16] Initial attempts to understand the feasibility of implementing PVAS into practice has showed promising results. Grant and colleagues[21] observed greater exercise-related progress note documentation and referrals, and increased physician exercise counseling when PVAS was implemented. In addition, when incorporated into electronic medical records, PVAS has demonstrated good face and discriminant validity.[22]

EXERCISE PRESCRIPTION AND EVALUATION

Current physical activity and exercise guidelines recommend engaging in $\geq$150 minutes per week of moderate-intensity or $\geq$75 minutes per week of vigorous-intensity aerobic activity, or some combination of both moderate- and vigorous-intensity aerobic activity.[2–4] It is also recommended that adults perform 2 days per week of strengthening activities involving moderate to high intensities for all major muscle groups.[2] Physical activity guidelines proposed for people with disabilities do not differ from those of the general population.[3] In the case when a person with a disability is unable to meet the physical activity guidelines, it is recommended that they engage in regular physical activity according to their abilities in an attempt to minimize time spent being physically inactive.[3]

According to the Centers for Disease Control and Prevention, from 2008 to 2018 the number of adults engaging in leisure-time physical activity has increased in the United States.[23] Similarly, an increase in the number of adults meeting the minimum and high aerobic physical activity guidelines for moderate- or vigorous-intensity activity (minimum: 43.5% in 2008– to 54.2% in 2018; high: 28.4% in 2008 and 37.4% in 2018) and resistance exercise (21.9% in 2008 and 27.6% in 2018) has been observed.[23] However, when comparing exercise type, the percentage of adults meeting the resistance exercise guideline was lower than those meeting the aerobic activity guidelines (27.6% vs 54.2% in 2018).[23] Finally, the percentage of adults meeting guidelines for the combination of aerobic physical activity and resistance exercise also increased from 18.2% in 2008 to 24% in 2018.[23] Therefore, despite levels of physical inactivity still being a major health and economic concern globally, the number of adults meeting the existing physical activity recommendations seems to be trending in a positive direction.

The benefits of regular physical activity and/or exercise include improved cardiovascular and respiratory function, reductions in cardiovascular disease risk factors, and decreased morbidity and mortality.[2] The dose-response relationship indicates that additional health benefits are obtained with 300 minutes per week or more of moderate-intensity aerobic activity or 150 minutes per week or more of vigorous-intensity activity.[2] However, any amount of moderate- to vigorous-intensity physical activity is better than none, and beneficial health effects of physical activity are seen even when meeting a modest percentage of the recommended guidelines (ie, one-third of the guidelines).[24] Regular physical activity is also important for cardiovascular, neuromuscular, and cognitive health as well as physical function in people with disabilities.[3]

Examples of moderate-intensity aerobic activities include walking at a brisk pace (ie, 2.5miles per hour or faster), leisure time and sports (ie, swimming, doubles tennis, golf, dancing), active forms of yoga (ie, vinyasa or power yoga), water aquatics, and general yard work and home repair work.[2,3] Vigorous-intensity activities include jogging or running, hiking at steep grades, heavy yard work (ie, digging or shoveling), jumping rope, tennis (singles), and cycling faster than 10 miles per hour.[2,3] Strengthening activities describe any activity that overloads the neuromuscular system to promote increases in neuromuscular health.[2] Examples of such activities include weight machines, free weights, resistance tubing, body-weight activities, aquatic activities, tai chi, and yoga.[2,3]

RISKS AND CONTRAINDICATIONS TO EXERCISE

Although the benefits of engaging in physical activity and exercise far outweigh the risks, there are some potential risks that health care professionals should be aware of when prescribing physical activity and exercise to ensure patient safety, especially when working with at-risk populations. For example, acute cardiovascular events are more likely to be triggered in response to vigorous-intensity activity as opposed to light- to moderate-intensity activity.[2] In addition, when performing strengthening activities, there is an increased risk for musculoskeletal injury and soreness.[2] Therefore, physical activity intensity and volume should be progressed in accordance with the tolerability of the individual, avoiding large increases in workload.[2] Key guidelines for safe participation in physical activity are presented in **Box 1**.

Preparticipation health screening can identify individuals who should receive medical clearance before initiating an exercise program or increasing the frequency, intensity, and/or volume of their current program; individuals with clinically significant diseases who may benefit from participating in a medically supervised exercise program; and individuals with medical conditions that may require exclusion from exercise programs until those conditions are abated or controlled.[2] The American College of Sports Medicine has developed a screening algorithm that classifies individuals by those who do or do not currently participate in regular exercise.[2] Individuals are also classified by the presence or absence of known cardiovascular or metabolic diseases or those with signs or symptoms suggestive of cardiac, peripheral vascular, or cerebrovascular diseases, type 1 and type 2 diabetes mellitus, and renal diseases.[2] Once an individual's disease status has been determined, further screening is

---

Box 1
Key guidelines for safe physical activity

To do physical activity safely and reduce risk of injuries and other adverse events, people should
1. Understand the risks, yet be confident that physical activity can be safe for almost everyone.
2. Choose the types of physical activity that are appropriate for their current fitness level and health goals, because some activities are safer than others.
3. Increase physical activity gradually over time to meet key guidelines or health goals. Inactive people should "start low and go slow" by starting with lower-intensity activities and gradually increasing how often and how long activities are done.
4. Protect themselves by using appropriate gear and sports equipment, choosing safe environments, following rules and policies, and making sensible choices about when, where, and how to be active.
5. Be under the care of a health care provider if they have chronic conditions or symptoms. People with chronic conditions and symptoms can consult a health care professional or physical activity specialist about the types and amounts of activity for them.

Data from U.S. Department of Health and Human Services. *Physical Activity Guidelines for Americans*. 2nd ed. Washington, DC; 2018. Available at: https://health.gov/our-work/physical-activity/current-guidelines. Accessed June 17, 2020.

completed to identify the presence or absence of signs and symptoms suggestive of undiagnosed cardiovascular, metabolic, and renal diseases.[2] An appropriate plan of action can then be established based on the information obtained from the preparation screening. The plan of action may include determining which activities or exercise to engage in and the associated intensities; however, this can also include the incorporation of an integrative approach to lifestyle change, which includes physical activity and exercise as well as other essential elements required for maintaining and improving overall health and wellness.

THE WHOLE HEALTH SYSTEM

WH is defined as an approach to health care that empowers and equips people to take charge of their health and well-being and live life to the fullest; thus, WH shifts the provider/patient conversation toward "what matters to you" and away from the traditional approach of "what's the matter with you." The health team personalizes the patient experience by understanding the person's values, needs, and goals and incorporates them into a personalized health plan.[7] This approach allows the patient to be actively engaged in the decision-making process of developing a plan of action while establishing a trusting relationship with the health care professional, both of which are critical for maximizing adherence and the overall success of the intervention plan.[25] WH incorporates all aspects of clinical care, including prevention, treatment, conventional, and complementary approaches, resulting in care for the whole person.[8]

The Whole Health System of Care (WHSC) is composed of 3 major components, all centered on the person's Personal Health Plan (**Fig. 2**). The 3 components include Empower, Equip, and Treat.[8] *Empower* is also referred to as the pathway and takes advantage of peer support to work with patients and develop their personal health plan. *Equip* focuses on self-care and uses Complementary and Integrative Health (CIH) modalities, including health coaching and skill-building classes. *Treat* extends the principles of WH into clinical care and involves both outpatient and inpatient treatment. The goal of WH within clinical care is to partner with clinicians to determine the most appropriate plan of care for the person, including both conventional and CIH approaches, oriented around the person's goals.

COMPLEMENTARY AND INTEGRATIVE HEALTH MODALITIES

The WHSC has identified 8 evidence-based (**Fig. 3**) CIH services to support interconnected areas of self-care and patient goals. These CIH modalities include Acupuncture, Massage Therapy, Tai Chi/Qigong, Yoga, Meditation, Guided Imagery, Biofeedback, and Clinical Hypnosis. A wide body of research and evidence supports the use of these CIH approaches as adjuncts or alternative nonpharmacologic approaches to care, thereby providing health care providers with additional treatment options.[8,27] Examples of diagnoses supported by the use of these CIH approaches include anxiety, cardiovascular disease, depression, falls prevention, fibromyalgia, hypertension, insomnia, irritable bowel syndrome, low back pain, migraine, nausea and vomiting, obesity, pain including postoperative pain, posttraumatic stress disorder, substance use disorder, and tobacco dependence.[28–33]

THE CIRCLE OF HEALTH

Eight key components of self-care to support health and well-being are outlined in the Circle of Health (**Fig. 4**). Patients are encouraged to participate in evaluation of these

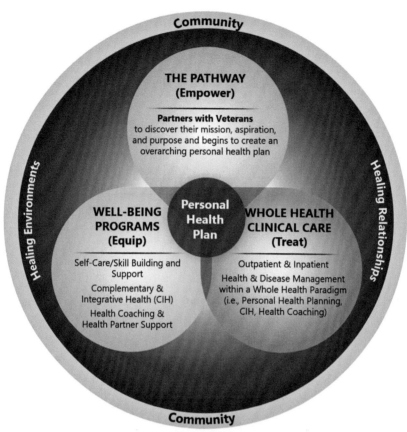

Fig. 2. The whole health system of care.[26] (*From* the U.S. Department of Veterans Affairs, Office of Patient Centered Care and Cultural Transformation; with permission.)

areas to formulate health goals based on strengths and perceived challenges. The components are supported by conventional and complementary approaches and include Moving the Body; Surroundings; Personal Development; Food and Drink; Recharge: Sleep and Refresh; Family, Friends, and Coworkers; Spirit and Soul, and Power of the Mind. The Circle of Health represents the interconnection between all areas of self-care and emphasizes the healing power of body and mind.[8]

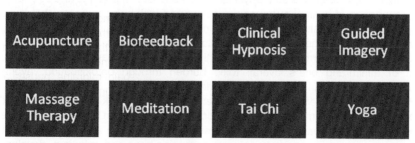

Fig. 3. Evidence-based CIH approaches offered at every Veterans Affairs Medical Center or to veterans through the community.[8] (*From* the U.S. Department of Veterans Affairs, Office of Patient Centered Care and Cultural Transformation; with permission.)

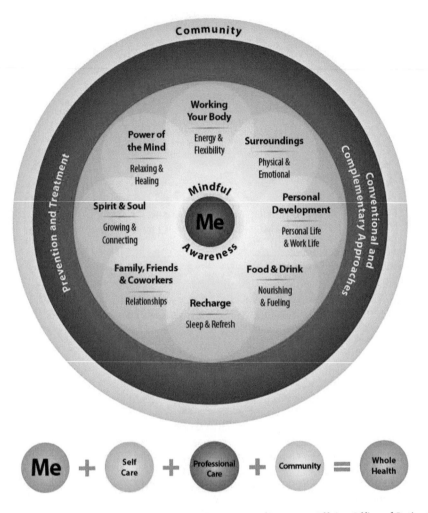

Fig. 4. The Circle of Health. (*From* the U.S. Department of Veterans Affairs, Office of Patient Centered Care and Cultural Transformation; with permission.)

Surroundings comprises both physical and emotional components and emphasizes the importance of healthy surroundings to support well-being in space that is safe, comfortable, and healthy. Surroundings may include home, work, neighborhood, emotional surroundings, climate and ecology, time in nature, and healing environments. Supporting surroundings in the clinical environment may include the component of minimizing one's overall toxic burden through detoxification, avoiding exposures, and focusing on healthy lifestyle choices.[26]

Personal Development includes both personal life and work life, emphasizing the importance of where time and energy are focused. The Passport to Whole Health identifies 14 essential areas of personal development, including Quality of Work Life, fostering resilience, improving happiness, cultivating hope and optimism, developing self-compassion, committing random acts of kindness, enhancing humor and laughter, building creativity, balance work and other areas of life, exploring lifelong learning, improving financial health, and practicing forgiveness and gratitude. Improving Quality of Work Life is particularly important for health care providers and other professions that experience a high risk of burnout and compassion fatigue.[26]

Food and Drink focuses on the impact of nutrition to nourish and strengthen, while impacting mood, energy, and physical health and performance. Nutrition-related choices are commonly included as goals using the health coaching model. Clinicians help with guiding patients toward appropriate, tailored nutrition plans. The component of food and drink comprehensively reviews macronutrient (carbohydrates, fats, and proteins) and micronutrient (vitamins and minerals) intake based on individual patient requirements. An anti-inflammatory diet, such as the Mediterranean diet, is commonly prescribed for rehabilitation patients with the intent of decreasing inflammation and related pain. The microbiome is included in the discussion about nutrition with a focus on the importance of a healthy microbiome for optimal health, and the role of prebiotics and probiotics.[26]

Recharge: Sleep and Refresh includes sleep, rest, and relaxation as critical components for physical, emotional, social, and mental functions. It is estimated that 30% of the American population experiences chronic insomnia.[26] This chronic lack of sleep has significant health implications, including increased risk of obesity, diabetes, hypertension, heart disease, stroke, impaired mood regulation, depression, and higher risk of suicidal ideation.[8] For example, sleeping less than 5 hours nightly is associated with a 152% increased risk of having a heart attack. As a component of WH, the focus is on improving sleep quantity and quality and using strategies to recharge, such as taking breaks. Recharge is an example of a self-care component integrally connected with several others, such as Moving the Body, Surroundings, Power of the Mind, Food and Drink, and Spirit and Soul.

Family, Friends, and Coworkers acknowledges the association of health and well-being with the strength of social connections. It emphasizes the importance of caring and supportive relationships in healing and maintaining health. The importance of healthy relationships goes beyond social connection. Studies show a significant impact of loneliness and poor social connection on the development of inflammation and chronic disease. Strong social connections have been associated with better surgical outcomes, decreased cancer recurrence, decreased depression, and improved hemoglobin A1c management. This component of self-care emphasizes the importance of the clinician relationship on patient outcomes.[26]

Spirit and Soul focuses on the importance of spirituality, meaning, and purpose. This component will be interpreted uniquely based on one's values and beliefs. Chaplains are well positioned to work with patients in exploring and developing spirit and soul skills, although these may be also be included as part of a health coaching plan when aligned with the patient's goals.[26]

Power of the Mind: Relaxing and Healing emphasizes the importance of mindfulness techniques on healing and coping. Mind-body approaches are used to enhance health and well-being; these may include psychotherapies, autogenic training, biofeedback, breathing exercises, clinical hypnosis, creative arts therapies, imagery, journaling, meditation, and progressive muscle relaxation. The collective purpose of these techniques is to move the patient out of sympathetic activation thereby positively impacting heart rate, blood pressure, stress hormone levels, and brain waves.[26] Many of these cost-effective techniques may be reproduced by patients to provide additional self-management strategies.

Moving the Body is an important area of engaged patient-driven self-care. Moving the Body focuses on energy and flexibility with the knowledge that exercise can improve mood, improve sleep, and increase one's sense of well-being. Examples of

Moving the Body may include yoga, tai chi/qigong, physical therapy, occupational therapy, recreation therapy, and general physical activity and exercise. A vast body of research supports physical activity for the prevention and treatment of multiple health conditions.[26] Moving the body is arguably one of the most impactful approaches to preventive health care with proven benefits of preventing or improving chronic health problems, reducing pain, facilitating better sleep, increasing lifespan, and decreasing symptoms of depression and anxiety.[26]

WHOLE HEALTH MODEL OF CARE RESEARCH

An evaluation of the WHSC by The Center for Evaluation Patient Centered Care (EPCC) in VHA suggests that there are significant patient and employee benefits to providing health care in this model, most notably a reduction of opioid use and pharmacy cost savings for patients using WH services. Recent evaluation of the WHSC found that veterans who used WH services demonstrated a threefold reduction in opioid use, with further reduction associated with increased use of services, compared with patients who did not use WH services.[34] Similarly, veterans with chronic pain who used increased WH services experienced larger decreases in opioid doses.[34] These data are critical for clinicians exploring alternate treatment methods to opioids and especially in the complex chronic pain population. In addition to patient impact, review of the data also suggests a significant positive impact for employees involved in the delivery of integrative health care. Employee benefits were greatest within primary care, mental health, rehabilitation, and home/community care. Employee satisfaction measures, including the Strategic Analytics for Improvement and Learning and the Survey of Healthcare Experiences of Patients, received higher ratings in facilities demonstrating higher employee WH involvement.[34] The EPCC report also demonstrated that greater employee improvement within WH also enhanced these ratings. WH care is good practice for patients, employees, and business. With its emphasis on personalized care and goal setting, the WH model naturally coalesces with traditional rehabilitative care.

INTEGRATIVE HEALTH COACHING

A challenging aspect of health care is promoting and successfully implementing behavior change, including in the areas of physical activity and exercise. IHC is an effective clinical tool used to set and support patient-driven goals, without judgment. A systematic review by Kivelä and colleagues[35] demonstrated significant improvements in adult patients' psychological, behavioral, psychological, and social life areas as a result of health coaching. The health coaching approach is designed to enhance motivation, accountability, self-awareness, and self-efficacy for the patient.[36] Health coaching is a proven, low-cost, low-risk, high-benefit intervention with significant potential positive implications on health factors. Multiple systematic reviews demonstrate that health coaching improves the management of chronic diseases.[35] Health coaching emerged from the concept of motivational interviewing and has been defined as the practice of health education and health promotion within a coaching context, to enhance the well-being of individuals, and to facilitate the achievement of their health-related goals.[34] IHC fits within the WH model of health care as a patient-centered, goal-oriented, and personalized modality.

Coaching Requirements and Certifications

Integrative health coaches work most effectively as part of an interdisciplinary patient care team and can be used in a variety of health settings. Health coaches partner with other clinical providers to support patient-centered, holistic care management. The principles of health coaching can be applied in a variety of health care settings to facilitate the achievement of health-related goals and behavior changes. Although certification is not a requirement, it is encouraged, and national board certification is available through organizations such as The National Board for Health and Wellness Coaching as a National Board-Certified Health and Wellness Coach.[37] Requirements for eligibility include completion from an approved training program, documentation of an associate's degree or higher in any field, and a written log of 50 health and wellness coaching sessions of at least 20 minutes in duration, and of which at least 75% of each session is devoted to coaching facilitation and not education.

Use of Health Coaching Tools to Achieve Goals

Health Coaches use specialized tools to promote and support behavior and lifestyle changes that impact health factors. These tools promote consistency and efficacy within the delivery of health coaching. Primary tools include the Personal Mission, Aspiration, and Purpose (MAP), Personal Health Inventory (PHI), and SMART Goals.[8] The MAP is the baseline tool that guides all recommendations and interventions based on the patients' input. Encouraging patients to identify their MAP for health care identifies what matters to them, thereby improving accuracy in establishing meaningful patient goals. The PHI (**Fig. 5**) is an assessment tool that is used to assess each of the 8 areas of self-care and informs the patient health plan. The PHI encourages patients to reflect on each area of self-care and identify strengths and opportunities for improvement within their own health and behavior. Health coaching goals are frequently linked to patient-driven motivations identified in the PHI. Health coaches create goals that are Specific, Measurable, Attainable, Relevant, and Time-Bound (SMART) in the health coaching relationship (**Fig. 6**). Goal setting is a key feature of an effective health coaching program. SMART goals are used to set goals, measure progress, and adjust goals and expectations as needed to encourage behavior changes and achievement of goals.

Outcomes of Integrative Health Coaching

IHC promotes patient-driven behavioral changes that support improved health and quality of life. Health coaching is shown to support body weight loss, increased physical activity, improvement in mental health status, improved medication adherence, improved social support, and improved physical health status, including HbA1c.[35,36] Telephone coaching is the most common delivery method; however, a combination of telephone, face-to-face, and Web-based coaching has been shown to yield good patient outcomes.[35] Olsen and Nesbitt[36] identified that key features of an effective health coaching program include the use of goal setting, collaboration with primary health care providers, and program durations of 6 to 12 months.

Impact on Rehabilitation

Incorporating IHC and other efforts to increase physical activity and exercise can have a significant impact on rehabilitation. The goal of all rehabilitation is to maximize an individual's overall level of independence and integration into the community, but extending the impact into the patient's home setting can be challenging because of the current health care system and reimbursement issues. Although rehabilitation has traditionally been a more patient-centered area of medicine because of its team-based approach, at times rehabilitation is very clinician focused with clinician-prioritized goals. Incorporation of Integrative Health Coaching and Whole Health is a unique opportunity to transition rehabilitation to be more patient-centric and to

Where You Are and Where You Would Like to Be

For each area below, consider "Where you are" and "Where you want to be." Write in a number between 1 (low) and 5 (high) that best represents where you are and where you want to be. You do not need to be a "5" in any of the areas now, nor even wish to be a "5" in the future.

Area of Self Care	Where I am Now (1-5)	Where I Want to Be (1-5)
Moving the Body: Our physical, mental, and emotional health are impacted by the amount and kind of movement we do. Moving the body can take many forms such as dancing, walking, gardening, yoga, and exercise.		
Recharge: Our bodies and minds must rest and recharge in order to optimize our health. Getting a good night's rest as well as recharging our mental and physical energy throughout the day are vital to well-being. Taking short breaks or doing something you enjoy or feels good for moments throughout the day are examples of ways to refresh.		
Food and Drink: What we eat and drink can have a huge effect on how we experience life, both physically and mentally. Energy, mood, weight, how long we live, and overall health are all impacted by what and how we choose to eat and drink.		
Personal Development: Our health is impacted by how we choose to spend our time. Aligning our work and personal activities with what really matters to us, or what brings us joy, can have a big effect on our health and outlook on life.		
Family, Friends, and Coworkers: Our relationships, including those with pets, have as significant an effect on our physical and emotional health as any other factor associated with well-being. Spending more time in relationships that "fuel" us and less in relationships that 'drain' us is one potential option. Improving our relationship skills or creating new relationships through community activities are other options to consider.		
Spirit and Soul: Connecting with something greater than ourselves may provide a sense of meaning and purpose, peace, or comfort. Connecting and aligning spiritually is very individual and may take the form of religious affiliation, connection to nature, or engaging in things like music or art.		
Surroundings: Our surroundings, both at work and where we live, indoors and out, can affect our health and outlook on life. Changes within our control, such as organizing, decluttering, adding a plant or artwork, can improve mood and health.		
Power of the Mind: Our thoughts are powerful and can affect our physical, mental, and emotional health. Changing our mindset can aid in healing and coping. Breathing techniques, guided imagery, Tai Chi, yoga, or gratitude can buffer the impact of stress and other emotions.		
Professional Care: "Prevention and Clinical Care" Staying up-to-date on prevention and understanding your health concerns, care options, treatment plan, and their role in your health.		

Fig. 5. PHI.[7,8,26] (*From* the U.S. Department of Veterans Affairs, Office of Patient Centered Care and Cultural Transformation; with permission.)

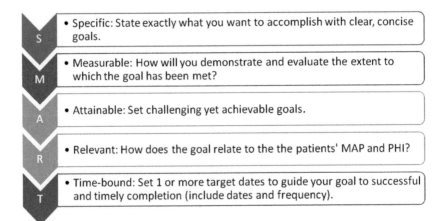

- S   • Specific: State exactly what you want to accomplish with clear, concise goals.
- M   • Measurable: How will you demonstrate and evaluate the extent to which the goal has been met?
- A   • Attainable: Set challenging yet achievable goals.
- R   • Relevant: How does the goal relate to the the patients' MAP and PHI?
- T   • Time-bound: Set 1 or more target dates to guide your goal to successful and timely completion (include dates and frequency).

Fig. 6. SMART goals.

increase patient's engagement in their rehabilitation plans. Using IHC can focus efforts toward meaningful goals and active engagement of the patient. Following inpatient rehabilitation, this can help ease the transition to home-based exercise programs and help build the individual's support system in the home setting. Studies have demonstrated poor compliance with home exercise recommendations, including less than half of patients in a sports medicine clinic completing recommended home exercises.[38] Following a course of skilled outpatient therapy, a more patient-centered approach with a more highly engaged patient will likely improve the impact of the skilled intervention.

SUMMARY

WH, physical activity, exercise, and IHC are all patient-centered, proactive approaches to achieving health outcomes. Rehabilitative specialists are well suited to practicing in a team-focused and goal-centered model. The WH model of care complements the rehabilitative process and provides additional tools to achieve patient goals. In addition to incorporating the MAP and PHI into clinical care, rehabilitative specialists may partner with integrative health coaches to achieve challenging behavior changes in the areas of physical activity and exercise.

CLINICS CARE POINTS

- Physical activity and exercise are primary preventative measures against many chronic diseases.
- Health care providers should view PVAS.
- Preparticipation health screening can be used to identify individuals who should receive medical clearance before initiating an exercise program or increasing the frequency, intensity, and/or volume of their current program.
- The WH model of care incorporates all aspects of care, including prevention, treatment, conventional, and complementary approaches resulting in care for the whole person.
- Health coaching supports body weight loss, increased physical activity, improvement in mental health status, improved medication adherence, improved social support, and improved physical health status, including HbA1c.
- IHC is an invaluable tool for clinicians seeking to achieve behavior changes for improved health, particularly in the areas of physical activity and exercise.
- IHC can effectively promote physical activity and exercise and is an important component of WH.

DISCLOSURE

None.

REFERENCES

1. Booth FW, Roberts CK, Laye MJ. Lack of exercise is a major cause of chronic diseases. In: Terjung R, editor. Comprehensive physiology. Hoboken (NJ): John Wiley & Sons, Inc.; 2012. p. c110025. https://doi.org/10.1002/cphy.c110025.
2. American College of Sports Medicine. ACSM's guidelines for exercise testing and prescription. 10th edition. Philadelphia: Wolters Kluwer; Department of Health and Human Services; 2018.
3. U.S. Department of Health and Human Services. Physical activity guidelines for Americans. 2nd edition. Washington [DC]: 2018.

4. World Health Organization. Global action plan on physical activity 2018-2030: more active people for a healthier world. Geneva (Switzerland): WHO; 2018.

5. Kraus WE, Bittner V, Appel L, et al. The National Physical Activity Plan: a call to action from the American Heart Association: a science advisory from the American Heart Association. Circulation 2015;131(21):1932–40.

6. Sallis RE, Matuszak JM, Baggish AL, et al. Call to action on making physical activity assessment and prescription a medical standard of care. Curr Sports Med Rep 2016;15(3):207–14.

7. Whole Health. Whole Health. Available at: http://www.va.gov/wholehealth/. Accessed July 24, 2020.

8. Whole Health Library. Advancing skills in the delivery of personalized, proactive, and patient-driven care. Available at: https://wholehealth.wisc.edu/. Accessed July 24, 2020.

9. Wolever RQ, Caldwell KL, Wakefield JP, et al. Integrative health coaching: an organizational case study. Explore (N Y) 2011;7(1):30–6.

10. Centers for Disease Control and Preventions. Adult physical inactivity prevalence maps. Physical activity. Available at: https://www.cdc.gov/physicalactivity/data/inactivity-prevalence-maps/index.html#overall. Accessed February 23, 2020.

11. Carroll DD, Courtney-Long EA, Stevens AC, et al. Vital signs: disability and physical activity–United States, 2009-2012. MMWR Morb Mortal Wkly Rep 2014; 63(18):407–13.

12. Hollis ND, Zhang QC, Cyrus AC, et al. Physical activity types among US adults with mobility disability, Behavioral Risk Factor Surveillance System, 2017. Disabil Health J 2020;100888. https://doi.org/10.1016/j.dhjo.2020.100888.

13. Jack K, McLean SM, Moffett JK, et al. Barriers to treatment adherence in physiotherapy outpatient clinics: a systematic review. Man Ther 2010;15(3):220–8.

14. World Health Organization, editor. Global health risks: mortality and burden of disease attributable to selected major risks. Geneva (Switzerland): World Health Organization; 2009.

15. Katzmarzyk PT, Powell KE, Jakicic JM, et al. Sedentary behavior and health: update from the 2018 physical activity guidelines advisory committee. Med Sci Sports Exerc 2019;51(6):1227–41.

16. Lobelo F, Rohm Young D, Sallis R, et al. Routine assessment and promotion of physical activity in healthcare settings: a scientific statement from the American Heart Association. Circulation 2018;137(18). https://doi.org/10.1161/CIR. 0000000000000559.

17. Ding D, Lawson KD, Kolbe-Alexander TL, et al. The economic burden of physical inactivity: a global analysis of major non-communicable diseases. Lancet 2016; 388(10051):1311–24.

18. Bowen PG, Mankowski RT, Harper SA, et al. Exercise is medicine as a vital sign: challenges and opportunities. Transl J Am Coll Sports Med 2019;4(1):1–7.

19. Pedersen BK, Saltin B. Exercise as medicine - evidence for prescribing exercise as therapy in 26 different chronic diseases. Scand J Med Sci Sports 2015; 25:1–72.

20. Cunningham C, O' Sullivan R, Caserotti P, et al. Consequences of physical inactivity in older adults: a systematic review of reviews and meta-analyses. Scand J Med Sci Sports 2020. https://doi.org/10.1111/sms.13616. sms.13616.

21. Grant RW, Schmittdiel JA, Neugebauer RS, et al. Exercise as a vital sign: a quasi-experimental analysis of a health system intervention to collect patient-reported exercise levels. J Gen Intern Med 2014;29(2):341–8.

22. Coleman KJ, Ngor E, Reynolds K, et al. Initial validation of an exercise "vital sign" in electronic medical records. Med Sci Sports Exerc 2012;44(11):2071–6.
23. Centers for Disease Control and Prevention. Trends in meeting the 2008 physical activity guidelines, 2008-2018. 2020. Available at: https://www.cdc.gov/physicalactivity/data/index.html. Accessed July 24, 2020.
24. Kraus WE, Powell KE, Haskell WL, et al. Physical activity, all-cause and cardiovascular mortality, and cardiovascular disease. Med Sci Sports Exerc 2019; 51(6):1270–81.
25. Martin LR, Williams SL, Haskard KB, et al. The challenge of patient adherence. Ther Clin Risk Manag 2005;1(3):189–99.
26. Rindfleisch A. Passport to whole health. vol. 3. Pacific Institute for Research & Evaluation with the University of Wisconsin - Madison; 2018.
27. Public law 114-198: comprehensive addiction and recovery act of 2016. Washington, DC: Sen. Whitehouse, Sheldon [D-RI]; 2016.
28. Rani Elwy A, Johnston JM, Bormann JE, et al. A systematic scoping review of complementary and alternative medicine mind and body practices to improve the health of veterans and military personnel. Med Care 2014;52:S70–82.
29. Nahin RL, Boineau R, Khalsa PS, et al. Evidence-based evaluation of complementary health approaches for pain management in the United States. Mayo Clin Proc 2016;91(9):1292–306.
30. Kearney DJ, McManus C, Malte CA, et al. Loving-kindness meditation and the broaden-and-build theory of positive emotions among veterans with posttraumatic stress disorder. Med Care 2014;52:S32–8.
31. Engel CC, Cordova EH, Benedek DM, et al. Randomized effectiveness trial of a brief course of acupuncture for posttraumatic stress disorder. Med Care 2014;52: S57–64.
32. van Dixhoorn J, White A. Relaxation therapy for rehabilitation and prevention in ischaemic heart disease: a systematic review and meta-analysis. Eur J Cardiovasc Prev Rehabil 2005;12(3):193–202.
33. Hayden JA, van Tulder MW, Tomlinson G. Systematic review: strategies for using exercise therapy to improve outcomes in chronic low back pain. Ann Intern Med 2005;142(9):776.
34. Bokhour BG, Hyde JK, Zeliadt S, et al. Whole Health System of Care Evaluation- A Progress Report on Outcomes of the WHS Pilot at 18 Flagship Sites. 2020. Veterans Health Administration, Center for Evaluating Patient-Centered Care in VA (EPCC-VA). Available at: https://www.va.gov/WHOLEHEALTH/professional-resources/clinician-tools/Evidence-Based-Research.asp.
35. Kivelä K, Elo S, Kyngäs H, et al. The effects of health coaching on adult patients with chronic diseases: a systematic review. Patient Educ Couns 2014;97(2): 147–57.
36. Olsen JM, Nesbitt BJ. Health coaching to improve healthy lifestyle behaviors: an integrative review. Am J Health Promot 2010;25(1):e1–12.
37. National Board for Health & Wellbeing Coaching. Available at: https://nbhwc.org. Accessed July 24, 2020.
38. Taylor AH, May S. Threat and coping appraisal as determinants of compliance with sports injury rehabilitation: an application of protection motivation theory. J Sports Sci 1996;14(6):471–82.

The Basics of Nutrition
A Primary Rehabilitation Intervention

David X. Cifu, MD[a,b,]*, William Carne, PhD[a,b], Hilary Pushkin, BA[a],
Isabelle Cifu, BA[c]

KEYWORDS

- Nutrition • Rehabilitation • Health maintenance • Diet

KEY POINTS

- Nutrition should be viewed as an active intervention to enhance rehabilitation programs and optimize long-term health maintenance for individuals with disability.
- Rehabilitation providers should have practical and actionable knowledge on the role of nutrition in the care of disability.
- Implementing and adopting basic, evidence-based nutritional approaches, such as a whole-food, plant-based 2000-calorie diet, to achieve long-term wellness should be prioritized rather than the use of fad diets, costly supplements, or other unsupported approaches.
- Individuals with disability and their families should learn and adopt healthy approaches to food shopping, meal preparation, and diet in order to optimize the impact of nutrition as a rehabilitation intervention.
- Extensive, readily available resources already exist to inform health care professionals and individuals with disability on the appropriate use of nutrition to enhance wellness and functional independence.

INTRODUCTION

Nutrition, the process by which a body nourishes itself through the transformation of food into energy and body tissues, is the most important factor in health maintenance, response to injury or illness, short-term and long-term rehabilitation, and longevity. It is also a key determinant of overall human health.[1–3] In a 2019 *Lancet* publication identifying causes of worldwide disease burden, an unhealthy diet was the top risk factor for the global burden of disease and was noted to require urgent attention.[4] However, most rehabilitation providers and the individuals they treat have limited training and knowledge on the basics of nutrition,[5] let alone as a rehabilitation, interventional, or

[a] Department of Physical PM&R, Virginia Commonwealth University School of Medicine, 1223 East Marshall Street, Richmond, VA 23298, USA; [b] Hunter Holmes McGuire Veterans Affairs Medical Center, Richmond, VA, USA; [c] Department of Anthropology, University of Virginia, 1223 East Marshall Street, Richmond, VA 23298, USA
* Corresponding author. Department of Physical PM&R, Virginia Commonwealth University School of Medicine, 1223 East Marshall Street, Richmond, VA 23298.
E-mail address: DCIFU@VCU.EDU

Phys Med Rehabil Clin N Am 31 (2020) 665–684
https://doi.org/10.1016/j.pmr.2020.07.001
1047-9651/20/© 2020 Elsevier Inc. All rights reserved.

even preventive tool, and much of what they think they know is based on pseudoscience, marketing (eg, diet of the month), and hearsay. Even the focus of the few clinicians and researchers with specialty expertise in nutrition seems to be on specialized and esoteric approaches to nutritional care, rather than on establishing a wholesome, lifelong nutrition plan that can be adjusted based on life events.[6–8] The term diet is being used to describe the sum total and type of food consumed by a person to maintain health and wellness. Importantly, the core diet that an individual maintains during rehabilitation plays a primary role in that person's ability to optimize the other key elements of care and lifestyle (ie, functional training, exercise, education, restorative sleep, stress management, social integration, health habits). During the critical phase of active rehabilitation, most health professionals' approaches to nutrition focus on adjusting supplemental factors (eg, novel approaches to hydration or micronutrients, perceived allergies, need for increased calories or protein, theoretic antiinflammatory characteristics) rather than the long-term benefits of a healthy and consistent baseline diet. Although there may be unique elements of rehabilitation care (eg, after extensive full-thickness burns, following polytrauma with open wounds and bony fractures, after a spinal cord injury, during a disorder of consciousness)[9–14] that will benefit from specialized additions to the standard diet for a period of time, in general, the overwhelming number of individuals undergoing rehabilitation care for a wide range of disabling conditions and injuries would benefit from a simple, core diet. This care would include hands-on training on how to achieve it (eg, healthful recipes, education on shopping, instruction on food preparation) and specific details on how patients can monitor their nutritional status (eg, pragmatic and disability-specific use of the body mass index [BMI]). This article outlines a practical, evidence-based nutritional approach to wellness, fitness, and optimal rehabilitative outcome that supports the fundamental knowledge of all rehabilitation providers and has applicability to all elements of care (eg, preventive, acute management, long-term sustenance).

OVERVIEW

Nutrition plays a vital role in people's maintenance, growth, reproduction, health maintenance, and response to disease and includes food intake, absorption, assimilation, biosynthesis, catabolism, and excretion. The diets of individuals are largely based on cultural and societal factors, perceived preferences, economic considerations, and availability. A healthy diet is influenced by the core choice of foodstuffs; the preparation and storage methods of the food; the timing, type, and quantity of food ingested; and the supplemental intake of additional nutritional elements. The healthiness of the diet can also be influenced by the foods or additives that are avoided or are used in significant moderation (eg, alcohol, salt, candy, processed foods). Importantly, although many people mistake dietary adjectives such as organic, genetically modified organism free, kosher, wild caught, cage free, free range, low sodium, gluten free, fat free, and sugar free with healthy or nutritious, in reality these terms are, at best, indicators of some degree of food cleanliness or purity in preparation rather than nutritional value, and at worst they are meaningless marketing terms. The most important elements, or the nouns, of nutrition that all clinicians must know and emphasize to their patients are understanding and achieving the basics of an individual's core diet (calories, balance of macronutrients, obtaining needed micronutrients, food preparation). Even the much discussed microbiome of the body, the normal microorganisms that live inside the gut and support digestion, the immune system, and brain health, is the direct result of a person's core diet and does not need additional supports (eg, prebiotics, probiotics, fermented cocktails) if balanced nutrition is maintained or is reestablished after illness. Only after a healthy, balanced core diet has been achieved in a sustainable way (ie, a diet the individual can afford, accept, and consistently follow) should the adjectives of food be discussed and applied to the nouns of diet.

Nutrition may be divided into macronutrients (chemical elements and compounds consumed in large quantities) and micronutrients (vitamins and minerals that support metabolism). The 7 major classes of nutrients are carbohydrates, fats, proteins, fiber, minerals, vitamins, and water, and these can be classified as either macronutrients or micronutrients. Although there are a range of common diet-related diseases related to nutritional scarcities seen in developing countries, including scurvy, kwashiorkor, beri-beri, marasmus, and blindness, there are also major diseases that are directly related to inappropriate diets and approaches to nutrition seen in the developed (or perhaps better known as overdeveloped) countries, such as obesity, metabolic syndrome, diabetes mellitus, cardiovascular disease, cerebrovascular disease, and osteoporosis. Diet and the direct effects of poor nutrition have also been repeatedly implicated as major factors in dementia and other neurodegenerative conditions.[15] In Dan Buettner's[16,17] approach to overall wellness, commonly known as the blue zones, he identifies a range of similarities in diet (ie, largely whole-food, plant-based diet focused on whole, unrefined, and unprocessed foods such as fruits, vegetables, whole grains, beans, legumes, nuts, and seeds) and other lifestyle elements (ie, stress management, life purpose, plant-based eating, socialization, family centric focus, activity mindedness, moderation, spirituality, healthy support network) among the oldest-living and healthiest cultures, including the importance of the approach to eating and dietary habits in these long-lived cultures. An example of one of them is the Okinawan term hara hachi bu, translated as, "Stop eating when you are 80% full." Although what is put on the plate is important, it is equally important in this clean-your-plate culture to recall the hara hachi bu philosophy that people should still be a little hungry when they push the plate away. In addition, individuals should be encouraged to eat intuitively, making food choices that honor their health and taste buds, while also making them feel good.

DIETARY COMPONENTS

An appropriate diet for individuals who are either in a health maintenance or an active program of rehabilitation includes 1500 to 2500 calories per day delivered via a balanced range of foodstuffs, optimally 40 to 50 g of protein, 250 to 300 g of carbohydrates with 35 to 45 g of fiber, and 60 to 70 g of fats, preferably in a whole-food, largely plant-based manner, made up of needed macronutrients and micronutrients. Macronutrients are composed of the elements carbon, hydrogen, nitrogen, oxygen, phosphorus, and sulfur, which make up the key compounds known as carbohydrates, proteins, and fats. Water and fiber are also key macronutrients that are necessary for optimal health. Certain minerals are required in large quantities and thus are also included in this category, including calcium, sodium, potassium, magnesium, and chloride. Micronutrients include minerals and vitamins that are needed in small amounts (eg, <100 mg/d) to support physiologic functions of metabolism.

Carbohydrates are compounds consisting of types of sugars and are classified according to their numbers of sugar units: monosaccharides (eg, glucose, fructose), disaccharides (eg, sucrose, lactose), oligosaccharides (ie, small chains of monosaccharides linked with lipids or amino acids), and polysaccharides (eg, glycogen, cellulose). Carbohydrates are a major energy source, are needed to build tissue structure, and have an energy content of 4 kcal/g. Healthy adults should consume approximately 250 to 300 g of carbohydrates (but <90 g of simple sugar) daily, and more than 97% of Americans exceed this amount. Importantly, when choosing carbohydrates, people should seek those with the highest complexity (ie, polysaccharides) and ones where the ratio of grams of carbohydrates to grams of dietary fiber is less than 5 (ie, The 5-to-1 fiber rule).[18]

Proteins are compounds consisting of amino acids joined by peptide bonds. The 9 essential amino acids are a subset that are made up of elements that must be supplied by the diet. Proteins are needed to build and maintain muscle mass and support the structure of the cells, and have an energy content of 4 kcal/g. Healthy adults should consume approximately 40 to 50 g of protein daily (ie, 10% of the daily dietary calories), and more than 97% of Americans, including vegetarians and vegans, exceed this amount. Importantly, all protein is initially produced by plants and fungi, and therefore all of the essential amino acids are found in plants. A whole-food (ie, nonprocessed), plant-based diet provides all of the amino acids and proteins needed for optimum health, without any cholesterol and with a lower proportion of fats than a meat-rich diet. Despite the familiar misbelief, soy, a common source of protein in Asian and vegan diets (eg, tofu, tempeh), has been repeatedly shown to have significant health benefits with no known risks (eg, cancer, heart disease, uterine fibroids).[19,20]

Fats are compounds consisting of a glycerin molecule with 3 fatty acids attached. These fatty acids may be classified as saturated (ie, they have single bonds in their structures) or unsaturated (ie, they have both single and double bonds in their structures). Essential fatty acids are a subset that have elements that must be supplied by the diet because they are not manufactured by the body. Fats are used for the construction and maintenance of cell structure, as an energy store, to maintain body temperature, and to sustain the health of the skin, and have an energy content of 9 kcal/g. Healthy adults should consume no more than 60 to 70 g of fats (<20 g saturated) daily, and more than 97% of Americans exceed this amount.

Fiber is a type of polysaccharide that is made up of parts of plant foods that cannot be digested by the body. Fiber is commonly classified as soluble or insoluble. Soluble fiber dissolves in water to form a gel-like material that assists with food absorption, including decreasing blood cholesterol and glucose levels. Insoluble fiber promotes the movement of material through the digestive system and increases stool bulk, thus it can be beneficial to people who struggle with constipation or irregular stools. Healthy adults should consume approximately 30 to 35 g of fiber daily, and less than 3% of all Americans consume this amount. Although the initiation of increased soluble and insoluble fiber into the diet is always followed by varying degrees of gastrointestinal issues or complaints (ie, bloating, gas, cramps) and an increase in bowel movements, individuals rapidly become accustomed to the needed increase and resume a regular, albeit greatly improved, pattern of gastrointestinal health.

Water is vital to the regulation of nearly all physiologic processes of the body and is essential to homeostasis and fluid regulation. Recommendations from European researchers, the Institute of Medicine, and the World Health Organization are that women should consume at least 240 mL (8 cups, or 8 US fluid ounces) of water from all sources (or at least 120 mL [4 cups] of actual water) and men 300 mL (10 cups) of water from all sources (or at least 180 mL [6 cups] of actual water) a day, assuming only moderate physical activity at moderate ambient temperatures. There are no specific benefits to enriched waters (eg, vitamin or mineral supplemented), juices (eg, electrolyte-containing energy and sport drinks), teas (eg, cleansing teas, hydrating teas), or other sources of hydration. These sources should be avoided because they predominantly contain an excess of simple sugars and physiologically meaningless trace electrolytes. The use of unsweetened teas and coffees has not been shown to significantly support or harm nutritional health and may be used as desired.

Mineral macronutrients, including calcium, sodium, potassium, magnesium, and chloride, are needed in significant quantities and help support various aspects of nutrition, building and maintaining body structures, regulation of fluid status, and physiologic properties. In general, American diets are deficient in calcium (1000 mg/d recommended) and potassium (4700 mg/d recommended) and supply a significant excess of sodium (2300 mg/d recommended). A daily calcium supplement (eg, a 1000-mg calcium carbonate antacid daily) is recommended for all individuals with a disability.

Mineral and vitamin micronutrients are organic compounds essential to the body that usually act as coenzymes or cofactors for various proteins in the body. Dietary minerals are generally 13 trace elements, salts, or ions, such as copper and iron, not synthesized by other living organisms. In general, American diets are deficient in iron and certain subtypes of vitamin B, and these may be easily addressed with a generic multivitamin supplement. Although vitamin D, a micronutrient readily made by the human body on exposure to as little as 15 minutes of sun daily, is frequently cited as a causal factor in a range of difficulties seen with rehabilitation, deficiencies are extremely rare (eg, in institutionalized individuals with no outdoor exposures), are easily overcome with simple multivitamin supplements, and are usually the result of inappropriate laboratory values or misperceptions. Although a well-balanced diet provides almost all needed micronutrients and macronutrients, it is highly recommended that all individuals, including those undergoing acute and chronic rehabilitation care, enhance their diets with a single, comprehensive vitamin and mineral supplement (eg, 1-a-day generic multivitamin/multimineral) and a calcium supplement (eg, a 1-g calcium carbonate antacid daily). There are no general (and nearly as few specific) indications for other supplements of minerals, vitamins, homeopathic agents, herbal agents, or other over-the-counter agents. Almost all ingredients in supplements are excreted in the urine and stool without supporting the nutrition of the individuals taking them, and should be avoided (supplements are discussed later and in **Table 1**).

TYPES OF DIETS

Although the term diet is often used to mean the time-limited, specific intake of nutrition for poor health or weight-management reasons, this more limited therapeutic definition is usually counterproductive to both short-term and long-term wellness and health, because these diets tend to have a negative connotation, are often significantly different from the individual's baseline intake, and are rarely maintained or successful for more than a few months. A more practical and effective approach is to understand diet as a lifestyle, or way of living, with an emphasis on the most appropriate nutritional intake for individuals over the course of their lifetimes, with specific modifications made based on an overall understanding of the ideal elements, needed alterations based on life events (eg, aging, injury, disease), and a mindset toward the recommendation of a stable and balanced diet and nurturing of healthy dietary habits. The Framingham Study, initiated in 1948, was the first population-wide investigation into a range of lifestyle factors (eg, diet, exercise, blood pressure control, medication use) performed in the modern era, and was the impetus for appreciating the major role that diet has in health and wellness.[21] Thousands of follow-up and additional large research studies have confirmed, expanded on, and clarified many of the findings, including examining the role of other lifestyle factors (eg, tobacco use, alcohol use, stress, sleep). Recently, the China Study[22] showed the serious health consequences

Table 1
Common supplements

Common Name	Scientific Name	Purported Mechanism/ Benefit	Evidence	Possible Side Effects	Economics
Echinacea	*Echinacea purpurea*	• Macrophage activation • Common cold resistance	Modest benefit reported by small methodically inadequate trials	• Allergic reaction • Autoimmune disorders • Interaction with conventional prescriptions	$300 million annually
Ginseng Dried root of *Panax ginseng*	Ginsenosides	• Targets multireceptor systems at the plasma membrane; enhanced nitric oxide synthesis in endothelium of lung, heart, and kidney and in the corpus cavernosum • Stress, fatigue, libido	Evidence limited by unregulated amount and type of ginseng; few double–blind RCTs available	• Possible interaction with warfarin • At higher doses, possible hypertension, gastrointestinal disturbances, insomnia, confusion, depression, and nervousness • Isolated reports of effect on neonates	$300 million annually
Fish oil	Omega-3 fatty acids Marine/plant derived	• Antithrombogenic Hypotriglyceridemia Antiatherosclerosis Antiinflammatory Relax endothelial • CHD • Psoriasis • Dry eye • Kidney disease • Rheumatic arthritis	Cochrane Review of 79 studies revealed little cardiac benefit Questionable: may retard IgA nephropathy	Some indication of adverse reactions in DM2 High doses: • Bleeding • GERD • HTN • Diarrhea • Vitamin A toxicity • Insomnia	$30 billion worldwide

		Uses/Claims	Evidence	Side effects	Market value
Ginkgo	Ginkgo biloba	Antioxidant • Depression/dementia • Anxiety • Heart health • Vision • Dementia • Headaches • Asthma/COPD • PMS	No RCT evidence of improved cognition healthy young people Cochrane Review showed inconsistent/no difference from placebo results for cognition, ADLs, mood	SDH case reported • Nausea • Diarrhea • Dizziness • Headaches • Stomach pain • Rash/allergic reaction	$1 billion in United States
Chondroitin/glucosamine	Chondroitin sulfate Glucosamine sulfate	Antioxidant • Osteoarthritis pain • Rheumatoid arthritis • Osteoporosis • Cataracts • Glaucoma • Bladder problems • CHD • High cholesterol level • TMJ	Inconsistent, modest effects on general OA, no support for spinal degeneration Possible benefit for knee OA but methodological limits	Rare: • Asthma exacerbation • Mild stomach pain/nausea • Bloating • Diarrhea • Constipation • Headache • Swollen eyelids • Leg swelling • Hair loss • Skin rash • Irregular heartbeat	$721 million
St John's wort	Hypericum perforatum	Inhibits uptake of various neurotransmitters • Depression • IBS • PMS	Mixed to inconclusive results; better than placebo in mild to moderate depression No head-to-head studies with SSRIs	Rare: • Nausea • Rash • Fatigue • Restlessness • Photosensitivity	>$200 million

(continued on next page)

Table 1
(continued)

Common Name	Scientific Name	Purported Mechanism/Benefit	Evidence	Possible Side Effects	Economics
Saw palmetto	*Serenoa repens*	• BPH • Chronic pelvic pain, decreased sex drive, migraine, hair loss	Some RCTs, but limited because of short duration, variable study design, different preparations, outcomes measurement Compared with finasteride, produces similar improvement in urinary symptoms and flow and associated with fewer adverse SEs	Mild gastrointestinal distress: infrequent	3594 metric tons used in United States annually
Green/black tea	*Camellia sinensis* Catechins (antioxidants)	• Anticancer • Cardiac health • Antiaging	Largely, observation studies; some controlled studies show reduced plasma serum amyloid alpha levels in subjects with metabolic syndrome	• Headache • Nervousness • Sleep problems • Vomiting • Diarrhea • Irritability • Irregular heartbeat • Tremor • Heartburn	14.4 billion liters (3.8 billion gallons) annually 84% of all tea is black, 15% is green

Abbreviations: ADLs, activities of daily living; BPH, benign prostatic hyperplasia; CHD, congestive heart disease; COPD, chronic obstructive pulmonary disease; DM2, diabetes mellitus type 2; GERD, gastroesophageal reflux disease; HTN, hypertension; IBS, irritable bowel syndrome; IgA, immunoglobulin A; OA, osteoarthritis; PMS, premenstrual syndrome; RCTs, randomized controlled trials; SDH, subdural hemorrhage; SEs, side effects; SSRIs, selective serotonin reuptake inhibitors; TMJ, temporomandibular joint.
Data from Refs.[23,35,36]

of a high consumption of proinflammatory foods, such as meat, dairy, and excessive fat and simple sugar (junk food) versus the low consumption of antiinflammatory plant foods, such as whole grains, vegetables, fruits, beans, split peas, chickpeas, and lentils. It was noted that the unnatural Western diet contributes to low-grade systemic inflammation, oxidative stress, tissue damage, and irritation, placing the immune system in an overactive state, a common denominator of conditions such as arthritis. However, despite the strength of these foundational research studies, few rehabilitation clinicians have used the knowledge gleaned in a practical and consistent manner. Similarly, most health care professionals either have limited insights on the specifics and importance of supporting their patients in developing an individualized diet, or are overwhelmed with the often contradictory recommendations of the many industry-supported dietary research publications, the challenges of the seemingly endless array of diets, food allergies, and supplements, or the growing complexities of their own medical practices. However, there are increasingly more balanced and reliable sources available in print and on the Web to help guide clinical providers and individuals with disability with both validated information on health effects and specific recipes and diet plans. Michael Greger[23] is a physician who provides nutritional information that is practical, evidence based, and consistent with a sustainable lifelong approach. Although most research supports the long-term benefits of a whole-food, plant-based diet for all individuals, including those undergoing acute and chronic rehabilitation interventions, it is important for practitioners to have a working knowledge of the diets that are most commonly described and used by individuals. As noted earlier, the goal of effective nutritional intervention is to establish a lifelong approach to diet and dietary habits that will support and enhance the other rehabilitation and lifestyle interventions used, thus there is no role for short-term diets; however, medical and/or disability-specific adjustments to the long-term diet may be appropriate. Specific diets are addressed in **Table 2**.[24–34]

SUPPLEMENTS

In general, dietary and herbal supplements contain ingredients such as vitamins, minerals, amino acids, herbs, and enzymes, and are sold as tablets, capsules, soft gels, gel caps, powders, and liquids. More than 1400 herbal supplements are available worldwide.[35] These herbal supplements have not been extensively scientifically studied, either with respect to effectiveness or adverse side effects. Only 10% are found in common foodstuffs, with the remaining not in the typical person's diet. Moreover, they are advertised as organic and with various benefits but no mention of possible side effects. In general, many people equate organic with natural/safe and may not be cognizant of or alert to side effects. Further, the US Food and Drug Administration is not authorized to review dietary supplement products for safety and effectiveness before they are marketed.[23,35] Dietary and herbal supplement manufacturers are therefore not motivated to conduct double-blinded randomized clinical trials, which are the standard with pharmaceutical manufacturers. Until dietary and herbal supplements are more thoroughly studied, caution should be encouraged. Even more importantly, patients should be regularly and consistently reminded to inform their physicians of all supplement use. Because of the tendency, promulgated by the supplement industry, to view these agents as benign, patients may forget to list them for their providers, exposing them to potential harmful medication interactions. Rehabilitation clinicians should encourage the individuals they treat to establish lifelong healthy diets and dietary habits to optimize nutrition, rather than considering the use of unproven, largely unneeded, and potentially risky supplements. Only after an

Table 2
Common diets

Common Name	Description	Consume	Eliminate	Benefits	Challenges
Vegan[24,27,28] (whole food/plant based)	Exclusively plant-based foods Excludes animal products and byproducts of any type	• Vegetables and fruits • Whole grains • Soy • Legumes and nuts • Plant-based dairy alternatives (nut-based milks, Daiya cheese substitutes) • Plant-based meat alternatives (tofu, Oumph, tempeh, seitan) • Sprouted or fermented plant foods	All animal products • Meat • Dairy • Poultry • Seafood • Fish • Eggs	Heart healthy Reduces inflammation and cholesterol level Improves blood sugar levels and kidney function Reduces risk of cancer, arthritis, dementia, Alzheimer disease Best diet for environmental sustainability Supports the ethical treatment of all species	Must supplement vitamin B$_{12}$ Must supplement calcium Although inexpensive, food preparation requires a period of transition and experience Alien to many and may provoke concerns
Mediterranean[31]	Foods that were eaten in the Mediterranean region during the nineteenth and twentieth centuries	• Vegetables, fruits, fish, whole grains, legumes, and olive oil • Limited poultry, eggs, cheese, and yogurt • Rarely consume meat	• Highly processed foods (meat included) • Sugar beverages • Added sugars • Refined grains and oils	Heart healthy Widely studied Many foods allowed, in moderation Meals prepared to enjoy and savor Easy to follow with many benefits	Less rigid and structured than most diets Healthy lifestyle more than simply a strict diet Excesses of unhealthy components is possible
Vegetarian[27,28] (lacto-ovo; dairy and eggs permitted)	Varying versions of meat-free eating • Lacto (no eggs) • Ovo (no dairy) • Pescatarian[a] (fish allowed) • Flexitarian[a] (most foods allowed)	• Vegetables • Fruit • Legumes • Nuts • Grains • Dairy • Eggs	• Meat • Poultry • Fish	May reduce risk of chronic disease Supports weight loss Better for the environment First step toward a vegan diet	Take a daily calcium supplement Dairy products (especially cheese) are high in fat and sodium Variants that include meats lose health benefits

DASH[24]	Vegetables, fruits, and low-fat dairy foods	• Fish • Poultry • Legumes • Small amounts of nuts and seeds a few times a week	• Whole grains • Fruit • Vegetables • Sodium • Low-fat dairy products	Reduction of blood pressure Heart healthy Reduces risk of multiple chronic conditions Improvements in mental health	Not food specific, more of an approach Particular about serving sizes of specific food groups
Diabetic[25,26]	Healthiest foods in moderate amounts Sticking to regular mealtimes Restricted fat and calories	• Vegetable • Fruit • Whole grains • Legumes such as beans and peas • Heart-healthy fish	• High-fat dairy products and animal proteins • Processed snacks • Baked goods • Sodium	Lower blood sugar levels Reduces risk of diabetic complications, cardiovascular diseases, and certain types of cancer	High risk of blood sugar level fluctuations if diet is not closely adhered to
Whole30[34]	30-d program designed to reset metabolism and reshape relationship with food	• Animal protein • Fruits • Vegetables (no peas, corn, lima beans) • Nuts and oils • Herbs/spices	• Soy • Dairy • Grains • Alcohol • Legumes • Processed foods • Added sugars	Gradually less strict after first month Antiinflammatory	Very specific lists of inclusions and exclusions to follow Not typically a long-term solution No available research to support claims
Paleo[29,32]	Whole, minimally processed foods Patterned after what human hunter-gatherer ancestors may have eaten	• Meat, fish, and eggs • Fruits and vegetables • Nuts and seeds • Herbs and spices • Certain oils • Wine and dark chocolate sparingly	• Processed foods • Dairy • Sugar • Grains • Legumes	Weight loss common (body is being starved of carbohydrates)	Increase in cholesterol intake Expensive Hunter-gatherer ancestors were likely largely vegetarian and tended to be short lived

(continued on next page)

Table 2
(continued)

Common Name	Description	Consume	Eliminate	Benefits	Challenges
Ketogenics[30,33]	High fat, normal protein, minimal carbohydrate Forces the body to burn fat rather than carbohydrates 80% fat 15% protein 5% carbohydrate	• Meat, bacon, sausage • Fish • Poultry • Cheese • Eggs • Butter and cream • Oils • Salt	• Fruits • Starch • Starchy vegetables • Legumes • Sweets • Most grains	Initially used for the treatment of epilepsy in children Lose weight quickly Challenging to remain on diet long term	Losing protein and water rather than body fat Weight improves but likely proinflammatory Increased cholesterol intake
Intermittent fasting/ calorie restricted[29]	Time-restricted feeding Alternate-day fasting 5:2 eating pattern Periodic fasting	Focus on when the eating occurs rather than what is being eaten Eating days unrestricted followed by hours/ days of fasting	Periods of time of eating (depending on the modification can be days or hours of restricted calories)	Lower cholesterol level, fasting glucose level, and blood pressure Decreases in levels of some inflammatory factors and thyroid hormones	More research is needed to its long-term effects

Abbreviation: DASH, Dietary Approaches to Stop Hypertension.

[a] Not vegetarian.

Data from Refs.[24-34]

individual has an established, long-term nutritional program in place should the use of any additional supplements be considered. See the commonly used supplements in **Table 1**.[36]

MONITORING NUTRITIONAL STATUS

The Health At Every Size (HAES) movement deemphasizes the specific weight of individuals and supports people of all sizes in addressing health directly by adopting healthy behaviors, including a wholesome diet. This inclusive movement recognizes that social characteristics, such as size, race, national origin, sexuality, gender, disability status, and other attributes, are assets, and acknowledges and challenges the structural and systemic forces that impinge on living well. The optimal approach to monitoring the nutritional status of individuals undergoing rehabilitation or on maintenance programs is to assess their dietary regimens (ie, diet, food preparation, food intake), monitor their weight (after establishing a healthy range), identify their urinary and bowel habits, and assess their overall state of wellness (eg, vital signs, sleep, pain, energy, mood). Although the BMI (weight [kilograms]/height2 [meters]) is a practical tool for many able-bodied individuals, with a healthy target being between 18.5 and 24.9, it does not necessarily measure body fat and has significant limitations in individuals who are wheelchair bound, have amputations, have muscle loss caused by paralysis, or are heavily muscled.[37,38] Waist/height ratio is superior to BMI or waist circumference alone in predicting body fat percentage and visceral fat mass, with a waist circumference that is less than half of the height being ideal. However, this measurement is also of limited validity in many disabled individuals. The mid–upper arm circumference may be a useful metric but is predominantly restricted to children. More exacting measurements can be taken via assessing the size of a range of skinfolds (peripheral and central) using calipers, but these may be impractical in a clinic setting. In short, the most practical approach for rehabilitation clinicians is to determine a baseline of overall wellness for individuals with disability that can be periodically monitored (preferably by the individuals themselves). This wellness baseline includes (1) a recommended weight that is within the BMI range (using the individual's premorbid height), (2) a recommended diet type and caloric intake (eg, 2000 calories), (3) an appropriate range of bowel and urinary habits, (4) a range of daily activity/exercise (eg, 4000–7000 steps or 3–6 km of travel distance per day), (5) a range of daily sleep and sleep quality (eg, 6–7 hours/night), and (6) a range of energy that allows the individuals to complete all of their needed functional and productivity (eg, work, leisure) activities.

DISABILITY-SPECIFIC ADJUSTMENTS TO NUTRITION

There are no physiologic or rehabilitation advantages to a diet high in carbohydrates (eg, so-called carbo loading) or fats (eg, ketogenic). The significantly increased risk of obesity, diabetes mellitus, hyperlipidemia, hypercholesterolemia, and metabolic syndrome of individuals with significant physical mobility restrictions supports advocating a low-carbohydrate and low-fat diet with no more than 250 to 300 mg/d and 40 to 60 mg/d for a 2000-calorie diet, respectively, for nearly all individuals with chronic disability. Even when the caloric needs of an individual may increase with the increased metabolic activities after acute illness or injury, the proportion of carbohydrates should remain no more than 40% to 50% and the proportion of fats should remain no more than 30% of the total caloric intake.[9–14] Rehabilitation clinicians should target at least 25% to 50% excess fiber (ie, 40–50 mg/d) in the diet of individuals with altered gastrointestinal motility as a result of their disability, advanced age, medication use, and decreased ambulation. Given the high prevalence of protein in the American diet, it is inappropriate to recommend a diet high in protein or the use of protein supplements for individuals during the chronic phases of rehabilitation. Individuals who are undergoing rehabilitation after significant acute physical impairment require a higher-calorie diet, with a proportional increase in protein of up to 15% to 20% of the total caloric intake, during the initial 4 to 12 weeks after injury or insult.[13,14] Similarly, individuals who are undergoing active rehabilitation interventions typically benefit from an increase in free-water uptake by up to 25%, unless they are on water restrictions because of renal or upper motor neuron–related bladder issues. There are countless products that are commonly being used or recommended under the general term of supplement, and these products should not be part of 99% of individuals' diets. At best, these are benign inexpensive products that make the individuals feel better psychologically and are then readily excreted by the body into the urine and stool. However, at worst, these are expensive and cleverly marketed products that do little for the individuals and may even cause significant harm if they convince the individuals to not consume a healthful and balanced diet or if they interact with therapeutically prescribed useful medications. Although it is notably easier to sip a tea, inhale incense, or swallow a glycerin pill than to purchase, prepare, and consume a balanced and nutritional diet, it is important for rehabilitation clinicians to make clear to these individuals that the core nutrition being consumed (ie, their diet) is the foundation for wellness and is of ultimate priority.

EDUCATION ON SHOPPING FOR, PREPARING, AND APPORTIONING FOOD

As important as an appreciation of the role that diet choice and related nutrition is, simply explaining the value of a healthy diet to an individual is unlikely to have significant impact. The analogy of the importance of using the most appropriate and highest-quality fuel to allow a race car to perform well may be more effective than talking about disease states. In addition to emphasizing the role that nutrition plays in the rehabilitation and health maintenance process, holistic rehabilitation professionals must also provide individuals with a disability (and their families) information, training, and resources on what is required to establish a healthy diet. A pictorial representation of the specific elements of the diet selected can be a useful tool. For individuals who have had limited formal training in the specifics of shopping for, preparing, and apportioning food in a healthy manner, simply identifying a diet or providing linkages to recipes may not be enough. In addition, there may be financial, cultural, religious, and logistical challenges that must be addressed. Although referral of individuals to a dietician may be helpful and an important step, it is equally important that rehabilitation clinicians work with disabled individuals and their families to ascertain obstacles, concerns, or unforeseen challenges that may arise once they have decided to modify their nutrition. Ideally, in addition to using a dietician to enhance the individual's practical knowledge, there should also be consideration to identifying both community (eg, therapeutic outing, home visit) and institutional (eg, therapy kitchen, meal preparation) services and facilities available to practice and implement the dietary decisions. The key skills include developing recipe and shopping lists, identifying accessible and appropriately stocked grocery stores, training on healthy diet preparation skills that are both functionally possible and produce palatable food, and learning the specifics of the portioning of the various foods of the diet. This requirement highlights the growing concern over food deserts: areas where access to healthy foods is geographically problematic. At present, 2.2% of the US population lives without a car and more than 1.6 km (1 mile) from a suitable grocery store. This issue is particularly heightened for the elderly and disabled and by the exodus of stores from urban centers. Even after the necessary knowledge and skills to obtain, prepare, and portion a healthy diet have been mastered, as with any acquired skill, there is always a need for intensive training, a role for periodic monitoring and reinforcement of skills, and a system in place to positively reward success. There are several easily accessible and practical resources available to provide healthy approaches to food preparation and recipes that should be made available by clinicians (**Figs. 1** and **2**).

MOTIVATION TO CHANGE

In addition to the specifics of nutrition, core diet, and disability-specific modifications, effective clinicians must also be cognizant of each individual's motivation to change. Nutritional deficits and excesses and poor health do not arise from 1 snack, 1 meal, or 1 day of eating. It is what is consumed consistently over time that matters, and an emphasis on progress, not perfection. A paradigm shift in the person's approach to food may be needed; eating to live, not living to eat. The focal point of life and socialization should not revolve solely around meals and eating; meals should not be about the food being consumed but the act of being together (eg, taking a walk with a friend may be a good alternative to sharing a midday snack).[16,17] The technique of motivational interviewing (MI)[39,40] has embedded within it an assessment of what stage the person is in and how to move the person to the action stage. This technique includes often helping people to identify barriers (eg, pros and cons, lack of factual knowledge, identifying intermediate reinforcers) to entering the action stage. MI also emphasizes partnering and collaborating with the individuals, rather than directing or forcing. The commonly identified stages of change[41,42] are precontemplation (unaware; no

Nutrition First Steps

Read: https://www.bluezones.com/books/

Register: https://nutritionfacts.org/register/

Watch: Forks Over Knives
                What The Health?

Recipes: https://www.bluezones.com/recipes/
                https://www.forksoverknives.com/recipes

Download: Dr. Greger's Daily Dozen APP

Consider: https://haescommunity.com/
                www.intuitiveeating.org

Fig. 1. Educational resources.

A Plateful of Wellness

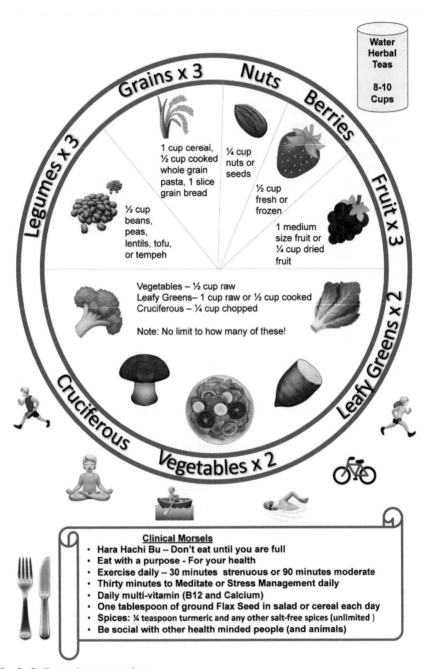

Water Herbal Teas

8-10 Cups

Grains x 3

Nuts

Berries

Legumes x 3

Fruit x 3

1 cup cereal, ½ cup cooked whole grain pasta, 1 slice grain bread

¼ cup nuts or seeds

½ cup fresh or frozen

½ cup beans, peas, lentils, tofu, or tempeh

1 medium size fruit or ¼ cup dried fruit

Vegetables – ½ cup raw
Leafy Greens– 1 cup raw or ½ cup cooked
Cruciferous – ¼ cup chopped

Note: No limit to how many of these!

Leafy Greens x 2

Cruciferous

Vegetables x 2

Clinical Morsels
- Hara Hachi Bu – Don't eat until you are full
- Eat with a purpose - For your health
- Exercise daily – 30 minutes strenuous or 90 minutes moderate
- Thirty minutes to Meditate or Stress Management daily
- Daily multi-vitamin (B12 and Calcium)
- One tablespoon of ground Flax Seed in salad or cereal each day
- Spices: ¼ teaspoon turmeric and any other salt-free spices (unlimited)
- Be social with other health minded people (and animals)

Fig. 2. Daily serving suggestions.

intention to take action within the next 6 months), contemplation (will start the healthy behavior within the next 6 months and recognize that the behavior may be problematic), preparation (ready to take action within the next 30 days, will start to take small steps toward the behavior change, and believe changing their behavior can lead to a healthier life), action (have changed behavior within the last 6 months and intend to keep moving forward with that behavior change), maintenance (have sustained the behavior change for >6 months and intend to maintain the behavior change going forward). In addition, the clinician's relationship with each individual is important. The individuals should trust the practitioner's knowledge and belief in the dietary changes being encouraged. It is also helpful if the practitioner has personally incorporated some of the changes and believes in the value of such changes. Given the amount of confusion that exists surrounding diet and nutrition, it often takes extensive discussion and time for information to be shared and plans of change formulated, which is rarely available in typical clinical settings. Identifying accessible and reliable resources to individuals is of vital importance. It is often difficult to give the time and attention to patient questions that is deserved. The complexity of these issues, the often-multimodal nature of these rehabilitation interventions (eg, diet, exercise, functional activity, restorative sleep), and the long time required to see many of the health benefits make these interventions challenging to fully implement and to be accepted. Although there may be a well-defined list of evidence-based lifestyle factors, including diet, that should be implemented to enhance rehabilitation outcomes, few individuals are motivated to make some, or even any, of these changes. In 1 study of dementias, Elwood and colleagues[43] found that, 30 years after study onset, less than 1% of all participants had followed all 5 recommended lifestyle factors, only 5% had followed 4, and 19% had followed 3. This finding is in spite of the fact that an estimated half of all dementia cases could be prevented by lifestyle modification.[15,44] In short, the effective adoption of modifiable lifestyle interventions depends on at least 2 factors: (1) a realistic assessment of individuals' ability to integrate these changes into their life patterns, and (2) the practitioner's relationship with the individual and ability to communicate the concepts.

SUMMARY

Nutrition should be viewed as a prioritized, active intervention to enhance rehabilitation programs and optimize long-term health maintenance for individuals with disability. Rehabilitation providers should have practical and actionable knowledge of the role of nutrition in the care of disability that is integrated into each patient's specific rehabilitation plan. Implementing and adopting basic, evidence-based nutritional approaches, such as a whole-food, plant-based, 2000-calorie diet, to achieve long-term wellness should be prioritized over the use of fad diets, costly supplements, or other unsupported approaches. Individuals with disability, together with their families, should learn and adopt healthy approaches to food shopping, meal preparation, and diet in order to optimize the impact of nutrition as a rehabilitation intervention. Extensive, readily available resources already exist to inform health care professionals and individuals with disability on the appropriate use of nutrition to enhance wellness and functional independence.

CLINICS CARE POINTS

- Although most individuals and clinicians desire to have improved nutrition as a part of their rehabilitation programs, common barriers include limited or inaccurate information, a temptation to use fad approaches, fiscal and logistical issues, and the belief that guidelines are not important during acute and chronic recovery.

- Nutritional interventions must be tailored to the cultural, personal, and physiologic needs of each individual to meet the individual's self-directed goals.
- Supporting individuals in implementing a whole-food, plant-based diet of 2000 calories in the acute and chronic rehabilitation stages after injury, insult, or disease is the primary nutritional intervention goal of rehabilitation clinicians.
- Information regarding nutrition must be holistic and include support in access to groceries, mindful recipe development, healthy food preparation, appropriate eating habits, adjusting to comorbid disease requirements, and a sensitivity to body image.
- Clinicians who are implementing nutritional interventions must be familiar with the use of MI and the stages of change: precontemplation, contemplation, preparation, action, and maintenance.

DISCLOSURE

The authors do not have any commercial or financial conflicts of interest or any funding sources.

REFERENCES

1. Micha R, Peñalvo JL, Cudhea F, et al. Association between dietary factors and mortality from heart disease, stroke, and type 2 diabetes in the United States. JAMA 2017;317:912, 912-924.
2. Ferlay J, Soerjomataram I, Dikshit R, et al. Cancer incidence and mortality worldwide: sources, methods and major patterns in GLOBOCAN 2012. Int J Cancer 2015;136:E359–86.
3. GBD 2015 Risk Factors Collaborators: Global, regional, and national comparative risk assessment of 79 behavioural, environmental and occupational, and metabolic risks or clusters of risks, 1990-2015: a systematic analysis for the Global Burden of Disease Study 2015. Lancet 2016;388:1659–724.
4. GBD 2017 Diet Collaborators: Health effects of dietary risks in 195 countries, 1990–2017: a systematic analysis for the Global Burden of Disease Study 2017. Lancet 2019;393(10184):1958–72.
5. Feinberg JL, Russell D, Mola A, et al. Developing an adapted cardiac rehabilitation training for home care clinicians: Patient perspectives, clinician knowledge, and curriculum overview. J Cardiopulm Rehabil Prev 2017;37(6):404–11.
6. Hicks K. Physician Nutrition Education Program (PNEP): survey and CME development to increase nutrition knowledge. Doctoral dissertation. College Station: Texas A & M University; 2017. Available at: http://hdl.handle.net/1969.1/165681.
7. Hicks K, Murano PS. Incorporation of online nutrition CME courses in state-level education libraries aid to improve physician knowledge. FASEB J 2017; 31(1suppl):957, 38.
8. Nyenhuis J. P209 Culinary medicine program improves physician resident's Nutrition knowledge and communication skills. J Nutr Educ Behav 2019; 51(7suppl):126–7.
9. Cork M. The role of nutrition in management of burns wounds. Deep Tissues: Wounds Australia newsletter. 2019. 11-14. Available at: https://search.informit.com.au/documentSummary. Accessed April 12, 2020.

10. Grangé C, Dépret F, Oueslati H, et al. Planned enteral nutrition over-prescription to cover caloric and protein requirements in severely-ill burn patients. Burns 2018;44(8):2106–7.

11. Chapple LS, Deane AM, Heyland DK, et al. Energy and protein deficits throughout hospitalization in patients admitted with a traumatic brain injury. Clin Nutr 2016;35(6):1315–22.

12. Kim H, Suh Y. Changes in the dysphagia and nutritional status of patients with brain injury. J Clin Nurs 2018;27:1581–8.

13. Silveira SL, Winter LL, Clark R, et al. Baseline dietary intake of individuals with spinal cord injury who are overweight or obese. J Acad Nutr Diet 2019;119(2):301–9.

14. Bigford G, Nash MS. Nutritional health considerations for persons with spinal cord injury. Top Spin Cord Inj Rehabil 2017;23(3):188–206.

15. Livingston G, Sommerlad A, Orgeta V, et al. Dementia prevention, intervention and care. Lancet 2017;390:2673–734.

16. Buettner D. The Blue Zones solution: eating and living like the world's healthiest people. Washington, DC: National Geographic Society; 2015.

17. Buettner D, Skemp S. Blue Zones: Lessons from the world's longest lived. Am J Lifestyle Med 2016;10(5):318–21.

18. Threapleton DE, Greenwood DC, Evans CE, et al. Dietary fibre intake and risk of cardiovascular disease: systematic review and meta-analysis. BMJ 2013;347: f6879.

19. Myung SK, Ju W, Choi H, et al. Soy intake and risk of endocrine-related gynaecological cancer: a meta-analysis. BJOG 2009;116:1697–705.

20. Ollberding NJ, Lim U, Wilkens LR, et al. Legume, soy, tofu, and isoflavone intake and endometrial cancer risk in postmenopausal women in the multiethnic cohort study. J Natl Cancer Inst 2012;104(1):67–76.

21. Hajar R. Framingham contribution to cardiovascular disease. Heart Views 2016; 17(2):78–81.

22. Campbell TC, Parpia B, Chen J. Diet, lifestyle, and the etiology of coronary artery disease: the Cornell China Study. Am J Cardiol 1998;82(10 Suppl2):18–21.

23. Greger M. How not to diet: the groundbreaking science of healthy, permanent weight loss. New York: Flatiron Books; 2019.

24. Appel LJ, Moore TJ, Obarzanek E, the Dash Collaborative Research Group. A clinical trial of the effects of dietary patterns on blood pressure. N Engl J Med 1997;336:1117–24.

25. Barnard ND, Cohen J, Jenkins DJA, et al. A low-fat vegan diet and a conventional diabetes diet in the treatment of type 2 diabetes: a randomized, controlled, 74-wk clinical trial. Am J Clin Nutr 2009;89(5):1588S–96S.

26. Choudhary P. Review of dietary recommendations for diabetes mellitus. Diabetes Res Clin Pract 2004;65(Suppl):S9–15.

27. Craig WJ. Health effects of vegan diets. Am J Clin Nutr 2009;89(5):1627S–33S.

28. Le LT, Sabaté J. Beyond meatless, the health effects of vegan diets: findings from the Adventist cohorts. Nutrition 2014;6(6):2131–47.

29. Obert J, Pearlman M, Obert L, et al. Popular weight loss strategies: A review of four weight loss strategies. Curr Gastroenterol Rep 2017;19:61.

30. Paoli A, Rubini A, Volek J, et al. Beyond weight loss: a review of the therapeutic uses of very-low-carbohydrate (ketogenic) diets. Eur J Clin Nutr 2013;67:789–96.

31. Sofi F, Cesari F, Abbate R, et al. Adherence to Mediterranean diet and health status: meta-analysis. BMJ 2008;337:a1344.

32. Tarantino G, Citro V, Finelli C. Hype or reality: Should patients with Metabolic Syndrome-related NAFLD be on the Hunter-Gatherer (Paleo) diet to decrease morbidity. J Gastrointestin Liver Dis 2015;24(3):359–68.

33. Westman EC, Mavropoulos J, Yancy WS, et al. A review of low-carbohydrate Ketogenic diets. Curr Atheroscler Rep 2003;5:476.

34. Available at: https://whole30.com/whole30-program-rules/. Accessed April 12, 2020.

35. Available at: https://www.fda.gov/food/buy-store-serve-safe-food/what-you-need-know-about-dietary-supplements. Accessed April 12, 2020.

36. Winterstein AP, Storrs CM. Herbal supplements: considerations for the athletic trainer. J Athl Train 2001;36(4):425–32.

37. Silveira S, Ledoux T, Robinson-Whelen S, et al. Methods for classifying obesity in spinal cord injury: a review. Spinal Cord 2017;55:812–7.

38. Yahiro AM, Wingo BC, Kunwor S, et al. Classification of obesity, cardiometabolic risk, and metabolic syndrome in adults with spinal cord injury. J Spinal Cord Med 2019. https://doi.org/10.1080/10790268.2018.1557864.

39. Brennan L. Does motivational interviewing improve retention or outcome in cognitive behaviour therapy for overweight and obese adolescents? Obes Res Clin Pract 2016;10(4):481–6.

40. Hardcastle SJ, Fortier M, Blake N, et al. Identifying content-based and relational techniques to change behaviour in motivational interviewing. Health Psychol Rev 2017;11(1):1–16.

41. Gersh E, Arnold C, Gibson SJ. The relationship between the readiness for change and clinical outcomes in response to multidisciplinary pain management. Pain Med 2011;12:165–72.

42. Şekerci YG, Kitiş Y. Effects of the stages of change model-based education and motivational interview on exercise behavior in diabetic women. Transl Behav Med 2019;9(2):256–65.

43. Elwood P, Galante J, Pickering J, et al. Healthy lifestyles reduce the incidence of chronic diseases and dementia: evidence from the caerphilly cohort study. PLOS One 2013;8(12):e81877.

44. Barnes DE, Byers AL, Gardner RC, et al. Association of mild traumatic brain injury with and without loss of consciousness with dementia in US military Veterans. JAMA Neurol 2018;75(9):1055–61.

The Use of Vitamins, Supplements, Herbs, and Essential Oils in Rehabilitation

Nathan D. Clements, MD[a], Brian Ryder Connolly, MD[a],
Madeline A. Dicks, DO[a], Rashmi S. Mullur, MD[b,*]

KEYWORDS

- Integrative medicine • Supplements • Herbal medicine • Herbs • Nutraceutical
- Essential oil

KEY POINTS

- It is critical for health care providers to understand the difference between micronutrient supplementation for therapeutic purposes and treatment and correction of a nutritional deficiency in patients with malnutrition syndromes.
- Micronutrient supplementation has been studied extensively in rehabilitation settings and has been shown to improve pain, bone density, falls, and biomarkers of inflammation.
- There is growing evidence to support the use of nutraceutical supplements in clinical rehabilitation, with improvements in muscle strength, decreased pain, and improved functional status.
- Evidence supporting the use of herbal supplements in clinical rehabilitation is small and larger clinical trials are warranted in this area, especially on the use of *Cannabis* and cannabinoid-related products.
- The topical use of essential (aromatic) oils may provide comfort and supportive care, but there is no current evidence on the use of these agents in therapeutic rehabilitation.

Dietary supplements represent a broad category of products taken orally that contain 1 or more ingredients, which include herbal, micronutrient, nutraceutical, and hormonal ingredients. The use of supplements and herbal remedies in integrative medicine can be challenging for both individuals and health care providers. Properly identifying and categorizing supplements is the key to demystifying the use of these products.

[a] Department of Rehabilitation Medicine, University of Texas Health Science Center at San Antonio, Mail Code 7798, 7703 Floyd Curl Drive, San Antonio, TX 78229-3900, USA;
[b] Department of Telehealth, David Geffen School of Medicine at UCLA, UCLA Integrative Medicine Collaborative, UCLA Health, 11301 Wilshire Boulevard, Los Angeles, CA 90073, USA
* Corresponding author.
E-mail address: rmullur@mednet.ucla.edu
Twitter: @rashmi2008 (R.S.M.)

Phys Med Rehabil Clin N Am 31 (2020) 685–697
https://doi.org/10.1016/j.pmr.2020.07.010
1047-9651/20/Published by Elsevier Inc.

pmr.theclinics.com

- A *nutraceutical* is a product isolated or purified from food that typically is used for medicinal and therapeutic purposes, such as polyunsaturated fatty acids (PUFAs) and carnitine.
- A *micronutrient* is a chemical element or substance that has been determined to be beneficial for normal growth and development and carries a recommended daily allowance, such as common vitamins and minerals.
- An *herbal supplement* is a plant-based product purified or extracted in different forms for therapeutic use, such as ginkgo and herbal tea blends.
- A *glandular supplement* or *hormonal supplement* is a compound created from animal or plant sources that contains 1 or more biologically active hormones, such as a bovine glandular supplement and bioidentical hormone.
- An *adaptogen* is a supplement that can augment the body's cellular response to stress. Adaptogens can be derived from plants (eg, herbs, such as ginseng, or certain mushroom species) and often have activity along immune and hormonal pathways.
- An *herbal compound*, typically used in traditional Chinese medicine and ayurvedic supplements, is sold as proprietary blends of herbs, micronutrients, nutraceuticals, and adaptogens.

Both individuals and health care professionals face several challenges when trying to discuss supplement use. The sheer number of available supplements, which has increased markedly over the past 2 decades, is overwhelming.[1] The paucity of controlled research trials on the potential benefits and harms of these products leaves a knowledge gap. Finally, understanding the role of drug-supplement interactions and the effect of supplements on laboratory assay interference remains unresolved.[2] Despite these challenges, it is important for the health care community to recognize that prior to modern medicine, cultures around the world used plant-based or herbal remedies for generations.[3] The therapeutic potential of plants is well established and knowledge of these benefits has resulted in several pharmaceutical treatments. It is critical, however, to also acknowledge that plant biochemistry is much more complex than a single active ingredient in a purified pharmaceutical product. Thus, it is naïve to view supplements as "natural drugs" and individuals should be counseled of this. Factors, such as diet, formulation, and the presence of various cofactors, can have an impact on bioavailability. Additionally, plants often contain several active ingredients and other biologic components that can interact with each other to enhance or augment therapeutic use; this phenomenon often is referred to as the *entourage effect*.[4] Importantly, basic nutritional support is an important therapeutic modality in individuals undergoing comprehensive rehabilitation, and up to half the people undergoing rehabilitation are malnourished.[5] Malnutrition is a predictor of adverse postacute rehabilitation outcomes, such as physical disability, falls, longer hospital stays, and lower quality of life.[6] It is important, therefore, to distinguish the repletion of essential micronutrients in malnourished patients from the use of supplements in patients whose baseline nutritional status is normal. This review focuses on the use of micronutrient supplementation and on role of medical nutrition therapy for patients with underlying dietary deficiencies.

MICRONUTRIENT SUPPLEMENTATION
Vitamin D

Vitamin D (calciferol) refers to vitamin D_2 (ergocalciferol) and vitamin D_3 (cholecalciferol). Both are produced from naturally occurring sterol precursors and are converted to 25-hydroxyvitamin D and 1,25-dihydroxyvitamin D. Because vitamin D can be formed in vivo in the presence of adequate amounts of ultraviolet light, it is more properly considered a hormone.[7] Dietary sources of vitamin D are clinically important because in some populations (eg, homebound and institutionalized) exposure to ultraviolet light may not be sufficient to maintain adequate production of vitamin D in the skin. The farther away from the equator, the shorter the period of the year during which the intensity of sunlight is sufficient to produce vitamin D_3.[8] Vitamin D is found in moderate to high concentrations in fish oils and fish liver and in lesser concentrations in eggs. Vitamin D is absorbed from the diet in the small intestine with the help of bile salts. Drugs that bind bile salts, such as colestipol and various malabsorption syndromes, reduce vitamin D absorption. Vitamin D promotes calcium absorption in the gut and, in conjunction with parathyroid hormone, maintains appropriate serum calcium and phosphate levels, allowing for normal bone mineralization, growth, and remodeling. Vitamin D deficiency can cause rickets in children and precipitates bone loss and fractures in adults. A circulating level of 25-hydroxyvitamin D of greater than 75 nmol/L, or 30 ng/mL, is required to maximize vitamin D's beneficial effects for health.[9]

Data on the use of vitamin D supplementation in rehabilitation is as follows: patients with suboptimal vitamin D levels can present with chronic musculoskeletal pain, and adequate treatment with vitamin D produced an increase in muscle strength and a marked decrease in back and lower limb pain within 6 months.[10] Vitamin D deficiency is a common occurrence in long-term stroke survivors that often leads to reduction in bone mineral density, altered calcium homeostasis, and an increase in hip fractures.[11] Vitamin D supplementation may provide several health benefits in poststroke patients, such as conserving bone, restoring muscle strength, and reducing falls.[12] Bischoff and colleagues[13] showed that vitamin D and calcium supplementation over a 3-month period reduced the risk of falling by 49% in elderly women. A meta-analysis conducted by Muir and Montero-Odasso[14] demonstrated that vitamin D supplementation improves muscle strength and body balance. Vitamin D has been established as a factor in the prevention of stress fractures, improving walking distance and decreasing general discomfort.[8] There is comprehensive evidence from epidemiologic, observational, and experimental studies that vitamin D may be beneficial in multiple sclerosis (MS). Vitamin D supplementation has been shown to reduce annual relapse rates in those who were supplemented.[15]

Vitamin A

Vitamin A refers to a group of organic compounds that includes retinol, retinal, retinoic acid, and several provitamin A carotenoids. It is absorbed in the diet via 2 main sources: β-carotene, which is found in plant-based sources, and retinol, including retinyl esters, which are found in animal tissues. Once absorbed, vitamin A is stored in the liver and adipose tissue as retinyl esters. Retinol, bound to retinol binding protein (RBP), is transported through the body, where it is oxidized to the activated form, retinoic acid, which is responsible for the neuroimmunological functions of this micronutrient. Vitamin A is a crucial component diverse biological functions, including reproduction, embryologic development, cellular differentiation, growth, immunity, and vision.[16] Vitamin A functions mostly through nuclear retinoic acid receptors, retinoid X receptors, and peroxisome proliferator-activated receptors and exerts significant cross-talk with other nuclear hormone pathways, including vitamin D. Vitamin A has been shown to be important for the maintenance of the immune system, wound healing, and vision.

Data on the use of vitamin A supplementation in rehabilitation is as follows: vitamin A supplementation has been shown as effective adjuvant therapy in supporting voice rehabilitation in patients with muscle tension dysphonia.[17] Emerging animal data suggest that treatment with retinoic acid stimulated alveolar formation and reversed emphysema in rat lungs. More research needs to be performed to determine whether retinoic acid could improve lung function in individuals with lung disease. Vitamin A has been studied extensively for its immunomodulatory role in MS and thought to have a dual role in both decreasing inflammation and increases tolerance of autoimmunity. Salzer and colleagues[18] evaluated RBP levels in prospectively collected biobank blood samples from MS cases and controls and concluded that suboptimal vitamin A levels may be associated with MS risk. A cohort study of 88 relapsing-remitting MS patients, followed prospectively for 24 months, revealed that higher serum retinol levels reduced the odds of developing new T1 gadolinium-enhanced lesions.[19]

Vitamin E

Vitamin E is the collective term given to a group of fat-soluble compounds that have distinct antioxidant activities essential for health. There are 8 naturally occurring forms of vitamin E, but α-tocopherols and γ-tocopherols are found in the highest concentration in the serum and red blood cells and are the most common forms of the vitamin used in supplementation. Vitamin E functions as an antioxidant by scavenging free radicals produced during lipid peroxidation.[20] Additionally, several tocopherol isoforms also influence immune function, cellular signaling, and cholesterol metabolism. As a result, vitamin E has been reported to have preventive effects against cardiovascular disease as well as a rationale for providing benefit for the treatment of Alzheimer disease. Nevertheless, randomized trials have found limited and inconsistent evidence of vitamin E supplementation as an effective clinical intervention for either disease process. Thus, despite a strong rationale in support of a beneficial role for vitamin E for therapeutic supplementation, evidence supporting clinical use inconclusive.[21,22]

Data on the use of vitamin E supplementation in rehabilitation is as follows: None available.

Vitamin K

Vitamin K exists naturally as vitamin K_1 (phylloquinone), found in green, leafy vegetables, and vitamin K_2 (menaquinone), found in small amounts in chicken, butter, egg yolks, and cheese. Vitamin K plays a role in the post-translational modification of proteins and also functions as a coenzyme to carboxylate glutamic acid residues in the production of vitamin K–dependent proteins, including coagulation factors, osteocalcin (a bone-forming protein), and matrix Gla protein, an anticalcification protein.[23] Although there are some data that support that use of vitamin K_2 supplementation in reducing hip, vertebral, and all nonvertebral fractures in postmenopausal women, several studies published in this area have since been retracted.[24] The benefit of vitamin K on bone is thought to be unrelated to increasing bone mineral density but rather to increasing bone strength.[25]

Data on the use of vitamin K supplementation in rehabilitation is as follows: none available.

Vitamin C

Vitamin C, or L-ascorbic acid, is a water-soluble vitamin that is obtained from a variety of food sources (eg, citrus fruits, tomatoes, potatoes, broccoli, and strawberries). It is required for the biosynthesis of collagen, L-carnitine and certain hormones.[26] In its role as an essential cofactor for collagen cross-linking, vitamin C is a key determinant of ligament, tendon, and bone quality. Data from the US National Health and Nutrition Examination Survey, 2003 to 2004, reveals suboptimal serum vitamin C concentrations were associated with the prevalence of neck pain, low back pain, and self-reported diagnosis of arthritis/rheumatism.[27] Vitamin C supplementation attenuates the oxidative stress and inflammation after a single bout of exercise.[28]

Data on the use of vitamin C supplementation in rehabilitation is as follows: preclinical animal data suggest that vitamin C supplementation may have stimulating effects on the recovery from Achilles tendon rupture.[29] Rabadi and Kristal[30] evaluated the use of vitamin C supplementation on functional recovery after stroke but found no significant benefit from supplementation on cognitive or motor impairment.

B-complex Vitamins

The B-complex vitamins are a group of water-soluble vitamins, including thiamine (vitamin B_1), riboflavin (vitamin B_2), niacin (vitamin B_3), pantothenic acid (vitamin B_5), pyridoxine (vitamin B_6), biotin (B_7), folate (vitamin B_9), and cobalamin (vitamin B_{12}). They are obtained from a variety of food sources and function as cofactors in energy-producing pathways. A diet rich in B-group vitamins is essential for optimal function, and B-vitamin deficiency is associated with higher levels of neural inflammation and oxidative stress and is marked by increased blood plasma homocysteine. Vitamin B_{12} deficiency also is a well-known cause of diabetic peripheral neuropathy and is associated with long-term metformin use. Preliminary evidence suggests that high-dose B-vitamin supplementation can reduce oxidative stress as measured by proton magnetic spectroscopy.[31]

Data on the use of B-vitamin supplementation in rehabilitation is as follows: Paulin and colleagues[32] demonstrated that vitamin B_{12} supplementation appears to improve exercise tolerance in participants with chronic obstructive pulmonary disease (COPD) undergoing pulmonary rehabilitation. Supplementation with thiamine supplementation has been shown to increase left ventricular function and improve functional status during a walk test in patients with chronic heart failure.[33] B-complex supplementation also has been shown to decrease the long-term risk of depression in poststroke patients.[34]

NUTRACEUTICAL SUPPLEMENTATION
Branched-Chain Amino Acids

Branched-chain amino acids (BCAAs), including leucine, isoleucine, and valine, modulate several key processes of energy homeostasis, nutrition metabolism, gut health, and immunity. BCAAs are substrates for synthesis of nitrogenous compounds and regulate glucose and lipid metabolism via activation of the phosphoinositide 3-kinase/protein kinase B/mammalian target of rapamycin (PI3K/AKT/mTOR) signaling pathway.[35]

Data on the use of BCAA supplementation in rehabilitation is as follows: a randomized controlled study of 68 patients revealed that supplementation with BCAA and vitamin D combined with low-intensity resistance training improves muscle-related outcomes in sarcopenic older adults undergoing hospital-based rehabilitation. It is not possible to conclude to what extent BCAA has an impact on the primary endpoint.[36] BCAA supplementation combined with muscle-strengthening exercises resulted in significant improvement in hip abductor muscle strength and knee extension strength of the contralateral side in elderly women recovering from total hip arthroplasty.[37] A small study of 40 participants with traumatic brain injury (TBI) and 20 healthy controls matched for age, sex, and sedentary lifestyle showed that supplementation with BCAA improved disability rating scale 15 days after admission to the rehabilitation department.[38] Larger trials and meta-analysis have shown that the efficacy of BCAA supplementation has been limited to patients with severe TBI.[39]

Polyunsaturated Fatty Acids

PUFAs are a type of dietary fat found in several food sources, including salmon, vegetable oils, nuts, and seeds, which have been shown to have several health benefits. Specifically, omega-3 PUFAs play an important role in the prevention of atherosclerosis, improvement of circulating triglyceride levels, and decrease platelet aggregation.[40] Omega-3 PUFAs have been shown to reduce the risk of developing arrhythmia, reduce triglycerides, and help lower blood pressure. High-dose omega-3 PUFA supplementation can increase risk of bleeding risk and gastrointestinal distress.

Data on the use of omega-3 PUFA supplementation in rehabilitation is as follows: King and colleagues[41] demonstrated that omega-3 PUFAs improve neurorecovery after acute spinal cord injury in adult rats, whereas omega-6 PUFAs have a damaging effect and worsen outcomes. Omega-3 fatty acid supplementation does not have an impact on on the chronic inflammation associated with spinal cord injury.[42] Preclinical studies suggest that omega-3 PUFA supplementation can improve brain remodeling, including generation of immature neurons, microvessels, and oligodendrocytes, and could be developed as a potential therapy to treat TBI victims in the clinic.[43]

α-Lipoic Acid

α-Lipoic acid (α-LA) is an organosulfur compound found in plants, animals, and humans that acts as a cofactor for the enzymatic reactions of oxidative metabolism. It has been shown to be an effective treatment of pain associated with diabetic peripheral neuropathy. Additionally, it has been associated with improved functional status in patients with progressive MS.[44]

Data on the use of α-LA supplementation in rehabilitation is as follows: α-LA supplementation has been studied extensively in poststroke management. Several studies have demonstrated that its antioxidant properties are neuroprotective and promote functional recovery after ischemic stroke by attenuating oxidative damage.[45,46] α-LA supplementation in combination with rehabilitation therapy improved neuropathic symptoms and deficits in patients with chronic back pain and radicular neuropathy.[47] A study of 98 patients with chronic low back pain treated for 60 days with 600-mg α-LA and superoxide dismutase showed an improvement in perceived pain, functional status, and decreased the use of analgesics.[48]

Coenzyme Q10/Ubiquinol

Coenzyme (Co) Q10, or ubiquinol, is a compound that is produced naturally in the human body, where it is stored within mitochondria. There, it acts as an antioxidant and is involved in the production of adenosine triphosphate. It can be found in foods, such as pork, beef, chicken organ meats, fatty fish, oranges, strawberries, spinach, broccoli, soybeans, lentils, soybean, and canola oil.

Data on the use of CoQ10 supplementation in rehabilitation is as follows: long-term CoQ10 supplementation in patients with chronic heart failure is safe, improves symptoms, and reduces major adverse cardiovascular events. It is considered a potential supplement for patients with heart failure undergoing cardiac rehabilitation.[49] Another study demonstrated that the oral administration of CoQ10, at 90 mg/d for 8 weeks, improved hypoxemia at rest, decreased heart rate, increased Pao_2 during exercise, and improved exercise performance in patients with COPD, suggesting that CoQ10 supplementation could be considered in patients undergoing pulmonary rehabilitation.[50]

HERBAL SUPPLEMENTATION
Cannabis

For more than 3000 years, *Cannabis,* a genus of plants comprising marijuana and hemp plants, has been used in ayurvedic medicine in India for a wide variety of ailments. In the early nineteenth century, Indian hemp was introduced to the Western world, where it was recognized for its ability to treat symptoms, such as muscle spasms, pain, and seizures. Nevertheless, *Cannabis,* in its many forms, has drawn intense scrutiny since its arrival in the United States, partially due to its psychoactive nature. Its use within Western medicine, although controversial, has been increasingly popular over the past few decades. More than 400 distinct chemicals have been extracted from *Cannabis* plants.[51] A group of more than 60 of these chemicals— known as the cannabinoids—are unique to *Cannabis* plants themselves. The term, *medical marijuana*, refers to the group of cannabinoids used to treat disease or improve symptoms. The 2 most well-known cannabinoids are cannabidiol (CBD) and tetrahydrocannabinol (THC).

CBD can be put into oils, tinctures, gummies, candies, beverages, or vaporized oil. Although there is not enough research to prove its efficacy on many of the conditions it is purported to treat, it commonly is used to treat conditions, such as pain, anxiety, seizures, inflammation, and nausea. It is not believed to have a psychoactive effect on the user. Currently, there are no established guidelines regarding dosing or delivery for treatment of medical conditions, as there are for classic prescription medications. Unlike CBD, which often is taken as an isolated extract, THC is taken more frequently with other compounds in its whole flower state and is known to have psychoactive properties. Its legality and methods to regulate its use vary widely throughout the United States. Further studies are needed to examine its potential for therapeutic use, but it is purported to treat many of the same conditions as CBD.

Data on the use of *Cannabis* and cannabinoid supplementation in rehabilitation is as follows: 1 study demonstrated that THC decreased the spasticity sum score in patients with spinal cord injuries. A minimum of 15 mg per day to 20 mg per day was required to have therapeutic effect.[52] CBD has been shown to reduce stroke injury in animal studies.[53] A survey taken in the United States found that 66% of CBD users believed CBD controlled their pain better than prescription medications, 54% of respondents used CBD for joint pain, 35% used it for muscle tension with cluster headaches, and 32% used it for chronic pain.[54] A survey consisting of *Cannabis* users in Colorado found that among individuals with TBIs, *Cannabis* most likely is to be used for recreation (67%), stress relief (62.5%), and as a sleep aid (59%). Among individuals with a spinal cord injury, the most common uses are to reduce spasticity (70%), for recreation (63%), and to improve sleep (55%). Smoking was the most common method used.[55] *Cannabis* should be used with caution in those with spinal cord injuries because evidence shows that they are disproportionately at risk for *Cannabis* use disorder.[56]

Ashwagandha

Withania somnifera, commonly known as ashwagandha or winter cherry due to its red fruit, is a shrub cultivated in India, Nepal, and China. For centuries, its root powder has been used in traditional Indian medicine as a stress-reducing agent. Although not commonly used in rehabilitation medicine, there is evidence to suggest that it may have utility in the rehabilitation process after brain injuries, muscle debility, and stroke.

Data on the use of ashwagandha supplementation in rehabilitation is as follows: a randomized, prospective, double-blind, placebo-controlled clinical study demonstrated that ashwagandha supplementation improved muscle strength on the bench-press exercise and leg extension exercise compared with placebo.[57] Ashwagandha has been shown to suppress the effects of sleep loss on learning and memory impairments, suggesting that supplementation may have a neuroprotective effect.[58] Supplementation with *W somnifera* was demonstrated to ameliorate neurodegeneration and memory impairment after hypobaric hypoxia in rats.[59]

Rhodiola

Rhodiola rosea, also known as golden or arctic root, is a perennial flowering plant that has been used in traditional medicine in Chinese, Russian, and Scandinavian medicine for centuries. In the wild, it grows in cold climates, particularly on mountains or sea cliffs. Within the field of herbal medicine, it has long been thought of as an adaptogenic herb that can increase an organism's resistance to stress.

Data on the use of *Rhodiola* supplementation in rehabilitation is as follows: *Rhodiola sacra* has been shown to improve exercise capacity in mice by enhancing mitochondrial quality control.[60] One study showed that 8-week Rhodiola crenulata and Cordyceps sinensis supplementation (20 mg/kg/d) faintly enhanced endurance training–induced positive adaptations in body composition in young sedentary individuals.[61] It has been proposed that *Rhodiola rosea* extract can improve function after stroke by lessening the effect stress has on synaptic plasticity, learning, and memory.[62] One study demonstrated that rats experienced less apoptosis and inflammation after acute spinal cord injury.[63]

Ginseng

Ginseng refers to a broad group of 11 species of perennial plants belonging to the *Panax* genus. In the wild, ginseng plants usually grow in cooler climates, usually on the sides of mountains. The dried roots of these plants have been used for thousands of years as a popular medicinal herb. Although ginseng has been used in traditional medicine in the Eastern world, the use of ginseng has been growing throughout the world. Ginseng has an antihypertensive effect that can improve and maintain cardiovascular health.[64] Ginseng products have high variability in their composition and overall quality and can have side effects, such as nausea, vomiting, diarrhea, constipation, and insomnia. Drug interactions, particularly with anticoagulants, such as warfarin, have been appreciated.[65]

Data on the use of ginseng supplementation in rehabilitation is as follows: it was observed that ginseng reduced edema and neuron degeneration in injured spinal cord segment in rats with acute spinal cord injuries, resulting in improvement in locomotor function following injury.[66] It has been proposed that ginseng may maintain homeostasis and prevent inflammation, oxidative stress, and apoptosis after brain injury.[67] Ginseng may reduce motor, sensorimotor, and cognitive deficits after stroke.[68]

ESSENTIAL OILS: AROMATHERAPY AND TOPICAL USE

Aromatic plants have been used in herbal medicine in many forms, including steams, smokes, inhalants, fumigants, snuffs, salves, lotions, colognes, perfumes, and baths.[69] Their popularity has increased in the twenty-first century, and essential oils currently are reported to be a $1 billion dollar industry within the United States alone.[70–72] Essential oils are extracted highly concentrated substances from flowers, leaves, stalks, fruits, and roots. They are complex structures, including mixtures of saturated and unsaturated hydrocarbons, alcohols, esters, ethers, ketones, phenols, and terpenes, which produce the specific fragrance of each oil.[71] There is reported to be more than 400 different oils in use, with 100 of those used in aromatherapy.[73] The therapeutic mechanism of aromatherapy relies on the theory that inhalation of the volatile aromatic compound can trigger changes in the limbic system, which secondarily stimulates physiologic responses in the nervous, endocrine, and immune systems.[74] This response can be either sedative or stimulatory.[75] Proposed benefits of essential oil inhalational and topical include inducing a state of relaxation, muscle relaxation, improved sleep, stimulation of lymph circulation, pain relief, reduced limb swelling, and desensitization, although controlled clinical trials on these outcomes are lacking.[76] Essential oils are associated with adverse effects related to skin irritation, photosensitization, and burns. Enteral consumption of essential oils consumed can result in nephrotoxicity, hepatotoxicity, and neurotoxicity and are not recommended.[77]

Data on the use of essential oils aromatherapy and topical use in rehabilitation is as follows: none available.

CLINICS CARE POINTS

- The use of supplements in clinical care requires clear communication from individuals and health care providers, with a focus on understanding the types of products being used and their potential effects on medications.
- It is critical for health care providers to understand the difference between micronutrient supplementation for therapeutic purposes and treatment and correction of a nutritional deficiency in patients with malnutrition syndromes.
- Micronutrient supplementation has been studied extensively in rehabilitation settings. Vitamin D has been shown to improve pain, bone density, falls, and biomarkers of inflammation. Additionally, B-complex supplementation has been shown to improve exercise tolerance and depression in patients recovering from stroke.
- Nutraceutical supplementation have been evaluated in several clinical settings. Supplementation with BCAAs and α-LA have been shown to improve muscle strength, decrease pain, and improve functional status.
- Evidence supporting the use of herbal supplements is small and larger clinical trials are warranted in this area, especially on the use of *Cannabis* and cannabinoid-related products.

DISCLOSURE

The authors have nothing to disclose.

REFERENCES

1. Dickinson A. History and overview of DSHEA. Fitoterapia 2011;82(1):5–10.
2. Luong JHT, Male KB, Glennon JD. Biotin interference in immunoassays based on biotin-strept(avidin) chemistry: An emerging threat. Biotechnol Adv 2019;37(5):634–41.
3. Adegbaju OD, Otunola GA, Afolayan AJ. Anti-inflammatory and cytotoxic evaluation of extracts from the flowering stage of Celosia argentea. BMC Complement Med Ther 2020;20:152.
4. Ribeiro S. Whole Organisms or Pure Compounds? Entourage Effect Versus Drug Specificity. In: Labate B, Cavnar C, editors. Plant Medicines, Healing and Psychedelic Science. Springer: Cham; 2018. p. 133–49.
5. Yoshimura Y, Wakabayashi H, Bise T, et al. Prevalence of sarcopenia and its association with activities of daily living and dysphagia in convalescent rehabilitation ward inpatients. Clin Nutr 2018;37(6 Pt A):2022–8.

6. Lieber AC, Hong E, Putrino D, et al. Nutrition, energy expenditure, dysphagia, and self-efficacy in stroke rehabilitation: A review of the literature. Brain Sci 2018;8(12):218.

7. Holick MF. Medical progress: Vitamin D deficiency. N Engl J Med 2007;357(3): 266–81.

8. Ogan D, Pritchett K. Vitamin D and the athlete: Risks, recommendations, and benefits. Nutrients 2013;28(6):1856–68.

9. Holick MF, Chen TC. Vitamin D deficiency: A worldwide problem with health consequences. Am J Clin Nutr 2008;87(4):1080S–6S.

10. Schilling S. Epidemic Vitamin D deficiency among patients in an elderly care rehabilitation facility. Dtsch Aerzteblatt Online 2012;109(3):33–8.

11. Poole KES, Loveridge N, Barker PJ, et al. Reduced vitamin D in acute stroke. Stroke 2006;37(1):243–5.

12. Bischoff-Ferrari HA, Dawson-Hughes B, Willett WC, et al. Effect of Vitamin D on falls: a meta-analysis. JAMA 2004;291(16):1999–2006.

13. Bischoff HA, Stähelin HB, Dick W, et al. Effects of vitamin D and calcium supplementation on falls: A randomized controlled trial. J Bone Miner Res 2003;18(2): 343–51.

14. Muir SW, Montero-Odasso M. Effect of vitamin D supplementation on muscle strength, gait and balance in older adults: A systematic review and meta-analysis. J Am Geriatr Soc 2011;59(12):2291–300.

15. Burton JM, Costello FE. Vitamin D in Multiple Sclerosis and Central Nervous System Demyelinating Disease—A Review. Journal of Neuro-Ophthalmology 2015; 35(2):194–200.

16. Polcz ME, Barbul A. The role of vitamin A in wound healing. Nutr Clin Pract 2019; 34:695–700.

17. Ruoppolo G, Longo L, Pescerelli P, et al. CoQ10 and Vitamin A supplementation support voice rehabilitation. A double-blind, randomized, controlled, three-period cross-over pilot study. Front Pharmacol 2019;10:939.

18. Salzer J, Hallmans G, Nyström M, et al. Vitamin A and systemic inflammation as protective factors in multiple sclerosis. Mult Scler J 2013;19(8):1046–51.

19. Løken-Amsrud KI, Myhr KM, Bakke SJ, et al. Alpha-tocopherol and MRI Outcomes in Multiple Sclerosis - Association and Prediction. PLoS One 2013;8(1): e54417.

20. Rizvi S, Raza S, Ahmed F, et al. The Role of Vitamin E in Human Health and Some Diseases. Sultan Qaboos University Medical Journal [SQUMJ] 2014;14(2): 157–65.

21. Browne D, McGuinness B, Woodside JV, et al. Vitamin E and Alzheimer's disease: What do we know so far? Clin Interv Aging 2019;14:1303–17.

22. Myung SK, Ju W, Cho B, et al. Efficacy of vitamin and antioxidant supplements in prevention of cardiovascular disease: Systematic review and meta-analysis of randomised controlled trials. BMJ 2013;346:7893.

23. DiNicolantonio JJ, Bhutani J, O'Keefe JH. The health benefits of Vitamin K, vol. 2. BMJ Publishing Group; 2015. Open heart.

24. Correction: Vitamin K and the prevention of fractures: Systematic review and meta-analysis of randomized controlled trials. JAMA Intern Med 2006;166(12): 1256–61, Vol. 178, JAMA Internal Medicine. American Medical Association; 2018. p. 875–6.

25. Knapen MHJ, Schurgers LJ, Vermeer C. Vitamin K2 supplementation improves hip bone geometry and bone strength indices in postmenopausal women. Osteoporos Int 2007;18(7):963–72.

26. Li Y, Schellhorn HE. New developments and novel therapeutic perspectives for vitamin C. J Nutr 2007;137(10):2171–84.

27. Dionne CE, Laurin D, Desrosiers T, et al. Serum Vitamin C and spinal pain: A nationwide study. Pain 2016;157(11):2527–35.

28. Yimcharoen M, Kittikunnathum S, Suknikorn C, et al. Effects of ascorbic acid supplementation on oxidative stress markers in healthy women following a single bout of exercise. J Int Soc Sports Nutr 2019;16(1):2.

29. Fusini F, Bisicchia S, Bottegoni C, et al. Nutraceutical supplement in the management of tendinopathies: a systematic review. Muscles Ligaments Tendons J 2016; 6(1):48.

30. Rabadi MH, Kristal BS. Effect of vitamin C supplementation on stroke recovery: a case-control study. Clin Interv Aging 2007;2(1):147–51.

31. Ford TC, Downey LA, Simpson T, et al. The effect of a high-dose vitamin b multivitamin supplement on the relationship between brain metabolism and blood biomarkers of oxidative stress: A randomized control trial. Nutrients 2018;10(12): 1860.

32. Paulin FV, Zagatto AM, Chiappa GR, et al. Addition of vitamin B12 to exercise training improves cycle ergometer endurance in advanced COPD patients: A randomized and controlled study. Respir Med 2017;122:23–9.

33. Schoenenberger AW, Schoenenberger-Berzins R, Der Maur CA, et al. Thiamine supplementation in symptomatic chronic heart failure: A randomized, doubleblind, placebo-controlled, cross-over pilot study. Clin Res Cardiol 2012;101(3): 159–64.

34. Almeida OP, Marsh K, Alfonso H, et al. B-vitamins reduce the long-term risk of depression after stroke: The VITATOPS-DEP trial. Ann Neurol 2010;68(4):503–10.

35. Nie C, He T, Zhang W, et al. Branched chain amino acids: Beyond nutrition metabolism. Int J Mol Sci 2018;19(4):954.

36. Takeuchi I, Yoshimura Y, Shimazu S, et al. Effects of branched-chain amino acids and vitamin D supplementation on physical function, muscle mass and strength, and nutritional status in sarcopenic older adults undergoing hospital-based rehabilitation: A multicenter randomized controlled trial. Geriatr Gerontol Int 2019; 19(1):12–7.

37. Ikeda T, Matsunaga Y, Kanbara M, et al. Effect of exercise therapy combined with branched-chain amino acid supplementation on muscle strength in elderly women after total hip arthroplasty: a randomized controlled trial. Asia Pac J Clin Nutr 2019;28(4):720–6.

38. Aquilani R, Iadarola P, Contardi A, et al. Branched-chain amino acids enhance the cognitive recovery of patients with severe traumatic brain injury. Arch Phys Med Rehabil 2005;86(9):1729–35.

39. Sharma B, Lawrence DW, Hutchison MG. Branched chain amino acids (bcaas) and traumatic brain injury: a systematic review. J Head Trauma Rehabil 2018; 33:33–45.

40. Ander BP, Dupasquier CMC, Prociuk MA, et al. Polyunsaturated fatty acids and their effects on cardiovascular disease. Exp Clin Cardiol 2003;8(4):164–72.

41. King VR, Huang WL, Dyall SC, et al. Omega-3 fatty acids improve recovery, whereas omega-6 fatty acids worsen outcome, after spinal cord injury in the adult rat. J Neurosci 2006;26(17):4672–80.

42. Norouzi Javidan A, Sabour H, Latifi S, et al. Does consumption of polyunsaturated fatty acids influence on neurorehabilitation in traumatic spinal cord-injured individuals? a double-blinded clinical trial. Spinal Cord 2014;52(5):378–82.

43. Pu H, Jiang X, Wei Z, et al. Repetitive and prolonged omega-3 fatty acid treatment after traumatic brain injury enhances long-term tissue restoration and cognitive recovery. Cell Transplant 2017;26(4):555–69.

44. Loy BD, Fling BW, Horak FB, et al. Effects of lipoic acid on walking performance, gait, and balance in secondary progressive multiple sclerosis. Complement Ther Med 2018;41:169–74.

45. Choi KH, Park MS, Kim HS, et al. Alpha-lipoic acid treatment is neurorestorative and promotes functional recovery after stroke in rats. Mol Brain 2015;8:9.

46. Lv C, Maharjan S, Wang Q, et al. α-Lipoic acid promotes neurological recovery after ischemic stroke by activating the Nrf2/HO-1 pathway to attenuate oxidative damage. Cell Physiol Biochem 2017;43(3):1273–87.

47. Ranieri M, Sciuscio M, Cortese AM, et al. The use of alpha-lipoic acid (ALA), gamma linolenic acid (GLA) and rehabilitation in the treatment of back pain: effect on health-related quality of life. Int J Immunopathol Pharmacol 2009;22(3 Suppl):45–50.

48. Battisti E, Albanese A, Guerra L, et al. Alpha lipoic acid and superoxide dismutase in the treatment of chronic low back pain. Eur J Phys Rehabil Med 2013; 49(5):659–64.

49. Mortensen SA. Overview on coenzyme Q10 as adjunctive therapy in chronic heart failure. Rationale, design and end-points of "Q-symbio" - A multinational trial. BioFactors 2003;18(1–4):79–89.

50. Fujimoto S, Kurihara N, Hirata K, et al. Effects of coenzymeQ10 administration on pulmonary function and exercise performance in patients with chronic lung diseases. Clin Investig 1993;71(8 Suppl):S162–6.

51. Richins RD, Rodriguez-Uribe L, Lowe K, et al. Accumulation of bioactive metabolites in cultivated medical Cannabis. PLoS One 2018;13(7):e0201119.

52. Hagenbach U, Luz S, Ghafoor N, et al. The treatment of spasticity with Δ^9-tetrahydrocannabinol in persons with spinal cord injury. Spinal Cord 2007;45:551–62.

53. Rodríguez-Muñoz M, Onetti Y, Cortés-Montero E, et al. Cannabidiol enhances morphine antinociception, diminishes NMDA-mediated seizures and reduces stroke damage via the sigma 1 receptor. Mol Brain 2018;11(1):51.

54. Cannabis in Pain Management (Nov 2018) Townsend Letter, Alternative Medicine Magazine. Available at: https://www.townsendletter.com/Nov2018/cannabis1118_2.html. Accessed April 27, 2020.

55. Hawley LA, Ketchum JM, Morey C, et al. Cannabis use in individuals with spinal cord injury or moderate to severe traumatic brain injury in Colorado. Arch Phys Med Rehabil 2018;99(8):1584–90.

56. Graupensperger S, Corey JJ, Turrisi RJ, et al. Individuals with spinal cord injury have greater odds of substance use disorders than non-sci comparisons. Drug Alcohol Depend 2019;205:107608.

57. Wankhede S, Langade D, Joshi K, et al. Examining the effect of Withania somnifera supplementation on muscle strength and recovery: A randomized controlled trial. J Int Soc Sports Nutr 2015;12:43.

58. Kaur T, Singh H, Mishra R, et al. Withania somnifera as a potential anxiolytic and immunomodulatory agent in acute sleep deprived female Wistar rats. Mol Cell Biochem 2017;427(1–2):91–101.

59. Baitharu I, Jain V, Deep SN, et al. Withania somnifera root extract ameliorates hypobaric hypoxia induced memory impairment in rats. J Ethnopharmacol 2013; 145(2):431–41.

60. Dun Y, Liu S, Zhang W, et al. Exercise combined with rhodiola sacra supplementation improves exercise capacity and ameliorates exhaustive exercise-induced

muscle damage through enhancement of mitochondrial quality control. Oxid Med Cell Longev 2017;2017:8024857.

61. Liao YH, Chao YC, Sim BYQ, et al. Rhodiola/cordyceps-based herbal supplement promotes endurance training-improved body composition but not oxidative stress and metabolic biomarkers: A preliminary randomized controlled study. Nutrients 2019;11(10):2357.

62. Concerto C, Infortuna C, Muscatello MRA, et al. Exploring the effect of adaptogenic Rhodiola Rosea extract on neuroplasticity in humans. Complement Ther Med 2018;41:141–6.

63. Lin YC, Chang CW, Wu CR. Anti-nociceptive, anti-inflammatory and toxicological evaluation of Fang-Ji-Huang-Qi-Tang in rodents. BMC Complement Altern Med 2015;15:10.

64. Irfan M, Kwak Y-S, Han C-K, et al. Adaptogenic effects of Panax ginseng on modulation of cardiovascular functions. J Ginseng Res 2020;44(4):538–43.

65. Bilia AR, Bergonzi MC. The G115 standardized ginseng extract: an example for safety, efficacy, and quality of an herbal medicine. J Ginseng Res 2020;44(2): 179–93.

66. Kim YO, Kim Y, Lee K, et al. Panax ginseng improves functional recovery after contusive spinal cord injury by regulating the inflammatory response in rats: an in vivo study. Evid Based Complement Alternat Med 2015;2015:817096.

67. Rastogi V, Santiago-Moreno J, Doré S. Ginseng: A promising neuroprotective strategy in stroke. Front Cell Neurosci 2015;8:457.

68. Liu L, Anderson GA, Fernandez TG, et al. Efficacy and mechanism of panax ginseng in experimental stroke. Front Neurosci 2019;13:294.

69. Cooke B, Ernst E. Aromatherapy: A systematic review. Br J Gen Pract 2000; 50(455):493–6.

70. What is aromatherapy?. 2015. 1–4. Available at: https://craighospital.org/uploads/Educational-PDFs/801.CAM.Aromatherapy.pdf. Accessed April 27, 2020.

71. Aziz ZAA, Ahmad A, Setapar SHM, et al. Essential oils: extraction techniques, pharmaceutical and therapeutic potential - a review. Curr Drug Metab 2018; 19(13):1100–10.

72. Lis-Balchin M. Essential oils and "aromatherapy": their modern role in healing. Journal of the Royal Society of Health 1997;117(5):324–9.

73. Ladas EJ, Kelly KM. Integrative strategies for cancer patients: A practical resource for managing the side effects of cancer therapy. Integrative Strategies for Cancer Patients: A Practical Resource for Managing the Side Effects of Cancer Therapy. 2011.

74. Buckle J. Clinical Aromatherapy: Essential Oils in Practice. Clinical Aromatherapy: Essential Oils in Practice. 2003.

75. Gaware V, Nagare R, Dhamak KB, et al. Aromatherapy: art or science. Int J Biomed Res 2013;4(2):74–83.

76. Buckle J. Clinical aromatherapy: Essential oils in healthcare. Clinical Aromatherapy: Essential Oils in Healthcare. 2014.

77. Buckle J. Essential Oil Toxicity and Contraindications. In: Clinical Aromatherapy. 2015.

Acupuncture

Evidence-Based Treatment in the Rehabilitation Setting

Joseph Walker III, MD[a], Freda L. Dreher, MD[b,c,d],*

KEYWORDS

- Acupuncture • Evidence-based • Rehabilitation medicine
- Physical medicine and rehabilitation • PM&R

KEY POINTS

- Acupuncture is supported as complementary treatment for the following diagnoses: knee osteoarthritis, low back pain, myofascial pain syndrome, neck pain, carpal tunnel syndrome, and chronic pain.
- Acupuncture is equivocal as complementary treatment for the following diagnoses: plantar fasciitis, complex regional pain syndrome, medial epicondylitis, lateral epicondylitis, shoulder pain, and hip osteoarthritis.
- Acupuncture is not supported as complementary treatment for the following diagnoses: neuropathic pain and traumatic brain injury.

According to the National Center for Complementary and Alternative Medicine, approximately 38% of US adults aged 18 years and over and approximately 12% of children used some form of complementary and alternative medicine (CAM).[1] Nearly $34 billion was spent on visits to CAM practitioners and purchases of CAM products, classes, and materials.[2] CAM has been used in numerous subspecialties of medicine, most notably oncology, mental health, and chronic pain management, in which optimal outcomes depend on addressing both the mental and the physical components of the patient's concerns.

Conventional medicine is defined by the National Cancer Institute at the National Institutes of Health (NIH) as a system in which medical doctors and other health care professionals (such as nurses, advanced practice providers, pharmacists, and therapists) treat symptoms and diseases using drugs, radiation, or surgery.

[a] Department of Orthopedics, University of Connecticut, 263 Farmington Avenue, Farmington, CT 06030, USA; [b] Private Practice, Physical Medicine & Rehabilitation and Medical Acupuncture; [c] American Academy of Medical Acupuncture; [d] Helms Medical Institute, The Acus Foundation
* Corresponding author. 20 West Park Street, Suite 214, Lebanon, NH 03766.
E-mail address: fdreher@comcast.net

Phys Med Rehabil Clin N Am 31 (2020) 699–717
https://doi.org/10.1016/j.pmr.2020.07.005
1047-9651/20/© 2020 Elsevier Inc. All rights reserved.

Alternative medicine refers to using a non–mainstream approach *in place of* conventional medicine. Because evidence-based findings and conclusions blur the line between conventional and alternative medicine, the distinction between conventional and alternative medicine has become less discrete, widening the "zone" of what is complementary (the amalgam between the two).

Complementary medicine generally refers to using a non–mainstream approach *together with* conventional medicine. It is the gestalt of the rational interaction of both approaches.

Acupuncture is an increasingly popular form of CAM with particular focus on cancer and cancer-related diagnoses, on mental health disorders, and in chronic pain, in part to help mitigate the well-established risks and side effects of purely "conventional" medicine. This article introduces the art and science of acupuncture, explains its keystone concepts and principles, and cites the literature regarding its efficacy across a wide spectrum of rehabilitation diagnoses.

HISTORY

Although the practice of acupuncture predates written records, the earliest known documentation is from approximately 100 years BCE. Early principles of acupuncture emphasized the importance of understanding, integrating, and abiding by the laws of nature, rather than resisting or altering them, in order to achieve health and wellness. The acupuncture practice is based on a holistic approach not only to the patient's bodily conditions but also to mental, emotional, and spiritual conditions at the time of treatment. The mental, emotional, spiritual, and environmental conditions play a part in how and where a disease or condition originates and how the ailment will manifest.

There are many styles of acupuncture practiced in the world today, all stemming from classic Chinese literature. These styles of acupuncture include practices that have been individualized in China, Korea, Japan, Vietnam, and other unique areas of Asia. In the sixteenth and seventeenth centuries, Jesuit missionaries brought Asian practices of language, art, science, philosophy, and medicine back to Europe. The terms *acupuncture* and *meridians*, the hypothetical energy channels that are contacted by acupuncture needles, are European terms derived from their studies of the Chinese classic literature. French meridian–style acupuncture is currently one of the more commonly practiced styles of acupuncture in America. The term Traditional Chinese Medicine (TCM) is not to be confused with Chinese traditional medicine. TCM was a term coined and a style advanced by the People's Republic of China within the past century. TCM calls from the classics of Chinese medicine, and this particular style became the predominant style of medical practice, including acupuncture and herbalism, during a time when unification of the country's medical practices was of utmost importance to the government. In the United States today, most physicians report using a neuroanatomical model in how they approach the acupuncture practice.

The way acupuncture is delivered varies depending on the style used: how practitioners evaluate the body for diagnostic purposes, acupuncture point selection and combination, needle size, depth of insertion, manipulation of the needles once inserted, and whether herbal medicines are used in conjunction with needling. Electro-acupuncture, which is a modern technique frequently used, introduces electrical frequencies through the needles to respective targets, neuromodulating pain locally, regionally, segmentally, and nonsegmentally. The NIH and the World Health Organization cite more than 52 common problems that acupuncture can successfully address. For example, acupuncture is one of the most widely used integrative treatments for pain conditions in an acute-care setting. Dusek and colleagues[3] showed that inpatient integrative medicine had a significant impact on pain scores for hospitalized patients, reducing self-reported pain by more than 50%, without placing patients at increased risk for adverse effects. The individual goals of a patient-focused integrative program for chronic pain varied in 1 study, resulting in significant improvements in pain as well as other unique outcome measures.[4] Acupuncture and its benefits are applicable to broad swaths of disability, many of which are seen during both the inpatient rehabilitation stay and the outpatient rehabilitation visit.[5,6]

EVIDENCE FOR THE TREATMENT OF CENTRAL NERVOUS SYSTEM DISORDERS

Neurologic disorders may be caused by dysfunction in the central or peripheral nervous systems. Central nervous system (CNS) disorders may emanate from anywhere within brain or spinal cord and manifest as a diverse assortment of signs, symptoms, and syndromes, including spasticity, dystonia, weakness, tremor, paresthesia, allodynia, and hyperalgesia. According to a 2017 estimate, nine of the most common neurologic disorders of the brain and spinal cord cost Americans a total of $789 billion. As the costs continue to grow, this cost has the potential to destabilize health care in the United States. Hence, an affordable and effective complementary therapy for treating CNS disorders is needed. In recent years, research studies have investigated the effectiveness of acupuncture on various CNS disorders. In this section, the authors discuss the evidence for using acupuncture in the management of stroke and associated symptoms and other neurologic disorders, such as spinal cord injury (SCI) and spasticity (**Table 1**).

Traumatic Brain Injury

Lucke-Wold and colleagues[7] noted that acupuncture is a popular treatment for TBI but that the current evidence was not adequate to support recommendations for acupuncture as a standard procedure for traumatic brain injury (TBI). Earlier, Wong and colleagues[8] noted similar results from their Cochrane database metaanalysis and systematic review of 4 randomized control trials (RCTs), which included 294 participants. The studies reported beneficial results of acupuncture, but the studies had low methodological quality. More high-quality studies are needed to understand the effects of acupuncture. Several on-going research studies related to acupuncture and TBI have published their protocols. Liu and colleagues[9] have proposed a study to assess the effects of auricular electroacupuncture to improve the consciousness of patients after TBI. Wang and colleagues[10] have proposed an RCT to examine the effects of acupuncture for hearing loss after TBI. The outcome of these studies will help advance the current knowledge of acupuncture as a treatment of TBI.

Spinal Cord Injury

Fan and colleagues[11] carried out a systematic review to assess the effectiveness of acupuncture for treating post-SCI complications. The outcome of their research suggests that acupuncture is effective in treating post-SCI complications, such as motor and sensory dysfunction, pain, neurogenic bowel and bladder, pressure ulcers, spasticity, and osteoporosis. Widrin[12] described a case study of a 25-year-old man with monoplegia resulting from an SCI after a motor vehicle accident. The patient was treated by scalp acupuncture in addition to intensive physical therapy and was able to make right hallux dorsiflexion and dorsiflexion of the paralyzed foot after 4 treatments. Apart from body acupuncture, auricular acupuncture has also shown beneficial results. Estores and colleagues[13] conducted a pilot study to investigate the effects of an auricular acupuncture protocol called battlefield acupuncture (BFA) on pain

Table 1
Neurologic disorders

Author, Year	Type of Study	Study Design	Number of Participants	Acupuncture Points Used	Summary	Citation
Stroke						
Xu et al,[16] 2018	Review	Systematic review	33 Trials (3946 participants)	Not available (NA)	6.2% participants reported adverse events. The quality of evidence is low, and hence larger trials are needed before including acupuncture as a treatment for acute stroke	Xu M, Li D, Zhang S. Acupuncture for acute stroke. Cochrane Database of Systematic Reviews 2018, Issue 3. Art. No.: CD003317. DOI: 10.1002/14651858. CD003317.pub3[16]
Tang et al,[17] 2019	Review	Metaanalysis	32 RCTs (1310 participants)	Scalp, tongue, Jin's 3 needles	As compared with traditional acupuncture and rehabilitation treatment, scalp/tongue/Jin's 3-needle acupuncture yield significantly better total effective rate	Tang HY, Tang W, Yang F, et al. Efficacy of acupuncture in the management of post-apoplectic aphasia: a systematic review and meta-analysis of randomized controlled trials. BMC Complement Altern Med. 2019;19(1):282. Published 2019 Oct 25. https://doi.org/10.1186/s12906-019-2687-1[17]

Data from Lee S, Shin B, Lee M, et al. Scalp acupuncture for stroke recovery: a systematic review and meta-analysis of randomized controlled trials. Eur J Integr Med. 2013;5(2):87–99 and You YN, Cho MR, Kim JH, et al. Assessing the quality of reports about randomized controlled trials of scalp acupuncture combined with another treatment for stroke. BMC Complement Altern Med. 2017;17(1):452.

intensity in chronic SCI and neuropathic pain. The study reported that the BFA group reported more improvement in the pain scores, that is, more pain reduction, than the delayed entry group. Recently, Lei and colleagues published a protocol for their proposed study. The researchers intend to conduct a systematic review to assess the effects of different types of acupuncture and moxibustion therapy, the practice of burning of a medicinal herb near an acupuncture point for a warming effect, to address neurogenic bladder after SCI.[14] In another study, Yang and colleagues[15] published the protocol of their on-going study to assess the effectiveness of the rehabilitation training combined with acupuncture for treating patients with neurogenic bladder secondary to the SCI. In summary, acupuncture is a promising treatment for SCI complications, and further research will help to develop clinical guidelines.

Stroke

Xu and colleagues[16] investigated the RCTs of acupuncture that started within 30 days from stroke onset compared with placebo or sham acupuncture or open control. The objective was to assess whether acupuncture could reduce the proportion of people who die or have dependency later. No difference was observed in death incidences, and 6.2% of participants reported adverse events. Tang and colleagues[17] evaluated the effectiveness of scalp, tongue, and Jin's 3-needle acupuncture for the improvement of postapoplectic aphasia, and compared with traditional acupuncture and rehabilitation therapies, scalp, tongue, and Jin's 3-needle acupuncture, yielded significantly better total effectiveness and better scores on oral expression, repetition, reading, and writing tests. Li and colleagues[18] conducted a metaanalysis to evaluate the effectiveness and safety of acupuncture in patients with post–stroke dysphagia that included 29 trials and revealed evidence for the efficacy and safety of acupuncture in the treatment of post–stroke dysphagia in short term as compared with rehabilitation or medication without adverse events. Thomas and colleagues[19] studied the effects of various interventions for treating urinary incontinence 30 days after stroke in 20 published RCTs. Five of these studies used acupuncture as a complementary treatment for incontinence, and the outcome suggested that the participants in the treatment group were 3 times more likely to be continent. Wang and colleagues[20] and Lee and colleagues[21] have documented scalp acupuncture as an effective treatment for stroke. You and colleagues[22] focused on assessing the quality and limitations of articles reporting RCTs of scalp acupuncture treatment for stroke and concluded that the overall quality of reporting on RCTs of scalp acupuncture for stroke was moderate to low.

Spasticity

Yi and colleagues[23] conducted a narrative review to assess the effects of acupuncture on spasticity occurring after upper motor neuron lesions, such as stroke, brain injury, SCI, cerebral palsy, and multiple sclerosis, and reported that electroacupuncture combined with routine care reduces spasticity and improves motor function and activities of daily living after stroke. However, there was not enough evidence to conclude that acupuncture could reduce spasticity with other CNS diseases. Yang and colleagues[24] conducted a systematic review of publications regardless of subtype of stroke, neurologic deficits, or needling style and reported that acupuncture had beneficial effects on reducing spasticity for people with stroke in the subacute or chronic stage. Gao and colleagues[25] assessed the effects of acupuncture on spasticity in children with cerebral palsy, and study revealed that adding scalp acupuncture as a treatment significantly improved gross motor function and the ability to perform activities of daily living in children with spastic cerebral palsy.

EVIDENCE FOR THE TREATMENT OF ORTHOPEDIC DISORDERS

In 2010, osteoarthritis (OA) was the most common joint disorder in the United States, affecting more than 10% of older adults.[26] There has been several scientific investigations into the effect of acupuncture on OA and a range of other musculoskeletal, soft tissue, and orthopedic disorders (**Table 2**).

Knee Osteoarthritis

Li and colleagues[27] conducted a metaanalysis of studies using acupuncture, electro-acupuncture, fire needle (a specific acupuncture needling technique), warm needle, and sham needle with education for the treatment of knee OA, and reported that fire needle and electro-acupuncture was effective in the short term to reduce the pain but not stiffness. The researchers recommended that acupuncture with heat might be a better choice. Another metaanalysis conducted by Li and colleagues[28] reviewed 12 studies to assess the effectiveness of acupuncture on pain relief and functional recovery in patients with knee OA, with a particular focus on the risk of bias and reporting quality. The study found that as compared with western medicine, acupuncture, and in particular, electroacupuncture, had greater total effective rate, greater short-term effective rate, and less adverse reactions. Chen and colleagues[29] assessed the effects of laser acupuncture on knee OA and, although laser acupuncture had short-term effects, it had no advantage over placebo in the follow-up.

Hip Osteoarthritis

Zhang and colleagues[30] described 23 recommendations from the Osteoarthritis Research International expert committee for knee and hip OA. For optimal results, a combination of pharmacologic and nonpharmacologic modalities was recommended, and acupuncture was one of the recommended nonpharmacologic modalities. Manheimer and colleagues[31] conducted a review for assessing the safety and effectiveness of acupuncture on hip OA that included 6 studies from Cochrane CENTRAL, MEDLINE, and Embase databases. They found there were little or no effects in reducing pain or improving function relative to sham acupuncture in hip OA. In 2019, the American College of Rheumatology/Arthritis Foundation Guideline for the Management of Osteoarthritis of the Hand, Hip, and Knee has conditionally recommended acupuncture only for knee OA but not hip OA,[32] stating that the greatest number of positive trials with the largest effect sizes have been carried out for knee OA.

Shoulder Pain

Although direct evidence is available for shoulder OA, there is evidence available for shoulder pain. Guerra de Hoyos and colleagues[33] compared the efficacy of electroacupuncture with placebo acupuncture for the treatment of shoulder pain. At 6-month follow-up, the electroacupuncture group showed a significantly greater improvement in pain intensity, range of motion, and functional ability compared with the control group (placebo acupuncture). Molsberger and colleagues[34] conducted an RCT for chronic shoulder pain with the acupuncture group, sham, and conventional treatment group undergoing 15 sessions over 6 weeks. The results are significant for acupuncture's effect compared with conventional treatment immediately after treatment and at 3-month follow-up. Vas and colleagues[35] examined the effects of acupuncture on painful shoulder using acupuncture with physiotherapy and physiotherapy-only groups. The participants received 15 physiotherapy sessions over 3 weeks plus 1 acupuncture session per week, and the single-point acupuncture and physiotherapy

Table 2
Orthopedic disorders

Author, Year	Type of Study	Study Design	Number of Participants	Acupuncture Points Used	Summary	Citation
Knee osteoarthritis						
Li et al,[27] 2018	Review	Metaanalysis	16 articles (2065 patients)	NA	Fire needle and electroacupuncture are effective in the short term to reduce the pain but not stiffness Acupuncture with heat might be a better choice.	Li S, Xie P, Liang Z, et al. Efficacy comparison of five different acupuncture methods on pain, stiffness, and function in osteoarthritis of the knee: a network meta-analysis [published correction appears in Evid Based Complement Alternat Med. 2019 Nov 20;2019:3713197]. Evid Based Complement Alternat Med. 2018;2018:1638904. Published 2018 Nov 1. https://doi.org/10.1155/2018/1638904[27]
Li et al[28] 2019	Review	Metaanalysis	12 articles	NA	As compared with western medicine, acupuncture had more total effective rate, short-term effective rate, and less adverse reactions	Li J, Li YX, Luo LJ, et al. The effectiveness and safety of acupuncture for knee osteoarthritis: An overview of systematic reviews. Medicine (Baltimore). 2019;98(28):e16301. https://doi.org/10.1097/MD.0000000000016301[28]

(continued on next page)

Table 2
(continued)

Author, Year	Type of Study	Study Design	Number of Participants	Acupuncture Points Used	Summary	Citation
Chen et al,[29] 2019	Review	Metaanalysis	7 articles	NA	Although laser acupuncture has short-term effect, it has no advantage over placebo in follow-up	Chen Z, Ma C, Xu L, et al. Laser acupuncture for patients with knee osteoarthritis: a systematic review and meta-analysis of randomized placebo-controlled trials. Evid Based Complement Alternat Med. 2019;2019:6703828. Published 2019 Nov 3. https://doi.org/10.1155/2019/6703828[29]

Data from Refs. [27–29]

group had improved shoulder function and reduced pain compared with physiotherapy control group.

Rotator Cuff Tear/Tendinitis

In a case report, Settergren[36] described a case of a 30-year-old woman with supraspinatus tendinopathy and achy pain at rest and sharp pain on movement, who was treated with dry needling acupuncture guided by ultrasound. After 10 days, her pain was reduced, and she resumed about 50% of her exercises. One of the underlying mechanisms of acupuncture is cellular proliferation and matrix synthesis, and a Cochrane Database Systematic review found 1 trial that concluded manual therapy and exercise may not be as effective as acupuncture plus dietary counseling and Phlogenzym supplement for symptoms.[37] In summary, the evidence for acupuncture as a treatment for rotator cuff tendinitis is statistically weak but compelling based on symptom relief.

Plantar Fasciitis

Thiagarajah[38] conducted a review study to assess the effectiveness of acupuncture in reducing pain caused by plantar fasciitis. Of the 17 studies available, four met the criteria for inclusion, and their analysis reported that 4 to 8 weeks of treatment acupuncture (in particular, electroacupuncture) resulted in pain reduction. In a multi-center RCT, Dunning and colleagues[39] included electricity added to dry needling to treat plantar fasciitis. After 3 months of treatment, individuals receiving electrical dry needling combined with manual therapy, exercise, and ultrasound showed greater improvements in pain and function than those receiving only manual therapy, exercise, and ultrasound. Lee and Marx[40] in a case study reported of a 43-year-old woman who presented with heel pain and difficulty in walking and who was managed with a multimodal approach using massage, gua sha (an acupuncture-related soft tissue technique), bleeding, acupuncture, and moxibustion. At 1-week follow-up, her pain had significantly reduced, and function was improved.

Medial and Lateral Epicondylitis

Medial epicondylitis is typically studied and reported in combination with lateral epicondylitis (LE). A review article by Dingemanse and colleagues[41] evaluated the effectiveness of electrophysical modalities for the treatment of medial and LE. These treatments included ultrasound, extracorporeal shock wave therapy (ESWT), transcutaneous electrical nerve stimulation, and laser therapy. The study noted that ultrasound and laser for the management of LE were effective, but no effects on medial epicondylitis were observed. Wu and colleagues[42] conducted an RCT to assess the efficacy of acupuncture plus fire needle therapy versus acupuncture alone in the treatment of LE. The results suggested that for immediate and intermediate term (3-month follow-up), acupuncture plus fire needle therapy proved to be more beneficial as compared with the control group. Wong and colleagues[43] also studied the efficacy of acupuncture versus ESWT. The acupuncture group was given a 3-week treatment with 2 sessions per week, and the ESWT group received a 3-week treatment with 1 session per week. Although pain was decreased at 2 weeks in both groups, there were no group differences. Valera-Garrido and colleagues[44] examined the efficacy of ultrasound-guided percutaneous needle electrolysis (a type of electrical stimulation) along with exercise and stretching for 6 weeks in patients with LE. After treatment and at 52-week follow-up, pain and structural tendon changes had improved.

Carpal Tunnel Syndrome

In an RCT, Maeda and colleagues[45] studied the effect of acupuncture on pain in carpal tunnel syndrome using 2 acupuncture (local and distal) and 1 sham control groups. At 3-month follow-up, the acupuncture groups showed a sustained reduction in pain scores as compared with the sham group. Furthermore, acupuncture also produced improvements in neurophysiologic outcomes local to the wrist (ie, median sensory nerve conduction latency) and centrally (ie, D2/D3 S1 cortical separation distance in the brain). Another RCT by Mohammadjavad and colleagues[46] showed similar results, with the acupuncture group demonstrating improvement in the global Boston Carpal Tunnel Questionnaire and visual analog scale (VAS) score as compared with the ibuprofen group. In addition, the acupuncture group showed improvements in electrophysiologic parameters, such as median distal sensory latency and median nerve conduction velocity.

Trigger Finger

Inoue and colleagues[47] studied the effects of acupuncture on the pain associated with trigger finger. Nineteen fingers were treated 5 times a day in 15 patients. After the second session, patients reported a significant improvement in pain and snapping severity. Acupotomy is a type of treatment that has been implemented for trigger finger treatment whereby acupuncture is done using a needle knife, that is, acupuncture is combined with modern surgical principles. However, evidence for this treatment is unclear. Jia and colleagues[48] have proposed to study this technique further.

EVIDENCE FOR ACUPUNCTURE IN THE TREATMENT OF PAIN CONDITIONS

The American Chronic Pain Association's (ACPA) resource guide defines chronic pain as pain persisting after the usual course of tissue healing, or after an injury for more than 3 to 6 months.[49] The ACPA resource guide acknowledges that CAMs, such as acupuncture, meditation, and yoga, have proven scientific validity. Pain (whether nociceptive or neuropathic) creates disability and interferes with rehabilitation process. Although acute pain is a warning signal, chronic pain is a disease; acute pain is a symptom, but chronic pain is a diagnosis[50] (**Table 3**).

Phantom Limb Syndrome

Tseng and colleagues[51] reported a 71-year-old woman amputee who had phantom limb syndrome (PLP) for 2 years after a road traffic accident. She received acupuncture treatment for 6 sessions, twice a week for 3 weeks, and at 6-month follow-up, she no longer experienced PLP. Trevelyan and colleagues[52] reported in a pilot study an RCT for acupuncture in patients with PLP that after 4 weeks of treatment; average pain scores for the acupuncture group were significantly lower, and in semistructured interviews patients reported feeling good about the treatment. DeMoss and colleagues[53] reported in a review article that acupuncture should be considered a complementary modality for treating PLP.

Complex Regional Pain Syndrome

Hommer[54] described a case report in which 2 soldiers with complex regional pain syndrome (CRPS) from post–upper limb injuries were treated with Chinese Scalp Acupuncture twice weekly for 1 to 4 weeks using acupuncture needles on the scalp. At 16 months' follow-up, the patients reported more than 80% improvement in the pain on the VAS or numeric rating scale. In another case report, Tae and Kyeong[55] provided acupuncture treatment to a 42-year-old woman with CRPS type I after an injury

Table 3
Pain disorders

Author, Year	Type of Study	Study Design	Number of Participants	Acupuncture Points Used	Summary	Citation
Phantom limb						
Tseng et al,[51] 2014	Prospective	Case report	1	EX-HN1, GV20, GB7	71-y-old woman with 2 y of PLP after a road traffic accident. PLP and PLS relieved after 6 mo of acupuncture	Tseng CC, Chen PY, Lee YC. Successful treatment of phantom limb pain and phantom limb sensation in the traumatic amputee using scalp acupuncture. *Acupunct Med.* 2014;32(4):356–358. https://doi.org/10.1136/acupmed-2014-010556[51]
Trevelyan et al,[52] 2016	Prospective	Pilot for RCT	15	LI4 + LR3, LR3, GV20, SP10	In the acupuncture group mean average pain decreased from 5.44 to 2.75 and in the usual care group from 5.43 to 4.43. The protocol is acceptable for full-fledged trial	Trevelyan EG, Turner WA, Summerfield-Mann L, et al N. Acupuncture for the treatment of phantom limb syndrome in lower limb amputees: a randomised controlled feasibility study. *Trials.* 2016;17(1):519. Published 2016 Oct 25. https://doi.org/10.1186/s13063-016-1639-z[52]
DeMoss,[53] 2018	Review	Theoretic review	NA	NA	In pediatric oncology, acupuncture is a complementary modality to manage PLP	DeMoss P, Ramsey LH, Karlson CW. Phantom limb pain in pediatric oncology. *Front Neurol.* 2018;9:219. Published 2018 Apr 9. https://doi.org/10.3389/fneur.2018.00219[53]
CRPS						

PLS, phantom limb syndrome.
Data from Refs.[51–53]

to the left forearm. Human placental extract was injected weekly into acupuncture points LI5, LU2, SI10, HT1, GB21, and SI11 in the left shoulder region. After the 45th session, the pain reports on VAS improved from an initial 8 to 0. Pai and Vas[56] reported similar results in a case report using dry needling.

Myofascial Pain

Myofascial pain can be treated by various forms of acupuncture, including dry (without injection) needling. A 2002 study reported that deep acupuncture stimulation of trigger points has a better analgesic effect when compared with superficial acupuncture stimulation in the treatment of myofascial pain syndrome.[57] Edwards and Knowles[58] found that superficial dry needling of trigger points followed by active stretching was more effective in deactivating trigger points and reducing subjective pain than both (1) stretching alone and (2) not performing any treatment. Itoh[59] concluded that trigger point acupuncture therapy may be more effective on chronic neck pain in older patients than the standard acupuncture therapy.

Migraine Headaches

A Cochrane review update of acupuncture for the prevention of episodic migraine reported that participants who received acupuncture treatment reported reduced frequency of migraine episodes. This evidence suggests that acupuncture is at least similarly effective as treatment with prophylactic drugs and thus useful in the prevention of episodic migraine. Jia and colleagues[60] conducted a systematic review and metaanalysis to examine the therapeutic and preventive effect of acupuncture treatment. The study also investigated safe acupuncture for migraines without aura and reported that acupuncture was tolerated better than medication because of fewer side effects. Acupuncture was also helpful in reducing the frequency of the migraine episodes. An RCT from Li and colleagues[61] used functional MRI (fMRI) to study the effects of acupuncture in migraines without aura. fMRI imaging showed that after longitudinal acupuncture treatment, the decreased amplitude of low-frequency fluctuations of the trigeminocervical complex (brainstem) was normalized in migraine patients.

Posttraumatic Headaches

A systematic review of 36 articles by Khusid[62] revealed the effectiveness of acupuncture is similar to that of drug treatment for migraine prophylaxis and neurovascular and tension-type headaches. The study also mentioned the safety, cost-effectiveness, and long-lasting benefits of acupuncture and recommended it as a treatment alternative for posttraumatic headache. In a pilot study, Jonas and colleagues[63] compared auricular acupuncture and traditional acupuncture with usual care in posttraumatic headaches and reported that both acupuncture groups had significant decreases in numerical rating scale scores, compared with the control group. Other outcome measures, such as the Pittsburgh Sleep Quality Index or SCL-90, did not show any changes, and the researchers recommend a large-scale clinical trial to confirm the findings of secondary measures.

Lower Back Pain with/Without Radiculopathy

The American College of Physicians (ACP) strongly recommended nonpharmacologic treatments, such as acupuncture, for patients with chronic back pain.[64] Converging scientific evidence indicated that acupuncture was found to lower pain intensity in chronic back pain and also improve function. Vickers and colleagues[65] conducted a metaanalysis of 13 randomized trials and concluded that acupuncture is an effective treatment for pain conditions, such as chronic musculoskeletal pain and headache. Hu and colleagues[66] conducted a metaanalysis of 16 articles and reported that dry needling reduces pain and disability at postintervention as compared with acupuncture and sham needling in chronic low back pain. However, during the follow-up period, dry needling and acupuncture showed similar results. Although the evidence for the efficacy of acupuncture in acute or subacute back pain is low quality, the ACP still strongly recommends nonpharmacologic treatments, such as acupuncture, because most patients improve over time regardless of the treatment.

Neck Pain with/Without Radiculopathy

An RCT conducted to assess the clinical efficacy of abdominal acupuncture (a style of acupuncture) for neck pain (Ho and colleagues[67]), whereby participants were assigned to an abdominal acupuncture group or the sham group, reported that the abdominal acupuncture group exhibited significantly improved scores on the neck pain disability and pain scores. Cerezo-Téllez and colleagues[68] assessed the effectiveness of deep dry needling of myofascial trigger points on health-related quality-of-life improvement whereby participants were randomly assigned to either deep dry needling and stretching group or to stretching-only groups. The intervention group improved on all dimensions of Short Form-36 after intervention and up to 6-months' follow-up. To address the question of whether the pain relief from acupuncture was related to placebo or therapeutic effect, researchers from the *Acupuncture Trialists' Collaboration* conducted an analysis of individual patient data from 29 high-quality RCTs that included 17,922 participants. These trials investigated the use of acupuncture for back and neck pain, OA, shoulder pain, or chronic headache. For all pain types studied, the researchers found modest but statistically significant differences between acupuncture versus simulated acupuncture approaches (ie, a variety of acupuncture-like approaches), and larger differences between acupuncture versus no-acupuncture controls (ie, nonspecific effects). The investigators noted that these findings suggest that the total effects of acupuncture, as experienced by patients in clinical practice, are clinically relevant. They also noted that their study provides the most robust evidence to date that acupuncture is more than just placebo and a reasonable referral option for patients with chronic pain.[69]

SUMMARY

Rehabilitation services and practitioners are most likely to provide global, holistic treatments resulting in restoration of human function. Acupuncture and its various related techniques not only add another therapeutic modality to the wide range of available interventions but also, by their very nature, incorporate a holistic approach toward the goals desired. Acupuncture both modulates pain at the spinal level via the gate phenomenon and facilitates brain neuroplasticity.[70,71] The neuromodulating effects of endorphins, enkephalins, dynorphin, GABA, and monoamine-dependent pathways by acupuncture have been well established.

It has taken time for western research to take an interest in non–western treatment modalities. Although the emergence of acupuncture occurred in America by 1971, the Food and Drug Administration did not approve of an acupuncture needle as a medical device until 1996. The NIH released a consensus statement regarding safe and effective use of acupuncture in 1997, stimulating interest and opportunity for expansion of valid research into acupuncture for various conditions.

Over the past 20 years, acupuncture research has grown in quantity, scope, and quality. Although most acupuncture practiced in the United States focuses on pain management, any primary care indication can be addressed with acupuncture. In 2014, the US Department of Veterans Affairs, after a systematic review of acupuncture research publications, published an *Evidence Map of Acupuncture* mapping literature size, confidence, and effectiveness in the realms of pain management, wellness, and mental health. Positive results were noted for chronic pain, headache, insomnia, and mood disorder, as well as many other conditions.

As the disconnect between the East and the West equilibrates, new studies will emerge that may mature into level 1A and other reliable high-level evidence upon which to earn the moniker "evidence based."[72] There are several confounding factors contributing to difficulties conducting quality acupuncture research and valid reviews of world literature that must be addressed. Simple nomenclature is a challenge, as the classics of Chinese medicine often used metaphorical rather than scientific terms. In review of world acupuncture literature, acupuncture terms are not always translated and used in uniform ways, thus making it difficult to compare 1 study to another. When acupuncture studies are published, the type or style of acupuncture that is practiced or details of the protocol used is not always documented. Because it is possible that some styles are more effective than others, this introduces a significant complicating factor. Acupuncture is an interactional practice, dependent on the skills, experience, and, theoretically, the health of the practitioner. Thus, it is difficult to standardize an acupuncture approach and still achieve an optimal or uniform outcome. According to the classic literature on acupuncture, the environment of the care provided is a variable influencing the treatment outcome and may not be considered in a research setting. Research to prove the validity of acupuncture is limited by the necessary human interaction of a treatment that makes it difficult to fully blind a patient to the treatment that they are receiving. Because most current studies are now focusing on pain reduction as a measurement of value, subjective reporting of pain further confounds outcome measurements. Sham needling devices have been developed to use for acupuncture research and have, in and of themselves, some effect on the patient, perhaps by influence on superficial and fascial tissues.

Despite confounding factors regarding acupuncture research, there is an emerging body of convincing evidence to support its use, and as a result, greater clinical acceptance is occurring. For example, as of 2020, the Centers for Medicare and Medicaid Services (CMS) agreed to cover acupuncture for Medicare patients with chronic low back pain. The evidence that CMS reviewed supported including acupuncture within the clinical strategy of nonpharmacologic therapies for chronic low back pain. Although many studies have demonstrated that acupuncture makes a significant improvement in clinical outcome, more research is needed.

DISCLOSURE

The authors have nothing to disclose.

CLINICS CARE POINTS

- Increasingly, medical institutions and medical insurance carriers are considering provision and coverage of acupuncture as part of overall patient management. Current research literature guidelines are important to help providers and patients with legitimate expectations of an acupuncture treatment.
- Although acupuncture is steeped in Traditional East Asian Medical theory, current research methods are increasingly supporting the benefits of acupuncture for specific conditions.

- Acupuncture should not be thought of as a specific treatment for TBI or SCI, but current studies looking into the value of acupuncture as part of the management of TBI and SCI complications are promising.
- Evidence supports the use of acupuncture, along with standard medical care, in the treatment of aphasia, dysphagia, and urinary incontinence following stroke.
- Most acupuncture being used in physician practices today is for the management of various pain conditions, and evidence supports the use of acupuncture for many orthopedic and neurologic pain conditions.

REFERENCES

1. Barnes PM, Bloom B, Nahin R. CDC National Health Statistics Report #12. Complementary and alternative medicine use among adults and children: United States, 2007. National Health Statistics Reports. No. 12. 2008. Available at: http://www.cdc.gov/nchs/data/nhsr/nhsr012.pdf. Accessed February 24, 2020.
2. Nahin RL, Barnes PM, Stussman BJ, et al. Costs of complementary and alternative medicine (CAM) and frequency of visits to CAM practitioners: United States, 2007. Natl Health Stat Report 2009;18:1–14.
3. Dusek JA, Finch M, Plotnikoff G, et al. The impact of integrative medicine on pain management in a tertiary care hospital. J Patient Saf 2010;6(1):48–51.
4. Abrams DI, Dolor R, Roberts R, et al. The BraveNet prospective observational study on integrative medicine treatment approaches for pain. BMC Complement Altern Med 2013;13:146.
5. Naeser MA. Neurological rehabilitation: acupuncture and laser acupuncture to treat paralysis in stroke, other paralytic conditions, and pain in carpal tunnel syndrome. J Altern Complement Med 1997;3(4):425–8.
6. Gould A, MacPherson H. Patient perspectives on outcomes after treatment with acupuncture. J Altern Complement Med 2001;7(3):261–8.
7. Lucke-Wold BP, Logsdon AF, Nguyen L, et al. Supplements, nutrition, and alternative therapies for the treatment of traumatic brain injury. Nutr Neurosci 2018; 21(2):79–91.
8. Wong V, Cheuk DKL, Lee S, et al. Acupuncture for acute management and rehabilitation of traumatic brain injury. Cochrane Database Syst Rev 2013;(3):CD007700.
9. Liu T, Lu Y, Yu J, et al. Effect of auricular electroacupuncture combined with body acupuncture in improving the consciousness of patients after traumatic brain injury: study protocol for a randomized controlled trial. Medicine (Baltimore) 2019;98(30):e16587.
10. Wang WF, Yang LH, Yu HJ, et al. Acupuncture for hearing loss after traumatic brain injury: a protocol for systematic review of randomized controlled trial. Medicine (Baltimore) 2019;98(30):e16553.
11. Fan Q, Cavus O, Lize X, Yun X. Spinal Cord Injury: How Could Acupuncture Help? Journal of Acupuncture and Meridian Studies 2018;11(4):124–32.
12. Widrin C. Scalp Acupuncture for the Treatment of Motor Function in Acute Spinal Cord Injury: A Case Report. Journal of Acupuncture and Meridian Studies 2018; 11(2):74–6.
13. Estores I, Chen K, Jackson B, Lao L, Gorman PH. Auricular acupuncture for spinal cord injury related neuropathic pain: a pilot controlled clinical trial. J Spinal Cord Med 2017;40(4):432–8.
14. Lei H, Fu Y, Xu G, Yin Z, Zhao L, Liang F. Different types of acupuncture and moxibustion therapy for neurogenic bladder after spinal cord injury: A systematic

review and network meta-analysis study protocol. Medicine (Baltimore) 2020; 99(1):e18558.

15. Yang GF, Sun D, Wang XH, Chong L, Luo F, Fang CB. Effectiveness of rehabilitation training combined acupuncture for the treatment of neurogenic bladder secondary to spinal cord injury. Medicine (Baltimore). 2019;98(39):e17322.

16. Xu M, Li D, Zhang S. Acupuncture for acute stroke. Cochrane Database Syst Rev 2018;(3):CD003317.

17. Tang HY, Tang W, Yang F, et al. Efficacy of acupuncture in the management of post-apoplectic aphasia: a systematic review and meta-analysis of randomized controlled trials. BMC Complement Altern Med 2019;19(1):282.

18. Li L, Deng K, Qu Y. Acupuncture treatment for post-stroke dysphagia: an update meta-analysis of randomized controlled trials. Chin J Integr Med 2018;24:686.

19. Thomas LH, Coupe J, Cross LD, et al. Interventions for treating urinary incontinence after stroke in adults. Cochrane Database Syst Rev 2019;(2):CD004462.

20. Wang Y, Shen J, Wang XM, et al. Scalp acupuncture for acute ischemic stroke: a meta-analysis of randomized controlled trials. Evid Based Complement Alternat Med 2012;2012:480950.

21. Lee S, Shin B, Lee M, et al. Scalp acupuncture for stroke recovery: a systematic review and meta-analysis of randomized controlled trials. Eur J Integr Med 2013; 5(2):87–99.

22. You YN, Cho MR, Kim JH, et al. Assessing the quality of reports about randomized controlled trials of scalp acupuncture combined with another treatment for stroke. BMC Complement Altern Med 2017;17(1):452.

23. Yi Z, Yujie Y, Jianan L. Does acupuncture help patients with spasticity? A narrative review. Ann Phys Rehabil Med 2019;62(4):297–301.

24. Yang A, Wu HM, Tang JL, et al. Acupuncture for stroke rehabilitation. Cochrane Database Syst Rev 2016;(8):CD004131.

25. Gao J, He L, Yu X, et al. Rehabilitation with a combination of scalp acupuncture and exercise therapy in spastic cerebral palsy. Complement Ther Clin Pract 2019;35:296–300.

26. Zhang Y, Jordan JM. Epidemiology of osteoarthritis [published correction appears in Clin Geriatr Med. 2013 May;29(2): ix]. Clin Geriatr Med 2010;26(3): 355–69.

27. Li S, Xie P, Liang Z, et al. Efficacy comparison of five different acupuncture methods on pain, stiffness, and function in osteoarthritis of the knee: a network meta-analysis. Evid Based Complement Alternat Med 2018;2018:1638904 [Erratum appears in Evid Based Complement Alternat Med 2019;2019:3713197].

28. Li J, Li YX, Luo LJ, et al. The effectiveness and safety of acupuncture for knee osteoarthritis: an overview of systematic reviews. Medicine (Baltimore) 2019; 98(28):e16301.

29. Chen Z, Ma C, Xu L, et al. Laser acupuncture for patients with knee osteoarthritis: a systematic review and meta-analysis of randomized placebo-controlled trials. Evid Based Complement Alternat Med 2019;2019:6703828.

30. Zhang W, Moskowitz RW, Nuki G, et al. OARSI recommendations for the management of hip and knee osteoarthritis, Part II: OARSI evidence-based, expert consensus guidelines. Osteoarthritis Cartilage 2008;16(Issue 2):137–62.

31. Manheimer E, Cheng K, Wieland LS, et al. Acupuncture for hip osteoarthritis. Cochrane Database Syst Rev 2018;5(5):CD013010.

32. Kolasinski SL, Neogi T, Hochberg MC, et al. 2019 American College of Rheumatology/Arthritis Foundation guideline for the management of osteoarthritis of the hand, hip, and knee. Arthritis Rheumatol 2020;72:220–33.

33. Guerra de Hoyos JA, del Andres Martin MC, Bassas y Baena de Leon E, et al. Randomised trial of long-term effect of acupuncture for shoulder pain. Pain 2004;112:289–98.

34. Molsberger AF, Schneider T, Gotthardt H, et al. German Randomized Acupuncture Trial for chronic shoulder pain (GRASP) - a pragmatic, controlled, patient-blinded, multi-centre trial in an outpatient care environment. Pain 2010;151: 146–54.

35. Vas J, Ortega C, Olmo V, et al. Single-point acupuncture and physiotherapy for the treatment of painful shoulder: a multicentre randomized controlled trial. Rheumatology (Oxford) 2008;47:887–93.

36. Settergren R. Treatment of supraspinatus tendinopathy with ultrasound guided dry needling. J Chiropr Med 2013;12(1):26–9.

37. Page MJ, Green S, McBain B, et al. Manual therapy and exercise for rotator cuff disease. Cochrane Database Syst Rev 2016;(6):CD012224.

38. Thiagarajah AG. How effective is acupuncture for reducing pain due to plantar fasciitis? Singapore Med J 2017;58(2):92–7.

39. Dunning J, Butts R, Henry N, et al. Electrical dry needling as an adjunct to exercise, manual therapy and ultrasound for plantar fasciitis: a multi-center randomized clinical trial. PLoS One 2018;13(10):e0205405.

40. Lee T, Marx B. Noninvasive, multimodality approach to treating plantar fasciitis: a case study. J Acupunct Meridian Stud 2018;4(11):162–4.

41. Dingemanse R, Randsdorp M, Koes BW, et al. Evidence for the effectiveness of electrophysical modalities for treatment of medial and lateral epicondylitis: a systematic review. Br J Sports Med 2014;48:957–65.

42. Wu SY, Lu CN, Chung CJ, et al. Therapeutic effects of acupuncture plus fire needle versus acupuncture alone in lateral epicondylitis: a randomized case-control pilot study. Medicine (Baltimore) 2019;98(22):e15937.

43. Wong CW, Ng EY, Fung PW, et al. Comparison of treatment effects on lateral epicondylitis between acupuncture and extracorporeal shockwave therapy. Asia Pac J Sports Med Arthrosc Rehabil Technol 2016;7:21–6.

44. Valera-Garrido F, Minaya-Muñoz F, Medina-Mirapeix F. Ultrasound-guided percutaneous needle electrolysis in chronic lateral epicondylitis: short-term and long-term results. Acupunct Med 2014;32(6):446–54.

45. Maeda Y, Kim H, Kettner N, et al. Rewiring the primary somatosensory cortex in carpal tunnel syndrome with acupuncture. Brain 2017;140(4):914–27.

46. Mohammadjavad H, Esmaeel B, Hadi M, et al. Efficacies of acupuncture and anti-inflammatory treatment for carpal tunnel syndrome. J Acupunct Meridian Stud 2015;8(5):229–35.

47. Inoue M, Nakajima M, Hojo T, et al. Acupuncture for the treatment of trigger finger in adults: a prospective case series. Acupunct Med 2016;34(5):392–7.

48. Jia Y, Qiu Z, Sun X, et al. Acupotomy for patients with trigger finger: a systematic review protocol. Medicine (Baltimore) 2019;98(42):e17402.

49. Feinberg S, et al. ACPA Resource Guide to Chronic Pain Management, an Integrated Guide to Medical, Interventional, Behavioral, Pharmacologic and Rehabilitation Therapies 2019 Edition.

50. Treede RD, Rief W, Barke A, et al. A classification of chronic pain for ICD-11. Pain 2015;156(6):1003–7.

51. Tseng CC, Chen PY, Lee YC. Successful treatment of phantom limb pain and phantom limb sensation in the traumatic amputee using scalp acupuncture. Acupunct Med 2014;32(4):356–8.

52. Trevelyan EG, Turner WA, Summerfield-Mann L, et al. Acupuncture for the treatment of phantom limb syndrome in lower limb amputees: a randomised controlled feasibility study. Trials 2016;17(1):519.

53. DeMoss P, Ramsey LH, Karlson CW. Phantom limb pain in pediatric oncology. Front Neurol 2018;9:219.

54. Hommer DH. Chinese scalp acupuncture relieves pain and restores function in complex regional pain syndrome. Mil Med 2012;177(10):1231–4.

55. Tae HC, Kyeong MP. Complex regional pain syndrome type 1 relieved by acupuncture point injections with placental extract. J Acupunct Meridian Stud 2014;7(3):155–8.

56. Pai RS, Vas L. Ultrasound-guided intra-articular injection of the radio-ulnar and radio-humeral joints and ultrasound-guided dry needling of the affected limb muscles to relieve fixed pronation deformity and myofascial issues around the shoulder, in a case of complex regional pain syndrome type 1. Pain Pract 2018;18(2):273–82.

57. Ceccherelli F, Rigoni MT, Gagliardi G, et al. Comparison of superficial and deep acupuncture in the treatment of lumbar myofascial pain: a double-blind randomized controlled study. Clin J Pain 2002;18(3):149–53.

58. Edwards J, Knowles N. Superficial dry needling and active stretching in the treatment of myofascial pain–a randomised controlled trial. Acupunct Med 2003; 21(3):80–6.

59. Itoh K, Katsumi Y, Hirota S, et al. Randomised trial of trigger point acupuncture compared with other acupuncture for treatment of chronic neck pain. Complement Ther Med 2007;15:172–9.

60. Jia X, Fu-qing Z, Jian P, et al. Acupuncture for migraine without aura: a systematic review and meta-analysis. J Integr Med 2018;16(5):312–21.

61. Li Z, Zeng F, Yin T, et al. Acupuncture modulates the abnormal brainstem activity in migraine without aura patients. Neuroimage Clin 2017;15:367–75.

62. Khusid MA. Clinical indications for acupuncture in chronic post-traumatic headache management. Mil Med 2015;180(2):132–6.

63. Jonas WB, Bellanti DM, Paat CF, et al. A randomized exploratory study to evaluate two acupuncture methods for the treatment of headaches associated with traumatic brain injury. Med Acupunct 2016;28(3):113–30.

64. Qaseem A, Wilt TJ, McLean RM, et al, for the Clinical Guidelines Committee of the American College of Physicians. Noninvasive treatments for acute, subacute, and chronic low back pain: a clinical practice guideline from the American College of Physicians. Ann Intern Med 2017;166:514–30.

65. Vickers AJ, Vertosick EA, Lewith G, et al. Acupuncture for chronic pain: update of an individual patient data meta-analysis. J Pain 2018;19(5):455–74.

66. Hu HT, Gao H, Ma RJ, et al. Is dry needling effective for low back pain? A systematic review and PRISMA-compliant meta-analysis. Medicine (Baltimore) 2018; 97(26):e11225.

67. Ho LF, Lin ZX, Leung AWN, et al. Efficacy of abdominal acupuncture for neck pain: a randomized controlled trial. PLoS One 2017;12(7):e0181360.

68. Cerezo-Téllez E, Torres-Lacomba M, Mayoral-Del-Moral O, et al. Health related quality of life improvement in chronic non-specific neck pain: secondary analysis from a single blinded, randomized clinical trial. Health Qual Life Outcomes 2018; 16(1):207.

69. Vickers AJ, Cronin AM, Maschino AC, et al. Acupuncture for chronic pain: individual patient data meta-analysis. Arch Intern Med 2012;172(19):1444–53.

70. Napadow V, Liu J, Li M, et al. Somatosensory cortical plasticity in carpal tunnel syndrome treated by acupuncture. Hum Brain Mapp 2007;28(3):159–71.
71. Napadow V, Kettner N, Liu J, et al. Hypothalamus and amygdala response to acupuncture stimuli in carpal tunnel syndrome. Pain 2007;130(3):254–66.
72. Burns PB, Rohrich RJ, Chung KC. The levels of evidence and their role in evidence-based medicine. Plast Reconstr Surg 2011;128(1):305–10.

Moving?

Make sure your subscription moves with you!

To notify us of your new address, find your **Clinics Account Number** (located on your mailing label above your name), and contact customer service at:

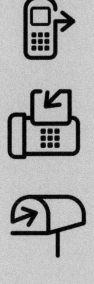

Email: journalscustomerservice-usa@elsevier.com

800-654-2452 (subscribers in the U.S. & Canada)
314-447-8871 (subscribers outside of the U.S. & Canada)

Fax number: 314-447-8029

Elsevier Health Sciences Division
Subscription Customer Service
3251 Riverport Lane
Maryland Heights, MO 63043

Printed and bound by CPI Group (UK) Ltd, Croydon, CR0 4YY

03/10/2024

01040407-0003